REUBEN M. CHERNIACK, M.D., F.R.C.P.(C), F.A.C.P., F.C.C.P.

Professor and Head, Department of Medicine, University of Manitoba,
Director, Joint Respiratory Programme, University of Manitoba,
Head, Section of Respiratory Diseases, Winnipeg General Hospital,
Director, Respiratory Division, Clinical Investigation Unit, Winnipeg General Hospital
Physician, Winnipeg General Hospital, and Rehabilitation Hospital—D. A. Stewart Centre

LOUIS CHERNIACK, M.D., F.R.C.P. (London), F.R.C.P.(C), F.A.C.P., F.C.C.P.

Associate Professor of Medicine, University of Manitoba,
Physician, Winnipeg General Hospital and Rehabilitation Hospital—D. A. Stewart Centre

ARNOLD NAIMARK, M.D., F.R.C.P.(C)

Dean of Medicine, Professor and Head, Department of Physiology, University of Manitoba,
Associate Director, Respiratory Division, Clinical Investigation Unit, Winnipeg General Hospital
Physician, Winnipeg General Hospital

With the Assistance of

VICTOR CHERNICK, M.D., F.A.A.P., C.R.C.P.(C)

Professor and Head,
Department of Pediatrics
University of Manitoba,
Physician, Winnipeg Children's Hospital and
Rehabilitation Hospital—D. A. Stewart Centre

Illustrated by

DOUGLAS LÀNE, B.F.A.

Head, Graphic Section, Instructional Media,
University of Manitoba

Respiration in Health and Disease

SECOND EDITION

W. B. SAUNDERS COMPANY PHILADELPHIA • LONDON • TORONTO

W. B. Saunders Company: West Washington Square
                           Philadelphia, Pa.   19105

                           1 St. Anne's Road
                           Eastbourne, East Sussex BN21 3UN, England

                           833 Oxford Street
                           Toronto, M8Z 5T9, Canada

Listed here is the latest translated edition of this book together with the language of the translation and the publisher.

Spanish (*2nd Edition*) — Ediciones Toray, Barcelona, Spain

Respiration in Health and Disease   ISBN 0-7216-2525-8

Print No.:   9   8

PREFACE TO
THE SECOND EDITION

In the original edition of this text emphasis was placed on the mechanisms of development of symptoms and physical signs and on the correlation of clinical, radiologic and morphologic manifestations with disturbances in respiratory function. Since then, several books stressing pulmonary function in respiratory disease have appeared, but none of them have been directed primarily toward the student in medicine and related health sciences. This, together with the fact that there have been many advances in our understanding of basic mechanisms of disturbed function has led to publication of a second edition. Therapy was not included in the initial edition because it was felt that an understanding of basic disturbances in respiratory disease would lead to the appropriate management. However, the absence of a discussion of the principles of management was soon recognized as a serious omission. The principles of management of patients suffering from acute or chronic respiratory failure have therefore been included. In addition, the defenses of the respiratory system, stress situations in which many of the respiratory symptoms occur, and special aspects related to the newborn infant and child have been added.

The authors wish to thank Drs. Earl Hershfield, Brian Kirk, Donal McCarthy, Shirley Parker, Ben Schoemperlen, Alex Sehon, Newman Stephens, Kam Tse, Carl Zylak, and the many students and residents in medicine for their helpful suggestions and criticisms. Special acknowledgement is due to Miss Nancy Joy, whose excellent illustrations were used in the first edition and have formed the basis of most of the figures in this book, and to Mrs. Laurayne Rusak, whose assistance in the preparation of the text and proofreading was immeasurable. The secretarial assistance of Mrs. Jean Zushman, Miss Elaine Dingwall, Mrs. Margaret Klaassen and Mrs. Sonya Olien is also gratefully acknowledged.

R. M. C.
L. C.
A. N.

v

CONTENTS

Chapter 8

Section Two
THE MANIFESTATIONS OF RESPIRATORY DISEASE

Chapter 9

Section Three
THE ASSESSMENT OF RESPIRATORY DISEASE

Chapter 10

Section Four
THE PATTERNS OF RESPIRATORY DISEASE

Section Five
RESPIRATORY FAILURE AND ITS MANAGEMENT

INTRODUCTION

The main functions of the respiratory system are to supply oxygen to the cells of the body and to remove carbon dioxide from them. Net movement of gases by diffusion occurs at two principal sites — in the lungs and in the tissues. In mammals the exchange of oxygen and carbon dioxide between the body and its environment cannot occur at a rate sufficient to sustain life by simple diffusion alone; therefore, a gas transport system for the conduction of oxygen and carbon dioxide between the atmosphere and lungs, on the one hand, and between the lungs and the tissues, on the other, is required. A schematic representation of this transport system is shown in Figure 1.

Bulk or convective transport occurs between the lungs and the tissues (circulation) and between the lungs and the environment (ventilation). In contrast to diffusion, which is passive, ventilation and circulation require that active work be done by the heart and the respiratory muscles in order to generate the mechanical energy needed to produce bulk flow of gas or blood. Since this energy is liberated as a result of muscular activity, it is possible to regulate convective transport by influencing the activity of cardiac and respiratory muscles.

In the tissues the oxygen diffuses from the blood to its intracellular binding site while the carbon dioxide diffuses from the cells to the blood. The blood entering the lungs comes from the tissues where oxygen has been extracted and carbon dioxide has been added, resulting in a low oxygen partial pressure (Po_2) and a high CO_2 partial pressure (Pco_2). The blood which enters the lungs is exposed to gas in the alveoli across the pulmonary capillary walls.

When the respiratory muscles contract, fresh air is inspired into the alveoli so that the alveolar Po_2 is raised and Pco_2 is lowered. Because of the differences between the partial pressures of oxygen and carbon dioxide in the alveoli and in the blood perfusing the lung, there is a net diffusion of oxygen into the blood and carbon dioxide into the alveoli. As the diffusion of oxygen from the lungs into the blood proceeds, there is a decrease in the alveolar Po_2, and the net diffusion of carbon dioxide from the blood into the alveoli results in an increase in the alveolar Pco_2. When the respiratory muscles relax, expiration occurs, and the oxygen-depleted and carbon dioxide-

1

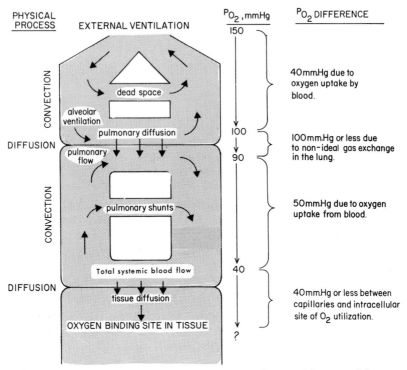

FIGURE 1.   Gas transport system between atmosphere and lungs, and lungs and tissues, and the fall in arterial partial pressure of oxygen along the transport system.

enriched alveolar gas leaves through the airway. With each succeeding inspiration, the alveolar gas is once again refreshed. Depending on the state of activity of the body, this cycle is repeated 10 to 50 times a minute.

The processes involved in the events which occur during respiration will be described in some detail in the following pages in order to set the stage for a discussion of the disturbances in function produced by disease and the functional interventions which constitute therapy.

Section One

BASIC CONSIDERATIONS

THE RESPIRATORY PUMP

THE PULMONARY CIRCULATION

OXYGEN AND CARBON DIOXIDE EXCHANGES
BETWEEN GAS AND BLOOD

THE CONTROL OF BREATHING

RESPIRATION UNDER STRESS

SPECIAL ASPECTS RELATED TO THE
NEWBORN INFANT

THE APPLICATION OF PULMONARY
PHYSIOLOGY TO CLINICAL PULMONARY
FUNCTION TESTING

THE DEFENSES OF THE RESPIRATORY
SYSTEM

Chapter 1

The Respiratory Pump

Expansion of the chest occurs when the inspiratory muscles contract and air enters the lungs and distends the tracheobronchial tree (Fig. 2). During inspiration, all portions of the tracheobronchial tree become enlarged, but the greatest relative expansion takes place in the distal portions of the bronchi. On fluoroscopic examination, both roots of the lungs are seen to descend during inspiration, owing to the elongation of the trachea. In addition, fluoroscopy with radiopaque media placed in the bronchi demonstrates that the bronchi lengthen and increase in diameter during inspiration, whereas during expiration they return to their original length and diameter.

The bronchi divide into successively smaller branches, down to the terminal bronchioles and the respiratory bronchioles, which can be recognized by their alveolar outpouchings. The respiratory bronchioles radiate into the alveolar ducts, which in turn give rise to

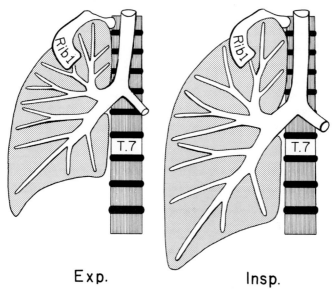

Exp.   Insp.

FIGURE 2. The change in size of the tracheobronchial tree during respiration.

5

the alveolar sacs. These sacs consist of groups of alveoli which have a radius of approximately 55 to 65 microns. It has been estimated that there are three to four billion alveoli in the human lungs and that they occupy an area of 70 to 100 square meters. During inspiration the alveolar ducts become elongated and widen, and the openings into the alveolar sacs increase in size.

THE SUPPORTING STRUCTURES – THE THORACIC CAGE

The human thorax is constructed in such a manner that it has sufficient rigidity to protect the vital organs it contains, and it provides the pliability which enables it to function as a bellows during the ventilatory cycle. The rigidity results from the bony composition of the ribs; there is pliability because each rib is attached to a resilient cartilage which is fixed to either the sternum or the seventh rib and, in addition, has moveable joints at its vertebral and sternal ends. The first seven ribs are attached to the sternum, and the cartilages of the next three ribs are attached to the cartilage of the seventh rib. The remaining two ribs, the "floating ribs," have no connection with the sternum or other ribs.

The sternum is held in position by its connection with the ventral ends of the ribs, which are under continuous elastic tension, even when the respiratory muscles are relaxed. The elasticity of the thoracic cage is also evident in that, when it is compressed in any direction, it always returns to its original position.

The chest increases in size with inspiration. This increase in the lung volume normally takes place in three dimensions: antero-posterior, transverse and longitudinal. This three-dimensional increase in volume occurs because the ribs are elevated as a result of the contraction of the scalene and intercostal muscles and because the diaphragm descends during inspiration. The degree and duration of movement of different portions of the chest are related to the shape of the ribs.

THE FORCE GENERATORS – THE RESPIRATORY MUSCLES

THE SCALENE MUSCLES

The scalene muscles, which arise from the transverse processes of the cervical vertebrae, raise the anterior end of the first rib, together with the manubrium sternum, when they contract during inspiration. This elevation of the first rib not only increases the anteroposterior diameter of the upper outlet of the thorax but also stabilizes the upper chest cage so that contraction of the intercostal muscles results in elevation of the remaining ribs.

THE INTERCOSTAL MUSCLES

The first to the sixth ribs are connected with one another by the intercostal muscles, whose fibers run downward and forward. Since the first rib is fixed by the scalene muscles, contraction of the intercostal muscles results in an upward and forward movement of the remaining five ribs. There is very little lateral movement of the first four ribs, which overlie the upper lobes of the lungs, and this portion of the chest cage increases in size primarily in an anteroposterior direction (Fig. 3, third rib).

The fifth and sixth ribs, which are situated approximately over the middle lobe of the right lung and the lingular segment of the left

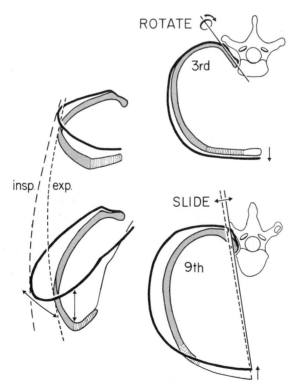

FIGURE 3. Anteroposterior and superior views of an upper and lower rib during inspiration and expiration.

lung, differ from the upper four ribs in having a greater radius of curvature. Because of this, inspiratory elevation of these two ribs increases both the anteroposterior and the transverse diameter of that portion of the thoracic cage.

The seventh to the tenth ribs, which overlie the lower lobes of the lung, differ from the ribs above them in both their shape and their direction of movement. The anterior ends of these lower four ribs are situated at almost the same level as their posterior ends. In addition, they are more sharply curved. The inspiratory movement of these ribs primarily increases the transverse diameter of this portion of the thoracic cage while the anteroposterior diameter decreases slightly (Fig. 3, ninth rib).

THE DIAPHRAGM

The diaphragm is the principal muscle of inspiration. Not only does contraction of the diaphragm increase the volume of the thoracic cage in a vertical direction, but it also tends to increase the transverse diameter of the lower thoracic cage. This increase in transverse diameter occurs because the muscular fibers of the diaphragm run in a vertical direction from their attachment at the costal margins. Since the diaphragm is normally dome-shaped, contraction of its fibers moves the lower ribs in an upward and lateral direction (Fig. 4). On the other hand, if the diaphragm is flattened and no longer dome-shaped, as in severe airway obstruction, it behaves like a flat sheet of muscles. Under such circumstances, contraction of the diaphragm is less effective in increasing the longitudinal dimension, and there may actually be narrowing of the transverse diameter of the lower thorax.

Apart from its function in normal breathing, the diaphragm also

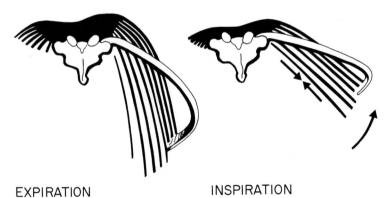

EXPIRATION   INSPIRATION

FIGURE 4.   Because of its dome shape, contraction of the diaphragm during inspiration results in elevation of the ribs with a consequent increase of the transverse diameter of the chest.

plays an important role in other respiratory acts such as coughing, sniffing and sneezing. In addition, contraction of the diaphragm, in conjunction with the contraction of the abdominal muscles, raises the intra-abdominal pressure. This influences the return of venous blood from the abdomen and also assists in defecation, vomiting and parturition.

Unlike the intercostal muscles, which are innervated from the corresponding thoracic segments of the spinal cord, the diaphragm derives its nerve supply from the third, fourth and fifth cervical segments via the phrenic nerves. The diaphragm, therefore, continues to function even when the intercostal muscles are paralyzed by either a lesion in the upper thoracic region or the administration of a spinal anesthetic. It has been shown that paralysis of both leaves of the diaphragm need not cause any disability, provided that the intercostal muscles are functioning normally and that the lungs are healthy. However, if the diaphragmatic paralysis is associated with underlying pulmonary disease, it can result in a considerable degree of difficulty in breathing.

THE MUSCLES OF THE ABDOMINAL WALL

During quiet respiration, the abdominal pressure rises during inspiration because of the descent of the diaphragm and falls during the first part of expiration. This results in protrusion of the upper abdominal wall during inspiration and recession during expiration. The muscles of the abdominal wall (the external oblique, the internal oblique, the transversus abdominis, and the rectus abdominis muscles) all arise from the superficial surfaces of portions of the lower eight ribs or their cartilages. Normally these muscles do not actively participate in the breathing act. However, if a maximum expiration is made voluntarily, they will contract and cause depression of the lower ribs of the chest cage. They are also important during coughing and sneezing in that by increasing the rigidity of the abdominal wall, the intrathoracic pressure can rise to high levels.

SECONDARY RESPIRATORY MUSCLES

The secondary respiratory muscles are those muscles which, although attached to the ribs, do not ordinarily partake in the respiratory act. However, they do come into play if there is marked hyperventilation, such as after severe exertion in a healthy person or in the breathlessness associated with cardiorespiratory diseases. In such circumstances, contraction of the trapezius muscle fixes the shoulder girdle so that the pectoral muscles can elevate the upper ribs.

THE DIMENSIONS — THE LUNG VOLUMES

The position of the chest cage when the muscles are relaxed is the situation at the end of a normal expiration and is called the *resting level* or *midposition.* The resting level is determined by the balance between the elastic forces of the lungs, which tend to reduce the volume of the lung and the elastic forces of the chest wall, which tend to increase it. Even after various maximal inspiratory and expiratory maneuvers, the lung volume normally returns to its original level. Nevertheless, this equilibrium volume is not constant but can be influenced by various conditions. For example, the resting level shifts to a more inspiratory position whenever there is obstruction to the expiratory flow of air or when the lung loses its elasticity, as in emphysema; it shifts to a more expiratory position in the supine position or when the lung becomes stiffer, as in fibrosis.

The changes in the volume of the lungs that can be produced by the action of the respiratory muscles may be studied by means of a recording spirometer. One generally thinks of the lung volumes as being divided into various components. Figure 5 illustrates these subdivisions as approximate proportions of the total lung capacity because their absolute values vary considerably, even in normal persons, and are dependent upon the age, sex and size of the person. Nevertheless, the proportion of the total lung capacity which each of the lung volume compartments occupies is remarkably similar in different healthy persons. The resting level or the *functional residual capacity* is about 40 per cent, the vital capacity is about 70 to 75 per

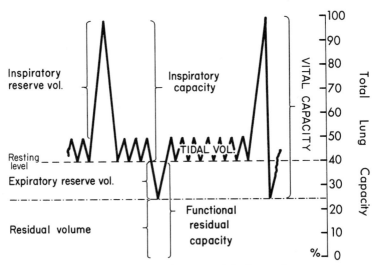

FIGURE 5.   The subdivisions of the lung volume.

TABLE 1

LUNG VOLUMES IN TWO MALES OF EQUAL AGE BUT DIFFERENT SIZE

LUNG VOLUME	HT., 180 CM.		HT., 150 CM.	
	ml.	% TLC	ml.	% TLC
Total lung capacity	7790	100	4680	100
Vital capacity	6030	77	3280	70
Inspiratory capacity	4100	53	2555	51
Functional residual capacity	3690	47	2115	49
Residual volume	1760	23	1400	30
Expiratory reserve volume	1930	24	715	19

cent and the residual volume is approximately 25 to 30 per cent of the total lung capacity. This principle is illustrated in Table 1, in which the values obtained in two males of the same age but of different size are shown.

The *total lung capacity* (TLC) is the total amount of air that is present in the lungs after a maximal inspiration. The *vital capacity* (VC) is the maximal amount of air that a subject is able to expire after a maximal inspiration. Its absolute value is limited by the strength of the respiratory muscles as well as by the elastic resistance of the lungs and the chest wall.

Almost all of the remaining lung volumes are estimated with reference to the normal end-expiratory position of the chest or its resting level. The *tidal volume* is the volume of air which is breathed in during inspiration or out during expiration. Although usually stated to be about 500 ml. in normal subjects under resting conditions, its absolute amount varies from one person to another as well as with the activity of each person. By multiplying the tidal volume by the respiratory rate, the *minute ventilation* may be determined.

The *inspiratory capacity* (IC) is the maximum volume of air which can be inspired from the resting level. It normally averages about 60 per cent of the total lung capacity. Since the tidal volume is included in this measurement, the *inspiratory reserve volume* (IRV) is the maximal volume of air which can be inspired over and above the tidal volume from the resting level.

The *functional residual capacity* (FRC) is the quantity of air which remains in the lungs after a normal expiration. Normally, it is about 40 per cent of the total lung capacity, but this also varies from person to person. It is smaller in the supine position or if the lungs become stiffer and is larger if there is an expiratory obstruction to the flow of air or a loss of lung elasticity.

The functional residual capacity has two components—the expiratory reserve volume and the residual volume. The *expiratory reserve volume* (ERV) is the maximal volume of air which can be expired beyond the resting level, when expiration is carried on to its fullest extent. It is limited by several factors: the extent of elevation of the diaphragm during expiration, the strength of the expiratory muscles, the resistance of the chest wall to a further decrease in volume, and the tendency for the smaller airways to close during a forced expiration.

The *residual volume* (RV) of the lungs is the amount of air which is still in the lungs at the end of a maximal expiration. The residual volume cannot be determined with an ordinary recording spirometer but may be estimated by special techniques employing a dilution principle or in a body plethysmograph. It is normally approximately 25 per cent of the total lung capacity. A ratio of the residual volume to the total lung capacity which is greater than 30 per cent may result because of either a loss of the elastic retractive force of the lung or an obstruction to expiratory airflow.

FORCES AND RESISTANCES INVOLVED IN BREATHING

The lung is invested with a serous membrane, called the visceral pleura, which reflects onto the chest wall, where it is called the parietal pleura. Only a thin film of fluid separates the two pleural surfaces. If a fine cannula were inserted between the parietal and visceral pleural layers and a small volume of air introduced, a pressure which reflects the forces exerted by the lungs or chest wall on the pleural space would be recorded. This pressure is variously called the intrapleural, pleural or intrathoracic pressure. Any force tending to move the chest wall away from the lungs or the lungs away from the chest wall is registered as a negative or subatmospheric pressure in the pleural space.

In the fetus, the lungs contain no air but nevertheless completely fill the thoracic cavity. With the first inspiratory effort, which occurs shortly after birth, the respiratory muscles contract powerfully and tend to expand the chest wall. The force is transmitted through the pleural fluid space to the lung surface, creating a negative pleural pressure which is as much as 80 cm. H_2O less than atmospheric pressure. Since the pressure acting on the inner surface of the lung (in the airways) is equal to atmospheric pressure (760 mm. Hg or 980 cm. H_2O), there is an outward force of 80 cm. H_2O which expands the lung and fills it with air.

With the ensuing expiration the lungs do not deflate completely, and some air remains at the end of the expiration (the functional residual capacity). Thus, from the first breath at birth to the last at death the lungs are never airless. The reason the lungs are not completely deflated at end-expiration is not because their elastic recoil energy has been totally expended but because in the intact chest at the functional residual capacity the tendency of the lungs to collapse is hindered by the pull of the chest wall. For example, if at functional residual capacity an opening were made into a pleural space so that it communicated freely with the atmosphere, the lung would collapse further and the chest cage would expand. Thus, at the functional residual capacity the lungs and chest wall are normally interacting in such a way that the tendency for the lung to collapse is balanced by the tendency for the chest wall to expand.

BALANCE OF FORCES BETWEEN THE LUNG AND CHEST WALL

Since there is no air moving at the end of an expiration, and since the gas inside the lung is in continuity with the atmosphere through the airways, the pressure at the airway opening, in the bronchi, in the alveoli and at the body surface are all equal to atmospheric pressure. The retractive force of the lungs which tends to pull them away from the chest wall is registered as a negative pleural pressure because it is opposed by the tendency of the chest wall to expand further.

The pressure difference between the inner and outer surfaces of the lungs is a measure of the net force acting on the lungs tending to inflate or deflate them. This is often referred to as the *transpulmonary pressure* and is represented in Figure 6 as $P_{alv} - P_{pl}$. The difference between the pleural pressure and that acting at the body surface is a measure of the net force acting on the chest wall tending to expand or collapse it and is represented as $P_{pl} - P_{bs}$.

At the end of a normal expiration when the lungs and chest wall are stationary it is clear that the net force acting on the lungs must be balanced by an equal and opposite force acting on the chest wall. In other words

$$P_{lung} = P_{wall}$$
$$\text{or} \quad P_{alv} - P_{pl} = P_{pl} - P_{bs}$$

The net force acting across the total respiratory apparatus, that is, across both the lungs and chest wall, is called the *transthoracic pressure* or P_{chest}:

$$P_{chest} = P_{lung} + P_{wall} = P_{alv} - P_{pl} + P_{pl} - P_{bs}$$

In a normal person at end-expiration the mean pleural pressure is about 5 cm. H_2O below atmospheric pressure (i.e., 975 cm. H_2O)

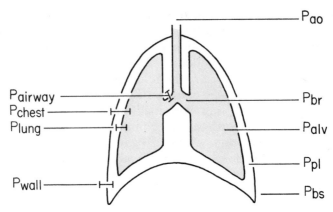

FIGURE 6.   Respiratory pressures:

P_{ao} = pressure at airway opening (usually atmospheric pressure)

P_{br} = pressure in the bronchi

P_{alv} = pressure in terminal air spaces (syn.: intrapulmonary pressure)

P_{pl} = pressure in pleural space (syn.: intrapleural pressure, intra-thoracic pressure)

P_{bs} = pressure at body surface (usually atmospheric pressure)

Transmural pressures in the chest:

$P_{airway} = P_{br} - P_{pl}$ = pressure tending to widen or narrow the airways

$P_{chest} = P_{alv} - P_{bs}$ = pressure tending to inflate or deflate lungs and chest wall together (transthoracic pressure)

$P_{lung} = P_{alv} - P_{pl}$ = pressure tending to inflate or deflate the lungs, depending on sign (transpulmonary pressure)

$P_{wall} = P_{pl} - P_{bs}$ = pressure tending to expand or collapse chest wall, depending on sign

so that

$$P_{lung} = P_{alv} - P_{pl} = 980 - 975 = 5 \text{ cm. } H_2O$$
$$\text{and } P_{wall} = P_{pl} - P_{bs} = 975 - 980 = -5 \text{ cm. } H_2O$$
$$\text{therefore } \quad P_{chest} = P_{lung} + P_{wall} = 5 - 5 = 0 \quad \text{(see Fig. 7)}$$

REGIONAL VARIATIONS IN PLEURAL PRESSURE

It has been clearly demonstrated that the pleural pressure is not the same at all points in the chest. It is most negative at the top of the pleural space and becomes progressively less negative toward the bottom. Thus, in the standing or seated position it is most negative at the apex of the lung and least negative in the basal (diaphragmatic) regions; in the supine position it is most negative at the sternal margin and least negative at the spinal margin.

There are several factors which may contribute to these differences in pleural pressure. At the top, the tendency for the lung to retract away from the chest wall is added to by the weight of the lung itself, which also tends to pull the lung away from the chest wall. At

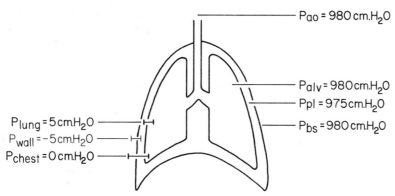

$P_{ao} = 980$ cm.H_2O

$P_{alv} = 980$ cm.H_2O
$P_{pl} = 975$ cm.H_2O

$P_{bs} = 980$ cm.H_2O

$P_{lung} = 5$ cm.H_2O
$P_{wall} = -5$ cm.H_2O
$P_{chest} = 0$ cm.H_2O

FIGURE 7.   The balance of forces acting in the chest at the end of a normal expiration (functional residual capacity).

the bottom, the retractive force of the lung tending to pull it away from the chest wall is now counteracted to some extent by the weight of the lung, which acts as a force tending to push the pleural surface of the lung against the chest wall. Thus, at the top of the lung the force of gravity (weight of the lung) and the retractive force of the lung act in the same direction so that the pleural pressure is more negative than it is at the bottom of the lung, where the force of gravity and the retractive force of the lung act in opposite directions. Regional variations of pleural pressure will also be affected by regional differences in the retractive forces of the lungs or the chest wall and, in the supine position, will also be influenced by the intra-abdominal pressure.

Because of the regional variations in pleural pressure, different parts of the lung are expanded to different degrees at functional residual capacity. If one recalls that at the end of an expiration, with the glottis open, the alveolar pressure is the same everywhere in the lung and is equal to atmospheric pressure, then clearly the trans-pulmonary pressure $(P_{alv} - P_{pl})$, or the force tending to expand the lung, is greater at the top of the lung than at the bottom. At the resting level, or functional residual capacity, therefore, the volume of the individual air spaces is greater at the top of the lung than at the bottom.

Since the pleural pressure varies in different areas of the pleural space, it is clear that a single measurement does not necessarily reflect the overall pressure required to overcome the resistances to breathing. For this reason, as well as the discomfort and inherent danger associated with the insertion of a needle into the pleural cavity, the changes in pressure within the esophagus during respiration have been used as an index of the changes in pleural pressure. Although the relationship between the esophageal and pleural pressures is not consistent and varies from one person to another, it may neverthe-less yield a better measure of the pressure at the surface of the lungs because it reflects the pressure over a larger area.

FORCES EXERTED DURING A RESPIRATORY CYCLE

Contraction of the respiratory muscles during inspiration results in the application of a force to the chest wall which tends to expand the chest. The outward movement of the chest wall is resisted by the lung, and it is this resistance which determines how much force must be applied in order to expand the lung. The greater the resistance offered by the lung, the more subatmospheric the pleural pressure must become in order to move a given volume of air into the lung; as pointed out earlier, the difference in pressure between the pleural surface and the alveolar surface is the force tending to expand the lung. This transpulmonary pressure is raised by decreasing the pleural pressure, as is the case during normal breathing, or by elevating the alveolar pressure (as in certain forms of artificial ventilation).

The relationship between pleural pressure and alveolar pressure during the respiratory cycle is shown in Figure 8. Simultaneous recordings of airflow in and out of the chest and the tidal volume

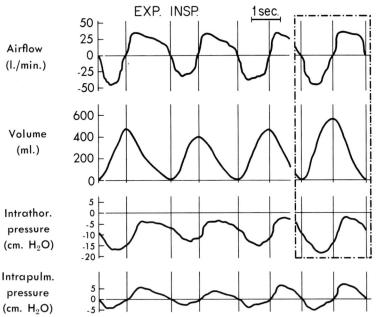

FIGURE 8.   The relationship between pleural pressure (P_{pl}) and alveolar pressure (P_{alv}) during breathing.

changes are also shown. With each inspiration the pleural pressure becomes more negative. If the alveoli communicated freely with the airway opening, then the only resistance to inspiration would be the elastic recoil of the lung, and we would not expect the alveolar pressure to change as pleural pressure fell. On the other hand, if the airway opening were completely occluded, the change in pleural pressure would be reflected almost completely by a similar change in alveolar pressure. In reality the alveoli do communicate with the atmosphere, but they do so through 23 generations of bronchial branchings; therefore, the communication is not completely free, and part of the pleural pressure change is reflected as a negative alveolar pressure. As a result there is a difference between the pressure at the airway opening, which is usually atmospheric, and that in the alveoli, which has become subatmospheric. This constitutes a driving pressure which causes air to flow into the alveoli through the bronchi. When enough air has entered the alveoli to raise its pressure to once again equal the pressure at the airway opening, there will no longer be a driving pressure; airflow ceases, the respiratory muscles relax and expiration proceeds. Under normal resting conditions, expiration is passive and is brought about by the elastic energy stored in the lung during inflation. Once again, the airways offer resistance to airflow so that the alveolar pressure will not remain equal to the pressure at the airway opening. The retractive force of the lung causes the alveolar pressure to exceed the pressure at the airway opening, thus generating a driving pressure, which will result in airflow out of the lung until the alveolar pressure is once again equal to the pressure at the airway opening.

There are two kinds of resistance which must be overcome during breathing: namely, the resistance offered by the elastic and viscous properties of the lung tissue (reflected in the pressure drop, $P_{alv} - P_{pl}$) and the resistance offered by the airways to the flow of gas through them (reflected by the pressure drop between the airway opening and the alveoli, $P_{ao} - P_{alv}$). Referring to Figure 6, it can be seen that during the acts of inspiration and expiration the total pressure difference between the pleural space and the airway opening ($P_{ao} - P_{pl}$) is made up of two components:

$$P_{ao} - P_{pl} = P_{gas} \pm P_{lung} = (P_{ao} - P_{alv}) \pm (P_{alv} - P_{pl})$$

At the end of inspiration or expiration, when there is no flow, the pressure in the airway opening is the same as that in the alveoli. Under these circumstances the equation becomes

$$P_{ao} - P_{pl} = P_{alv} - P_{pl}$$

The viscous resistance of lung tissue and the resistance of the airways have two important characteristics. First, they are only

encountered when the volume of the lung is in the process of changing, and second, the energy expended in overcoming them is dissipated as heat because of friction. Elastic resistance differs from
these so-called nonelastic resistances in that (1) it is dependent on
the lung volume and not on airflow and (2) the force which is required
to overcome the elastic resistance is stored during expansion of the
lung.

The chest wall also offers elastic and nonelastic resistances to
expansion. Part of the resistance is offered by the thoracic cage itself
and part by other structures which are deformed or displaced during
breathing, such as the abdominal wall and the abdominal contents.

ELASTIC BEHAVIOR OF THE RESPIRATORY APPARATUS

The elastic resistances which the tissues of both the lungs and
chest wall offer during breathing are perhaps best understood if
one imagines the lung-thorax system to be in the form of a two-plate
piston within a container, as illustrated in Figure 9.

The opposing surfaces of the two plates are attached to a rubber
balloon, the interior of which represents the pleural space. The
plates are attached to springs which are pulling in opposite directions.
The springs attached to the plate on the left represent the elastic
resistance of the lung, and the springs attached to the plate on the
right represent that of the chest wall. The total capacity of the container is indicated as 100 per cent (the total lung capacity). When the
piston is at its resting position, which is 40 per cent of the total lung
capacity, the forces exerted by the two sets of springs are equal. This

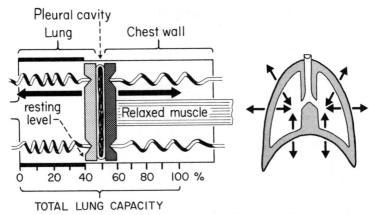

FIGURE 9.   The elastic forces of the lungs at "the resting level" in a mechanical
analogue (*left*) and within the thorax (*right*). The elastic forces of the lung and the chest
wall are pulling equally in opposite directions.

situation is analogous to that at the resting level or midposition of the lungs and the chest wall when the elastic forces exerted by the lung and chest wall are equal and opposite, as is shown in Figure 9.

The elastic behavior of the respiratory apparatus can be described by its force-displacement characteristics; in a three-dimensional system, it is considered conveniently in terms of pressure and volume. By changing the volume of the chest and noting the change in pressure required to maintain the new volume, or by changing the pressure and noting the change in volume which results, information about the elastic properties of the chest may be obtained. In either case, the elastic behavior can be described accurately only if the values of pressure and volume are those recorded when there is no airflow.

If a subject inflates his lungs to a given level and then relaxes his respiratory muscles while airflow is obstructed at the mouth, the pressures developed inside his chest will reflect the elastic forces which are operating at that particular lung volume. The pressure recorded just proximal to the obstructed airway opening under these circumstances (P_{ao}) now reflects the balance of elastic forces in the chest. By repeating this maneuver at different degrees of lung distension and recording the pressures in the airway (*relaxation pressure*) and in the pleural space midway in the chest, it is possible to describe the pressure-volume behavior of the total respiratory apparatus and its components.

If the values for the various lung volumes are plotted against their corresponding pressures, a pressure-volume diagram of the respiratory apparatus and its components can be constructed, as is shown in Figure 10.

As we have seen from Figures 7 and 9, the elastic forces of the lung and chest wall are equal and opposite at the FRC, or about 40 per cent of total lung capacity. The relaxation pressure at this volume is therefore equal to atmospheric pressure, since the gas in the lungs is neither compressed nor decompressed. Let us now look at three other levels of lung volume: 100 per cent of total lung capacity, approximately 67 per cent of total lung capacity, and residual volume or approximately 25 per cent of total lung capacity. The basis for the pressures obtained (i.e., forces developed) at these volumes is illustrated in Figure 11.

When the piston is pulled out as far as possible, it tends to recoil because the spring representing the elastic force of the lung is stretched. The spring representing the elastic force of the chest wall is compressed and actually attempts to re-expand (Fig. 11, A). This situation is analogous to that which exists when a maximum inspiration is made, that is, when the lung volume is at 100 per cent of capacity. The elasticity of the chest wall is exerting a small force in an

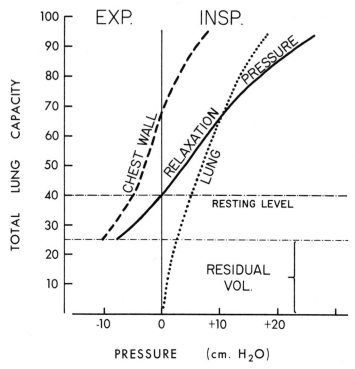

FIGURE 10.   The relaxation pressure curve. The pressure at any lung volume is the resultant of the elastic forces of the lung and chest wall. (From Rahn, H., Otis, A. B., Chadwick, L. E., and Fenn, W. O.: The pressure-volume diagram of the thorax and lung. Am. J. Physiol. *146*:161, 1946. By permission.)

expiratory direction, thereby assisting the lung elasticity, which is exerting a strong force in the same direction. At this lung volume, then, the two forces, acting in series, are additive and result in a high relaxation pressure ($P_{ao} = 1006$ cm. H_2O).

As the piston is allowed to return to its original position, the stretch on the spring which represents the lung elasticity diminishes (Fig. 11, *B*). The spring which represents the chest wall is no longer compressed but has reached a balance point at which it is not exerting an elastic force inwardly or outwardly.

When a lung volume which corresponds to about 67 per cent of the total lung capacity is reached, the chest wall is in its resting position and is exerting no force in either direction. At this level of lung volume the relaxation pressure is positive entirely because of the retractive force of the lung ($P_{ao} = 990$ cm. H_2O).

As the piston is pushed past its resting position, showing the action of the expiratory muscles, the spring representing the pulmonary elasticity exerts even less retractile force, while that of the

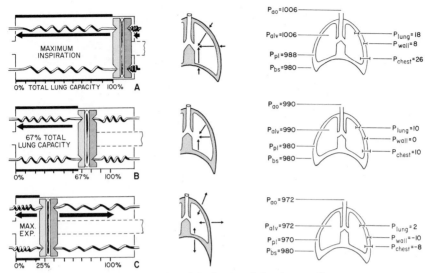

FIGURE 11. The elastic forces of the lung and the chest wall at maximum inspiration (A), at approximately 67 per cent of total lung capacity (B), and at maximum expiration (C). The relaxation pressure, equal to P_{ao} under these circumstances, is positive (i.e., greater than atmospheric) at the high lung volumes and negative at maximum expiration.

chest wall increases (Fig. 11, C). At a position of maximum expiration (i.e., at the residual volume or 25 per cent of total lung capacity), the outward force of the chest wall (in an inspiratory direction) exceeds the retractive force of the lung so that alveolar pressure, and hence the relaxation pressure, is subatmospheric ($P_{ao} = 972$ cm. H_2O).

ELASTIC BEHAVIOR OF THE LUNGS

Since it is impossible to empty the lungs completely, one cannot describe the total pressure-volume behavior of the lungs in intact man. Nevertheless, much important information has been gained by studying the elastic behavior of excised lungs, as is shown in Figure 12. If the excised lung is made completely airless and then increments of pressure are applied, the lung does not begin to inflate until the applied pressure reaches 15 to 20 cm. H_2O. With further increase in pressure the lung inflates but in an uneven manner. Areas of the lung are seen to pop open here and there until, finally, at a pressure of about 40 cm. H_2O the lung is completely inflated. When the pressure around the lung is reduced again, the lung deflates along a pressure-volume curve which differs from that inscribed during the application of pressure. The lung deflates uniformly, and it also remains slightly inflated even when the inflation pressure has fallen

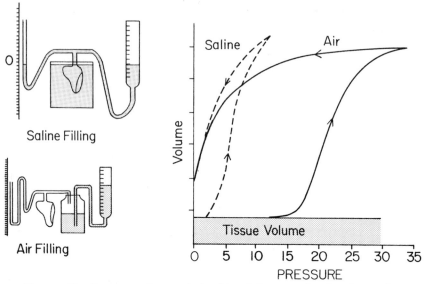

FIGURE 12. Pressure-volume relationship of the excised airless lung when inflated with air and with saline. With saline filling the lung is immersed in saline to counter-balance the effects of hydrostatic pressure. The "deflation limbs" of the air and saline curves diverge at high lung volumes as a result of surface tension at the air tissue interface.

to zero. This difference between the inflation and deflation curves and the failure of the lung to return to its original state after deformation is called *hysteresis*. Subsequent inflations and deflations result in pressure-volume curves which exhibit much less hysteresis and follow closely the deflation limb of the initial pressure-volume curve.

When the lungs are inflated with saline instead of air, they begin to expand at a low pressure, fill uniformly and require less pressure to fill them completely. When the lungs empty under these circumstances little hysteresis is noted. The difference between air and saline filling is attributed to the fact that the surface tension which exists at the air-tissue interface during inflation with air is much greater than the negligible amount of surface tension existing between the liquid-tissue interface during saline filling.

These pressure-volume characteristics demonstrated with air and saline filling indicate that the retractive force of the lung has two components: that due to elastic elements in the tissue and that due to surface tension.

SURFACE FORCES

Consideration of the deflation limb of the two pressure-volume curves indicates that at high lung volumes almost half of the retractive force of the lung is due to surface tension, whereas at low lung volumes the effect of surface tension is negligible. This low surface tension at low lung volumes is the result of the presence in the lung of surface active material (surfactant) which has special physical and chemical characteristics. Surfactant is formed in the terminal units of the lung, and it is generally believed to be a product of a large granular epithelial cell, the type II cell. Surfactant appears during the latter stages of gestation in association with the appearance of these type II cells. The surface of the terminal lung units (i.e., the alveoli, alveolar ducts, respiratory bronchioles) is lined with this material, which is rich in disaturated lecithins. These phospholipids account for the surface tension-lowering effects of the lining material.

The surface tension exerted by a liquid may be measured in an apparatus such as that shown in Figure 13 in which the pull of the liquid surface on a platinum strip is registered. Saline exerts a surface tension of about 70 dynes/cm. and this value does not vary with

Plan View

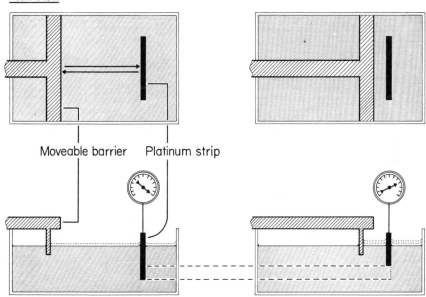

FIGURE 13. Measurement of surface tension. The apparatus consists of a trough containing an aqueous solution, which is shown in two views. On the surface, lung washings form a film; a barrier moves horizontally to increase or decrease the area of the surface film. Surface tension pulls down the platinum strip. As the barrier compresses the surface film, the tension drops (*right*) and rises again when the barrier is moved back (*left*).

expansion or contraction of the surface. When surfactant is added to the saline the surface tension falls; and when the surface film is compressed by movement of the barrier, the tension falls even further and may reach values as low as 1 to 2 dynes/cm., probably because surfactant molecules become concentrated in the surface. Such behavior may explain why the difference between air and saline pressure-volume curves is greater at high lung volumes than at low lung volumes. When the surface area (volume) is great, the surface tension is high, and when the surface area (volume) is small, the surface tension is low.

The physiological importance of surfactant may be appreciated by considering the factors which affect the pressure inside an alveolus. The law of LaPlace states that the pressure (P) inside a spherical structure is directly proportional to the tension (T) in the wall and inversely related to the radius of curvature (r).

$$P = \frac{2\,T}{r}$$

It will be seen that, for a given tension, the pressure which is required to keep a structure from collapsing will become greater as its radius of curvature becomes smaller. Assuming that this relationship is true in the alveoli of the lung, it is apparent that surfactant, by decreasing the value of T, contributes to the stability of the lung by

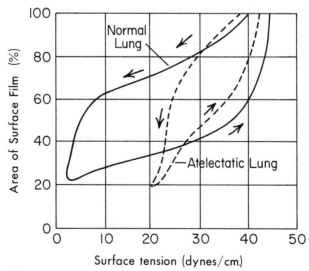

FIGURE 14.   Surface area tension diagrams obtained on compression and decompression of the surface of a saline extract of the lungs of a normal infant and of lungs from an infant with hyaline membrane disease.

allowing small air spaces to remain open at relatively low transpulmonary pressures. Furthermore, the fact that surfactant lowers the surface tension when the surface area is small means that the ratio 2T/r may have the same value in alveoli of different sizes, and as a result, they may be stable at the same transpulmonary pressure.

The production of surfactant depends on an adequate blood supply. A deficiency of surfactant would be expected to render the lung unstable and to promote collapse (atelectasis). Impaired surface activity has been found in lungs of children dying of hyaline membrane disease, in patients following open heart surgery and in a wide variety of experimental conditions, including exposure to high concentrations of oxygen. In all of these situations atelectasis is a prominent feature. Figure 14 demonstrates measurements of surface tension of extracts of lung tissue obtained from a normal and an atelectatic lung. Since many substances can interfere with pulmonary surfactant, notably certain factors in the fibrinolytic system, it is not possible at present to be certain whether abnormal surface activity is due to a primary effect on surfactant production or is secondary to inhibition of surfactant by interfering substances.

TISSUE ELASTICITY

Comparison of air and saline pressure-volume curves indicate that over the tidal breathing range of lung most of the retractive force of the lung is due to the elastic behavior of the tissue elements in the lung. Tissue elasticity is influenced by nutritional factors, at least in young growing animals, and changes in the collagen and elastin content of the lung have been demonstrated in disease in both animals and man. Tissue retractive forces are increased in pulmonary fibrosis and decreased in emphysema. In fibrosis the increase is due to a greater than normal amount of fibrous connective tissue in the lung, and in emphysema the decrease is due to destruction of alveolar walls and a loss of elastic elements. The stiffness or retractive force of the lung may also be increased when the pulmonary vessels are engorged with blood or when the interstitial spaces are filled with fluid.

Contraction of smooth muscle in large airways results in bronchoconstriction and an increase in nonelastic resistance. It is now known that muscle elements are present even in the small alveolar ducts. Contraction of the alveolar duct smooth muscle increases the elastic rather than the nonelastic resistance. The alveolar ducts contract when histamine is injected into the pulmonary circulation and when blood clots lodge in the pulmonary vascular bed. Like the smooth muscle in large airways, the alveolar duct smooth muscle is relaxed by epinephrine and isoproterenol.

COMPLIANCE

The slope of each of the curves representing the pressure-volume characteristics of the chest, the chest wall and the lungs in Figure 10 can be expressed in terms of the compliance of each part of the system; compliance has the dimensions of change in volume per unit change in pressure. The formula for compliance is

$$\text{Compliance} = \frac{\text{Change in volume (in l.)}}{\text{Change in pressure (in cm. } H_2O)}$$

$$C = \frac{\Delta V}{\Delta P}$$

Thus, the compliance of the chest is $\Delta V/\Delta P_{chest}$; the compliance of the lungs is $\Delta V/\Delta P_{lung}$; and the compliance of the chest wall is $\Delta V/\Delta P_{wall}$.

Clearly, the pressure required to overcome the elastic resistance of the chest and its lung and chest wall components is the sum of the pressure across the lung and across the chest wall:

$$\Delta P_{chest} = \Delta P_{lung} + \Delta P_{wall}$$

From the compliance formula we may say that

$$\Delta P_{chest} = I/C_{chest} \times \Delta V$$

$$\Delta P_{lung} = I/C_{lung} \times \Delta V$$

$$\Delta P_{wall} = I/C_{wall} \times \Delta V$$

$$\text{and} \quad I/C_{chest} \times \Delta V = I/C_{lung} \times \Delta V + I/C_{wall} \times \Delta V$$

If we divide by ΔV we see that

$$I/C_{chest} = I/C_{lung} + I/C_{wall}$$

Chest Compliance. From the above equations, it is clear that the compliance of the chest (or the total compliance) must necessarily be less than that of either the lung or the chest wall. This is indicated in Figure 10, which shows that the slope of the relaxation pressure (P_{chest}) curve, which reflects the elastic behavior of the chest, is less than the slope of the pressure-volume curves for either the lung or chest wall.

The total compliance of the chest may also be determined by measuring the changes in the functional residual capacity or resting level. These changes result when a pressure is applied to the external surface of the chest while the subject is breathing spontaneously. Under such circumstances, the compliance of the total respiratory system in normal subjects is approximately 0.12 l./cm. H_2O. It is reduced by any alteration of the compliance of the lung or the chest wall.

Although it would appear to be comparatively simple to determine the total elastic resistance involved in breathing by utilizing the above techniques, it should be pointed out that the respiratory muscles must be in a state of either complete relaxation or paralysis in order to obtain an accurate assessment. Complete relaxation of the respiratory muscles is extremely difficult to attain except in a well-trained subject; therefore, this method is not always practical. Similarly, although the compliance of the lungs and chest wall (either together or separately) can be measured when the respiratory muscles are paralyzed, one is never certain that the resistances of the chest are similar to those which occur in a subject who is breathing spontaneously.

Lung Compliance. It is evident that the pressure-volume curve of the lung is alinear. Thus, the value for the compliance of the lung will vary, depending upon the part of the curve over which the ratio of volume change to pressure change is determined. A person breathing near his total lung capacity will have an apparently stiffer lung than another person breathing near his functional residual capacity, even though the intrinsic elastic properties of the lungs of the two persons may be identical. Ideally one would like to be able to obtain the complete pressure-volume relationship for any person. However, this is not possible, even in normal subjects, because the lungs cannot be emptied completely. In patients with lung disease it may be particularly difficult because they are often unable to carry out the maneuvers required to obtain truly static measurements.

The compliance of the lung can be assessed in the spontaneously breathing subject by measuring the changes in pressure across the lungs from end-expiration to end-inspiration and the tidal volume. Although either pleural or esophageal pressure may be measured, it is usually the esophageal pressure which is determined.

Examples of the elastic behavior or the compliance of three different types of lung are plotted in Figure 15. Figure 15, *A* shows that a change in the intrathoracic pressure of 5 cm. H_2O results in an inspiration of 1 liter of air into the normal lung. Its compliance is therefore 0.20 l./cm. H_2O. When the lung loses its elasticity, as in emphysema, it becomes easier to distend; in other words, it is more compliant. Figure 15, *B* illustrates that a change in the intrathoracic pressure of 5 cm. H_2O now results in an inspiration of 2 liters of air. The compliance of these lungs is 0.40 l./cm. H_2O. If the lungs are stiff, as in pulmonary fibrosis or congestion, the same change in the intrathoracic pressure results in a change of volume of only 0.5 liter, and the compliance is only 0.10 l./cm. H_2O (Fig. 15, *C*).

When lung compliance is measured over the normal range of tidal volume during spontaneous breathing in clinical laboratories, the results are often expressed in relationship to the lung volume at which it was measured. "Compliance per unit lung volume" is termed *specific compliance*.

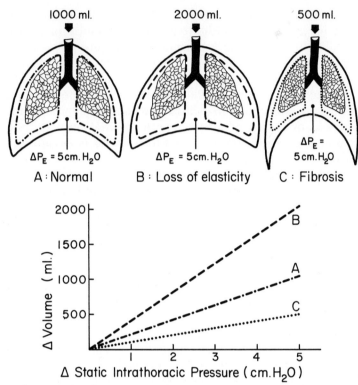

FIGURE 15. The distention produced by a change in intrathoracic pressure (pleural pressure) of 5 cm. H_2O in a normal lung (A), a lung which has lost elasticity (B), and a lung which has become fibrosed (C).

Compliance measured during spontaneous breathing is called *dynamic compliance* and may be significantly influenced by the non-elastic resistance of the lung. This will be considered in more detail after the factors determining nonelastic resistance are discussed.

When the lungs of animals or man are ventilated artificially with a fixed tidal volume the compliance tends to decrease with time. This has been attributed to progressive closure of air spaces which may in part be related to "aging" of the alveolar surface material. The decrease in compliance can be reversed by single large inflations which open the collapsed alveoli. It is clear that compliance depends on the " volume history" of the lungs which determines the number of spaces that are open and participating in volume change. When one lung is surgically removed, the compliance as it is ordinarily measured falls, not because the retractive force of the remaining lung is abnormally high but merely because there are fewer alveoli responding to a given change in transpulmonary pressure and the volume change is correspondingly less.

There is some hysteresis in the pressure-volume relationship of the lung, indicating that the compliance measured during inspiration might differ from that measured during expiration. Such a difference between the respiratory phases may be related to differences in the number of alveoli participating, in the alveolar surface tension and in tissue elastic elements. Such quasi-static hysteresis is negligible at normal breathing frequencies and tidal volumes but may be appreciable at very slow frequencies or during deep breathing.

Chest Wall Compliance. In order to measure the compliance of the chest wall it is necessary to determine both the total compliance of the chest and the lung compliance simultaneously. As pointed out previously, this entails measurement of the change in pleural pressure along with the functional residual capacity resulting from a pressure applied to either the upper airway or the external surface of the chest or airway pressure when the respiratory muscles are relaxed while airflow is obstructed at the mouth. By means of these techniques, the compliance of the chest wall has been estimated to be approximately 0.22 l./cm. H_2O in normal subjects. In obese subjects, on the other hand, the compliance of the chest wall has been found to be greatly reduced, averaging 0.77 l./cm. H_2O.

NONELASTIC RESISTANCE

There are two main types of nonelastic resistances which must be overcome during breathing. These resistances are illustrated by the mechanical analogue in Figure 16 which demonstrates that, in

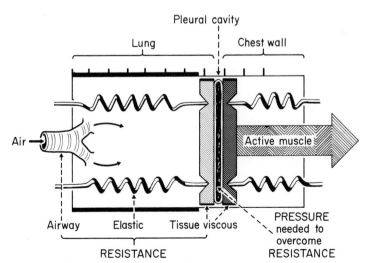

FIGURE 16. Resistances which must be overcome in order to move air into the lungs during breathing.

addition to the elastic resistance, both an airway resistance and a tissue resistance must be overcome while the piston is being pulled out or pushed in. A third type of nonelastic resistance is due to the inertia which must be overcome during acceleration and deceleration of the gas or tissues, but this is generally considered to be negligible. The pressure which is necessary to overcome the resistance to the flow of air in the tracheobronchial tree has been defined previously as the pressure difference between the airway opening and the alveoli ($P_{ao} - P_{alv}$). The nasal passages, the nasopharynx, the larynx and the trachea have been shown to contribute about 20 per cent of the nonelastic resistance at low rates of airflow and as much as 45 per cent at higher rates of flow. Tissue viscous resistance is due to the friction of tissue structures sliding over one another during movement of the lungs. Of the total nonelastic resistances in normal subjects, airway resistance accounts for 90 per cent or more, and tissue viscous resistance accounts for less than 10 per cent.

ESTIMATION OF TOTAL NONELASTIC RESISTANCE OF THE LUNG

The pressures which must be generated to overcome the elastic and nonelastic resistances to breathing are summarized in the following equation:

$$P_{total} = P_{elastic} + P_{nonelastic}$$

The pressure needed to overcome nonelastic resistance is then merely the difference between P_{total} and $P_{elastic}$.

Since flow resistance may be defined as the pressure required to produce a given rate of flow:

$$R_{nonelastic} = \frac{P_{nonelastic}}{Flow} = \frac{P_{total} - P_{elastic}}{Flow}$$

The usual units used for $R_{nonelastic}$ are cm. $H_2O/l./sec.$

The nonelastic pressure may be determined from simultaneous measurements of changes in pleural pressure, tidal volume and the rate of airflow, such as those shown in Figure 17, which is an excerpt from Figure 8. The change in pleural (intrathoracic) pressure during the respiratory cycle has the two components mentioned above: an elastic component and a nonelastic component.

The elastic pressure curve during a breath can be constructed as follows. Since at end-inspiration and end-expiration there is no airflow, the nonelastic pressure is zero and the pleural pressure is equal to the elastic pressure. The remainder of the elastic pressure curve between these points may be interpolated by assuming that the elastic pressure is linearly related to the volume change. However,

Airflow (l./min.)

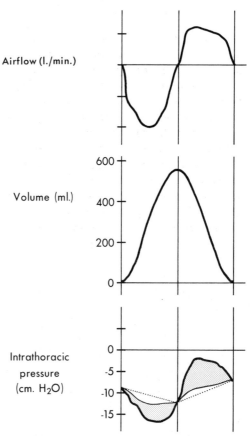

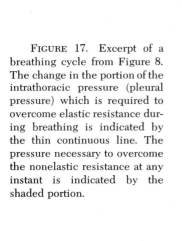

FIGURE 17. Excerpt of a breathing cycle from Figure 8. The change in the portion of the intrathoracic pressure (pleural pressure) which is required to overcome elastic resistance during breathing is indicated by the thin continuous line. The pressure necessary to overcome the nonelastic resistance at any instant is indicated by the shaded portion.

Volume (ml.)

Intrathoracic pressure (cm. H₂O)

reference to the total pressure volume curve (Fig. 10) indicates that this assumption is only valid for changes in volume over the tidal breathing range. Even in this range one cannot simply join the points of zero flow by a straight line, as is shown by the interrupted line in Figure 17, unless the rate of airflow is constant and the volume changes uniformly throughout the respiratory cycle. The shape of the elastic pressure curve during the respiratory cycle depends upon the rate of change in lung volume; one must interpolate the elastic pressure for many small increments or decrements in volume in order to obtain the true elastic pressure curve as is indicated by the thin continuous line in Figure 17. The pressure which is necessary to overcome the nonelastic resistance at any moment in the respiratory cycle equals the difference between the value for pleural pressure and the value for elastic pressure at that instant in the respiratory cycle.

THE PRESSURE-VOLUME LOOP

An analysis of the elastic and nonelastic components of the intrathoracic pressure curve, such as has been described, is a time-consuming procedure. In a simpler method, the simultaneous changes of the volume and the pleural pressure are plotted against one another. In this way the time element is removed from the relationship between the two measurements. By this method a loop is formed, its boundaries being derived from the pleural pressure changes at different degrees of lung inflation during the respiratory cycle. A pressure-volume loop determined in a normal subject is illustrated in Figure 18, A. Since the elastic resistance is linearly related to the state of lung distension over the tidal volume range, a line joining the points of end-expiration and end-inspiration, when there is no flow of air, represents the pressure which is required to overcome the elastic resistance at any given instant during the breathing cycle. The difference between the intrathoracic pressure and that portion required to overcome the elastic resistance at any given moment during the breathing cycle is, therefore, the pressure necessary to overcome the nonelastic resistance at that particular moment.

Similarly, one can see from the pressure-volume loop that if the airway distal to the pressure measurement is suddenly obstructed during breathing so that there is no flow of air, the pleural pressure will change to that which is required to overcome the elastic resistance at that particular lung volume. The interruption of airflow at intervals while a maximum inspiration and expiration is carried out will thus provide an assessment of the relationship between the elastic retractive force and lung volume. The change in pleural pres-

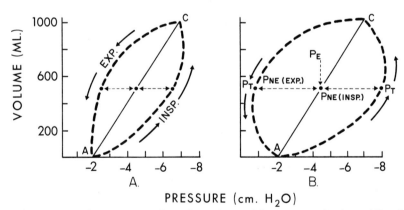

FIGURE 18.   The pressure-volume loop obtained from a normal subject (*A*) and a patient with airway obstruction (*B*). Note that if airflow were interrupted at points PT the pressure at zero flow would change to PE and the pressure change would equal the PNE required to overcome flow resistance just prior to interruption.

sure which occurs when airflow is interrupted is also important. It represents the pressure which was required to overcome the non-elastic resistance which happened to be present just prior to the interruption of airflow.

When there is airway obstruction, the pressure-volume loop is considerably widened, and there is a great increase in the pressure required to overcome the nonelastic resistance during both inspiration and expiration. This is demonstrated in Figure 18, *B* which shows a pressure-volume loop which was determined in a patient suffering from obstruction of the airway due to bronchospasm.

PRESSURE-FLOW RELATIONSHIP

When the nonelastic component of the intrathoracic pressure is plotted against the simultaneous rate of airflow, a pressure-flow plot is derived. This is illustrated in Figure 19 in which the inspiration is shown in the upper right quadrant and expiration in the lower left quadrant. It can be seen that the pressure change is linearly related to the airflow up to a certain point. After this there is a disproportionate increase in the pressure required to produce a further increase in airflow. The linear portion of the curve is due to the laminar resistance, and the horizontal portion of the curve is due to the addition of turbulent resistance. In the normal subject the total nonelastic resistance is approximately 1.8 cm. $H_2O/l./sec.$ of airflow, and only about one-tenth of the resistance at this rate of airflow is due to turbulence.

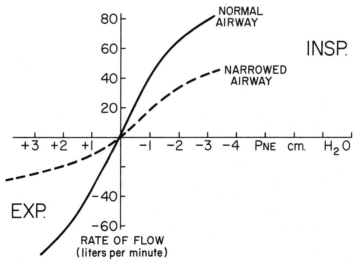

FIGURE 19. The pressure-flow relationship in a normal subject and in a patient with airway obstruction.

Figure 19 also shows the pressure-flow plot derived from the pressure-volume loop in Figure 18, *B* which was obtained from a patient suffering from airway obstruction. It can be seen that a given flow of air requires a greater than normal pressure, indicating that the resistance to airflow is increased. In patients suffering from obstruction of the airway, the total nonelastic resistance is increased and may be considerably greater than 5 cm. $H_2O/l./sec.$ of airflow. In these patients, this resistance is predominantly due to turbulence. When the ventilation is increased above normal, as it is during exertion, this turbulent resistance becomes exceedingly high.

TISSUE VISCOUS RESISTANCE

Using techniques which measure nonelastic resistance during the inhalation of gases which have a greater or lesser viscosity than that of air, it is possible to calculate by extrapolation the resistance which would be present if a gas possessing no viscosity whatsoever were being inhaled. The pressure required to overcome the tissue viscous resistance can then be derived. This pressure has also been determined by the simultaneous estimation of the pressure required to overcome the airway resistance and that which is necessary to overcome the total nonelastic resistance. The tissue viscous resistance has been found to form only a small part of the total nonelastic resistance; the major resistance is that which occurs in the airways. Therefore, it is the airway resistance or total nonelastic resistance which is usually determined.

AIRWAY RESISTANCE

The airway resistance component of total nonelastic resistance is given by the formula

$$R_{airway} = \frac{P_{ao} - P_{alv}}{Flow}$$

The pressure at the airway opening can be easily measured, but alveolar pressure is more difficult to measure. Two methods have been used to determine airway resistance. The interruptor method makes use of a device which obstructs airflow at the mouth for a split second many times during the respiratory cycle. Upon interruption of airflow, the pressure behind the obstruction will equal alveolar pressure. If it is assumed that this pressure is the same as that which was present the instant before interruption, one can, by relating it to the flow just before interruption, obtain an estimate of airway resistance. There is reason to believe, however, that this assumption is not always valid.

Another method for estimating alveolar pressure which is more widely used employs a body plethysmograph. The subject enters an airtight chamber and breathes through a tube containing a shutter while pressure inside the chamber and at the airway opening are continuously recorded. The shutter is then closed so that the airway is completely obstructed. Under this circumstance, pressure at the airway opening is identical to pressure in the alveoli. The subject makes inspiratory and expiratory efforts against the closed shutter, which decompresses and compresses the air in the lungs and has the opposite effect on the gas in the chamber. The changes in alveolar pressure and chamber pressure which result are noted, and the ratio of alveolar pressure to chamber pressure is determined. To determine airway resistance the subject breathes through an unobstructed airway while airflow and changes in chamber pressure are recorded. Using the previously determined ratio of alveolar pressure to chamber pressure, changes in alveolar pressure are calculated and are related to airflow in order to yield a value for airway resistance. The advantage of this technique is that it is simple to determine lung volume as well.

When the lungs inflate, airway caliber and length increase, resulting in a fall in the frictional resistance to flow. The relationship between the inverse of the flow resistance, which is called airway conductance, and lung volume is nearly linear so that conductance per unit volume, or *specific conductance*, is, as a useful approximation, independent of body size or the lung volume at which the subject is breathing.

Partitioning of Airway Resistance. It has already been mentioned that a substantial proportion of the total airway resistance is present in the upper respiratory tract. In the tracheobronchial tree most of the remainder of the resistance to airflow resides in airways greater than 2 mm. in diameter. The small peripheral airways, because of their vastly greater number, provide a large cross-sectional area for airflow and therefore contribute less than 20 per cent to the total airway resistance. As a result, the small peripheral airways may be the site of disease which severely impairs ventilation of the air spaces distal to them, and yet the effect of this disease on total airway resistance may be slight. Fortunately there are other ways in which such defects may be recognized, and they will be discussed later.

Factors Affecting Airway Resistance. Under normal circumstances airway resistance is determined by the cross-sectional area available for flow, the velocity of airflow and the physical properties of the gas being breathed.

CROSS-SECTIONAL AREA. The cross-sectional area available for airflow is determined by the balance of forces tending to narrow the airways and those tending to widen them. The forces tending to narrow airways include peribronchial pressure and the force exerted by contraction of bronchial smooth muscle; the forces tending to keep the airways open include the intraluminal pressure and the tethering action of the surrounding connective tissue. As lung volume increases and pleural pressure becomes more subatmospheric, those parts of the tracheobronchial tree which are exposed to pleural pressure will increase in size because of the increase in transbronchial pressure. During passive expiration the airways decrease in size again as transbronchial pressure falls.

The influence of peribronchial and intraluminal pressures on airway caliber during a forced expiration is particularly important and may be illustrated conveniently with the aid of a model of the lung, such as that shown in Figure 20. During active expiratory efforts of sufficient force both pleural and alveolar pressure become greater than atmospheric pressure. The intrabronchial pressure varies along the airways because of flow resistance, and it decreases from values

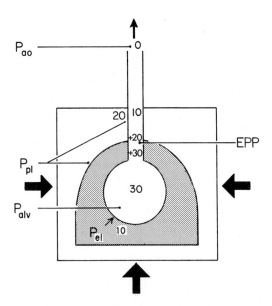

FIGURE 20.　Forces acting in the chest during a forced expiratory effort. The heavy arrows indicate compression of the thorax by contraction of the expiratory muscles.

P_{pl} equals the pleural pressure, in this case 20 cm. H_2O.

P_{el} equals elastic recoil pressure of the lung, in this case 10 cm. H_2O.

P_{alv} equals pressure in the alveolus = P_{pl} (20) + P_{el} (10) = 30 cm. H_2O.

Note that the pressure in the airways drops from the alveolar pressure (30 cm. H_2O) to the mouth or P_{ao} (or atmospheric pressure).

EPP indicates the "equal pressure point," i.e., the point in the airway at which the intramural and extramural pressures are equal, in this case 20 cm. H_2O. Further downstream from the equal pressure point, toward the airway opening, there is a transmural pressure tending to narrow or close the airway.

near alveolar pressure in the peripheral airways to atmospheric pressure near the airway opening. At some point in the airway the bronchial pressure may be equal to the pleural pressure. This has been called the equal pressure point (EPP). Toward the airway opening, the intrabronchial pressure will be less than the peribronchial pressure, and therefore there will be a net force tending to narrow the airway.

When a normal subject is asked to perform a series of active expirations of increasing force, and the airflow rate at the same lung volume in each of them is plotted against the corresponding transpulmonary pressure, so-called "isovolume pressure-flow curves" are obtained. Examples of such curves at three lung volumes are shown in Figure 21. At high lung volumes the airways are widely open so that very high flows can be achieved. A maximum flow is not observed during maximum effort, but rather the flow appears to be related to the amount of effort exerted. At low lung volume, airflow rate increases with increasing transpulmonary pressure up to a certain point at which flow reaches a maximum. Further effort produces no further increase in flow presumably because the increased compression of alveolar gas is offset by compression of airways which are exposed to the coincident increase in pleural pressure. At midlung

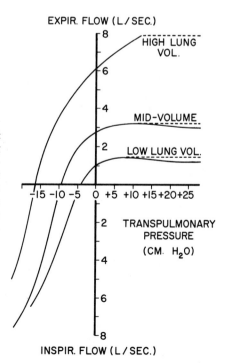

FIGURE 21. Isovolume pressure-flow curves obtained in a normal subject at three levels of lung inflation. At high lung volume, maximum expiratory flow increases with increasing effort. At lower lung volumes increasing pressure raises airflow rate up to a maximum and further effort produces no further increase in flow, presumably because of airways compression (see Fig. 20).

volume the airways are more distended, offer less resistance and hence a greater flow is achieved before increasing effort prevents further increases in flow by airway compression.

Patients with lung disease who have airways which are abnormally collapsible or who have lost lung elastic recoil exhibit flow limitation at much lower levels of transpulmonary pressure than is seen in normal subjects.

VELOCITY OF FLOW. As mentioned previously the relationship between airflow and driving pressure is not a simple one. At low levels of airflow gas moves in a streamline or laminar fashion, and flow and pressure are linearly related. At higher levels of flow, the flow pressure relationship departs from linearity (see Fig. 19) because turbulence is created, and this increases resistance. The laminar component of airflow is proportional to the velocity of airflow, and the turbulent component is related to the square of velocity of the airflow.

THE PHYSICAL CHARACTERISTICS OF THE RESPIRED GAS. Since airway resistance is the result of friction between the flowing gas and the walls of the airways and within the air stream itself, it is evident that any property of the gas tending to increase friction will increase airway resistance, and any property tending to decrease friction will decrease airway resistance. Thus, as originally proposed by Rohrer, the pressure drop between the alveolus and the mouth can be represented by the following equation:

$$P_{alv} - P_{ao} = K_1 \dot{V} + K_2 \dot{V}_2$$

Where $\dot{V}$ is flow, K_1 is a constant containing gas viscosity and airway geometry, and K_2 is another constant containing gas density and airway geometry.

Gases with low density, such as helium, reduce airway resistance; and gases with high density, such as sulfur hexafluoride, increase airway resistance. The density of gases is also determined by the barometric pressure. In divers exposed to increased barometric pressure the increased density of the gas may increase airway resistance sufficiently to interfere with breathing. Conversely, at higher altitudes airway resistance is decreased.

INTERACTION BETWEEN AIRWAY RESISTANCE AND COMPLIANCE

The rate at which a given part of the lung can fill or empty depends on both its airway resistance and compliance. This can be illustrated by reference to an electrical analogue. The emptying of an elastic reservoir such as the lung through a resistive conduit resembles the discharging of a capacitor through a resistor. If the charge (I) on the capacitor as a fraction of the initial charge (I_o) is plotted against time, then an exponential curve is obtained whose equation is

$$\frac{I}{I_o} = e^{-K_t}$$

The constant K is equal to 1/RC where R is the resistance and C the capacitance. When the exponent has a value of unity ($K_t = 1$) the equation becomes

$$\frac{I}{I_o} = e^{-1} = \frac{1}{e} = .37$$

$$\text{and} \quad t = \frac{1}{K} = \frac{1}{1/RC} = RC$$

Thus, the time it takes the charge to reach 37 per cent of its initial value is called the time constant and is equal to the product of the resistance and capacitance. Similarly, the time it takes a lung unit to fill or empty depends on its time constant or the product of its resistance and compliance.

When two or more parallel units are subjected to the same inflation or deflation pressure they will each fill or empty at a rate determined by their individual time constants. If their time constants are equal, the units will fill or empty uniformly. Conversely, if their time constants are unequal, the units will fill or empty nonuniformly. In normal subjects, the time constants are relatively uniform throughout the lung.

By influencing the distribution of gas in the lung, inequality of time constants can affect the measurement of compliance if it is determined during breathing (i.e., dynamic compliance). During breathing, local alterations in the mechanical properties of the lungs, such as may occur in unequally distributed bronchial obstruction, can alter the changes in pressure which are necessary to produce a given lung inflation. Figure 22 illustrates the change in the pleural pressure which is normally necessary to bring a liter of air into the lung as compared to that which is required when there is a local obstruction to airflow. It can be seen that when there is no airway obstruction, the tidal volume is equally distributed to all areas of the lung. When an airway obstruction is present, however, there is an increase in the resistance to the flow of air into the lung distal to the obstruction. During very slow breathing it is likely that the air is almost equally distributed, even in the presence of bronchial obstruction, so that the calculated value for the compliance is little altered. During rapid breathing, however, the air tends to move into areas of the lung which offer the least resistance. In order that the same volume of air may be inspired, a greater intrathoracic pressure must develop, and this results in a fall of the calculated (dynamic) com-

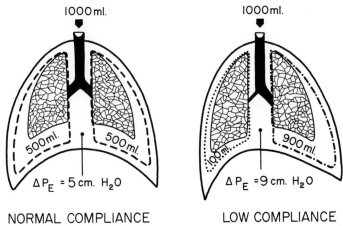

NORMAL COMPLIANCE   LOW COMPLIANCE

FIGURE 22.   The effect of a local airway obstruction on the pressure-volume relationship of two lungs with the same elastic properties when 1000 ml. of air is inhaled during breathing.

pliance. In addition, the measured compliance will fall with increasing respiratory frequency. This frequency dependence of compliance is a reflection of the inequality of the time constants throughout the lung. When the overall elastic properties of the lung are studied, therefore, it is extremely important that all the measurements of pressure should be truly static and that sufficient time is allowed for all areas of the lung to become inflated. Nevertheless, it should be pointed out that the dynamic compliance measured during breathing is important because it indicates the elastic resistance that is actually overcome while breathing at that respiratory rate, which clearly may be far greater than that which is reflected in static measurements. This is particularly true in obstructive disease involving the smaller airways. In such circumstances the frequency dependence of compliance may be the only abnormality detected.

DISTRIBUTION OF INSPIRED GAS IN THE LUNG

Even in young healthy persons, and particularly in older persons, the inspired air is not distributed uniformly throughout the lungs. This has been shown clearly with radioactive gas techniques involving scanning of the thorax, as demonstrated in Figure 23. As mentioned earlier, because of regional differences in transpulmonary pressure, the air spaces at the top of the lung are expanded to a greater degree than those at the bottom. Similarly, the various regions will be at different levels of the pressure-volume curve. Thus the distribution of the inspired air to the various regions will depend upon the lung volume at which one is breathing. The air spaces at the top of

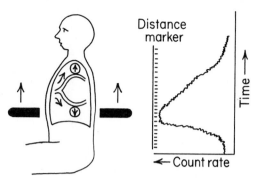

FIGURE 23.   Measurement of regional pulmonary blood flow and ventilation by the "poorly soluble radioactive gas method." Radioactive gas is injected intravenously to measure blood flow and inhaled to measure distribution of ventilation. The radioactive gas injected into the circulation is evolved into the alveolar gas when it reaches the lungs. By scanning the lung with counters during breath-holding the radioactivity over each lung region is measured and is found to be proportional either to blood flow or to ventilation distribution when the observed value is corrected for the amount injected or inhaled and for the dimensions of the chest. (From West, J. B.: Regional differences in blood flow and ventilation in the lung. Advances in Respiratory Physiology. Edited by Caro, C. G. Edward Arnold Publishers Ltd., London, 1966. By permission.)

the lung tend to fill less on inspiration during ordinary breathing at FRC (Fig. 24, *B*). When a person breathes at a low lung volume the upper part of the lung is ventilated more than the lower part (Fig. 24, *A*), and if he breathes near his residual volume, the lower part of the lung may receive almost no ventilation. Conversely, at a very high lung volume close to total lung capacity the change in volume in both regions will be similar (Fig. 24, *C*).

In·addition to the nonuniformity of gas distribution, which can be attributed to the regional differences in pressure, the distribution of the inspired gas is also affected by regional alterations in the mechanical resistances offered by the lung, the airways and the extrapulmonary structures (i.e., regional variations in mechanical time constants). The effect of a local airway resistance on distribution of gas is illustrated in Figure 25, which illustrates the moment-to-moment concentration of nitrogen in the expired air following a single inspiration of pure oxygen. Where there is no obstruction (Fig. 25, *A*), the inspired gas enters both lungs almost synchronously and equally, and expiration takes place in the same fashion. Initially the nitrogen concentration in the expired gas will be zero as pure oxygen is exhaled from the dead space. Then it will rise in a curvilinear fashion as oxygen from the dead space is mixed with gas containing nitrogen from the alveolar spaces. The last portion of the curve is an almost definite plateau in the curve of the nitrogen concentration as an equal amount of nitrogen comes from each lung. The very slight rise in the plateau is probably due to sequential ventilation of different areas of the lungs. In Figure 25, *B*, the inspired oxygen is asyn-

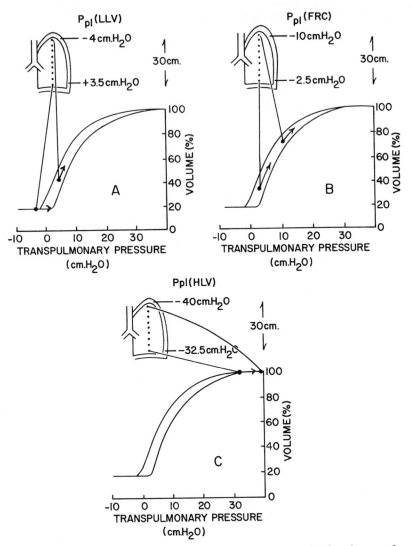

FIGURE 24. The effect of a pleural pressure gradient on the distribution of ventilation (the pressure is assumed to fall at a rate of 0.25 cm. of water per centimeter of vertical distance).

At low lung volumes (A) the pleural pressure at the base may exceed airway pressure so that this region is not ventilated and the initial part of inspiration is delivered to the apex of the lung.

During an inspiration from FRC (B) air is distributed to upper and lower parts of the lung. Because the pressures at the apex and base are taken to be −10 and −2.5 cm. of H_2O respectively, the two regions are on different parts of the pressure-volume curve, and the lung units at the base are smaller than those at the apex. On inspiration the lung units at the base have a greater change in volume than do those at the apex. At FRC, therefore, ventilation decreases with vertical distance up the lung.

At high lung volumes (C) both upper and lower lung regions are on the flat part of the pressure-volume curve and exhibit changes in volume that correspond to changes in transpulmonary pressure. (Modified from Emili, M., in West, J. B.: Ventilation: Blood Flow and Gas Exchange. London, Blackwell, Scientific Publications, 1965.)

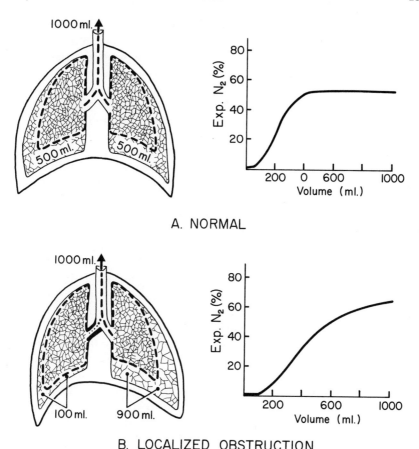

A. NORMAL

B. LOCALIZED OBSTRUCTION

FIGURE 25. The effect of a localized airway obstruction on the distribution of air. Normally (A) air is distributed synchronously and equally, and expiration takes place in the same manner. With localized airway obstruction (B), inspired oxygen predominantly moves into areas of lung which offer least resistance. During expiration air moves out of the unobstructed lung first and the asynchronous delivery of air results in a rising nitrogen concentration curve.

chronously and unequally distributed because the oxygen moves into and distends those areas of lung which offer the least resistance before it enters the others. The nitrogen in the unobstructed lung is, therefore, well diluted by the oxygen, but that in the obstructed lung is not. During expiration, air moves out of the unobstructed lung first, but that from the obstructed lung is delayed. The asynchronous delivery of air from the two lungs results in a rising nitrogen concentration curve, and in addition, the record suggests an enlarged dead space. Obviously other factors affecting the regional distribution of time constants, such as regional alterations of the elastic resistance or the tissue viscous resistance, will alter the distribution of gas in a similar manner.

Clearly then, the uniformity of the distribution of time constants in the lung can be assessed by study of the distribution of a gas such as oxygen. The uniformity of distribution of inspired gas may also be assessed by measuring the efficiency of gas mixing in the lung. In general, a relatively insoluble reference gas, such as helium or hydrogen, is inspired so that any variations in the pulmonary blood flow or in the diffusion of gas across the alveolocapillary membrane do not influence the measurement. The rate at which the nitrogen in the lung is diluted during the inhalation of oxygen or helium or the rate at which the lung and a spirometer reach equilibrium with respect to a foreign gas, such as helium or hydrogen, provides an index of the uniformity of gas distribution and therefore of the uniformity of distribution of time constants in the lung.

An abnormal distribution of inspired gas is encountered clinically in a variety of diseases in which the lesions are not uniformly distributed so that the mechanical time constants vary throughout the lung. A regional loss of elasticity with a resultant inequality of elastic properties in different areas of the lung occurs in emphysema; regional increases in elastic resistance occur when there is pulmonary congestion, an exudate in the alveoli or alteration in the architecture of the lung by fibrosis, tumors or kyphoscoliosis. In addition, the distribution of gas is altered by regional variations in airway resistance (as in bronchial asthma, chronic bronchitis, bronchiectasis and emphysema), in the smaller peripheral airways, or in the forces applied to the chest wall by the respiratory muscles (as in muscular dystrophy, local muscular weakness or paralysis).

WORK OF BREATHING

In order to overcome the resistances which are offered by the lung and the chest wall during breathing, work must be performed by the respiratory muscles. Three aspects of the work of breathing are of extreme importance in understanding pulmonary disability: (1) the total mechanical work which is done during breathing, (2) the relationship between the amount of work that is done and that portion of the total ventilation which is actually taking part in gas exchange, or the alveolar ventilation, and (3) the amount of oxygen which is consumed by the respiratory muscles while they are performing this work.

TOTAL WORK OF BREATHING

Work is usually defined as force acting through a distance and is expressed as dynes·cm. In the respiratory system it is convenient to consider the product of pressure and volume, which also has the units of work (dynes/cm² × cm³). In order to measure the mechanical work which is done during breathing, it is therefore necessary to obtain simultaneous measurements of both the volume change and the pressure which is exerted across the respiratory system.

The work which is necessary to overcome the elastic resistance of the total respiratory system may be estimated from the relaxation pressure curve. However, there does not seem to be any method available for measuring the total amount of work being done on the lung, the respired gases, the chest wall, the diaphragm and the abdominal contents while a subject is breathing because no technique has as yet been devised for the determination of the nonelastic resistance of the chest wall. Nevertheless, there are two techniques which measure indirectly the total amount of mechanical work which is carried out during breathing. In the first method, a respirator is substituted for the respiratory muscles of a paralyzed or "completely relaxed" subject. It is presumed that movements of the chest induced by the respirator are similar to those resulting from the action of the respiratory muscles during breathing. In the second method, the total mechanical work is calculated by measuring the change in oxygen consumption brought about by an increase in ventilation as well as the efficiency with which added respiratory work loads are handled. It is possible to calculate the total work of breathing by the latter techniques because the efficiency of the respiratory muscles would appear to be constant over a large range of added work loads, suggesting that their efficiency is the same when there is no added work load.

MECHANICAL WORK DONE ON THE LUNGS

The mechanical work which is carried out solely on the lungs during a breathing cycle can be estimated by simultaneously measuring the changes in the intrathoracic pressure, utilizing either the esophageal or pleural pressure, as well as the volume displacement which takes place. When these pressure measurements and volume alterations over the period of a complete breathing cycle are plotted against one another, a pressure-volume loop is obtained which is similar to that which has been described previously.

Figure 26 demonstrates the information which can be derived from such a loop. The mechanical work necessary to overcome the elastic resistance is calculated from the area of the trapezoid (OACD), and the mechanical work required to overcome the nonelastic resistance during both inspiration and expiration is calculated from the area of the loop (AB^{1}CB^2). The portion of the loop which falls to the right of the line ABC represents the mechanical work necessary to

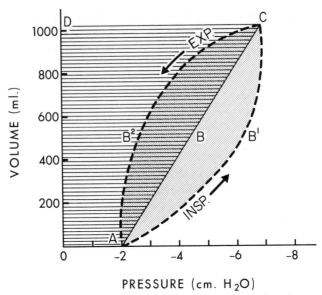

FIGURE 26.   The mechanical work done on the lungs during a breathing cycle. The work necessary to overcome elastic resistance equals the area of trapezoid OACD. Mechanical work necessary to overcome inspiratory nonelastic resistance equals area AB^1CB. Mechanical work necessary to overcome expiratory nonelastic resistance equals $ABCB^2$.

overcome the nonelastic resistance during inspiration. That portion of the loop which falls to the left of the line ABC represents the mechanical work required to overcome the nonelastic resistance during expiration.

During quiet breathing almost all of the muscular work is carried out during inspiration because the elastic recoil of the lungs is sufficient to overcome the nonelastic resistance of both the air and the tissues during expiration. The expiratory portion of the nonelastic loop does not usually fill the entire trapezoid representing the elastic work, indicating that some of the elastic energy which was built up during inspiration is dissipated in the form of heat. If the expiratory portion of the nonelastic work loop falls entirely within the trapezoid, it indicates that the intrathoracic pressure has been less than that of the atmosphere throughout expiration and that no extra work has been performed by the respiratory muscles during expiration. If a portion of the expiratory nonelastic work loop falls outside the trapezoid, it signifies that the intrathoracic pressure was greater than that of the atmosphere during expiration and that expiratory muscular work was required for that part of the expiration.

The total mechanical work which is carried out on the lungs during a breath is calculated from the sum of the inspiratory work necessary to overcome the elastic resistance and the inspiratory non-elastic resistance plus, when applicable, the expiratory work necessary to overcome that portion of the expiratory nonelastic work loop which falls outside of the trapezoid, representing the elastic work area. The total amount of mechanical work carried out on the lungs per minute may be determined by multiplying the work done during each breath by the respiratory rate.

In normal subjects the total mechanical work performed on the lungs has been estimated to be approximately 0.3 to 0.7 kg.m./min. In a patient suffering from diffuse bronchial obstruction, such as bronchial asthma or emphysema, the mechanical work necessary to overcome the nonelastic resistance is increased so that the pressure-volume loop becomes widened in a manner similar to that illustrated in Figure 18. In pulmonary fibrosis, the work required to overcome the nonelastic resistance may be only slightly altered. On the other hand, much more work must be performed in order to overcome the high elastic resistance of these "stiff lungs," and the result is that the area of the elastic work trapezoid is increased. In addition, in patients suffering from respiratory disease this work may increase disproportionately when the ventilation increases. It is probable that the disturbances in the mechanical properties of the lung and the resultant increase in mechanical work are operative in limiting the activity of a patient.

THE RELATIONSHIP BETWEEN MECHANICAL WORK AND ALVEOLAR VENTILATION

There would also appear to be a relationship between the mechanical work of breathing and the rate and depth at which a person breathes. It can be shown mathematically that for any given alveolar ventilation there is an optimum respiratory rate and tidal volume at which the total mechanical work of breathing is minimal. This is illustrated in Figure 27, *A*. It would appear that this is applicable to both normal subjects and patients with respiratory disease; they breathe at a rate and depth at which the work of breathing is least. When the elastic resistance becomes increased, as in pulmonary fibrosis or kyphoscoliosis, the respirations tend to become rapid and shallow (Fig. 27, *B*), probably because of the increase in mechanical work which is required to overcome the elastic resistance as a result of even small increases in tidal volume. On the other hand, when the nonelastic resistance becomes increased, as in bronchial obstruction, the respirations tend to become slower and deeper (Fig. 27, *C*) because a faster respiratory rate would entail higher flow rates and an increase in the amount of work required to overcome the resistance to airflow.

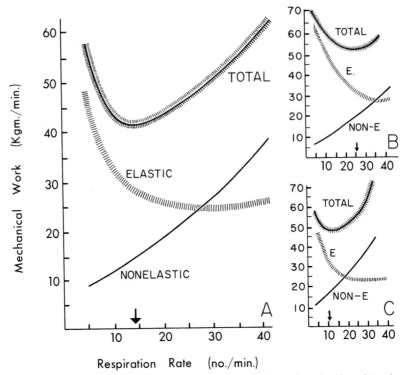

FIGURE 27.   The effect of respiratory rate on the mechanical work of breathing for a particular alveolar ventilation: normally (*A*), when the elastic work is increased (*B*), and when the nonelastic work is increased (*C*). The arrows indicate the respiratory rate at which total work is minimal.

THE OXYGEN COST OF BREATHING

In order to perform the mechanical work necessary for breathing, the respiratory muscles require oxygen. During quiet breathing the total oxygen consumption of the body is between 200 and 300 ml./min. The oxygen consumption of the respiratory apparatus has been estimated by determining the difference in the oxygen consumption during breathing at rest and during increased ventilation. In such an experiment, the nonrespiratory oxygen consumption is estimated by extending the calculation backward to a situation in which there is no ventilation at all. The difference between the total oxygen consumption and the nonrespiratory oxygen consumption at any level of ventilation, therefore, represents the oxygen consumption of the respiratory apparatus at that ventilation.

Figure 28 illustrates the change in oxygen consumption associated with increases in ventilation in a normal subject and in patients with respiratory insufficiency. It can be seen that in the normal sub-

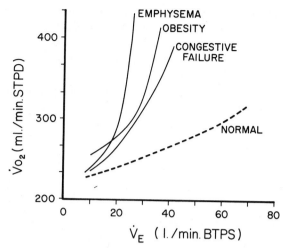

FIGURE 28. The change in oxygen consumption associated with increases in ventilation in a normal subject and patients with respiratory insufficiency.

ject the ventilation can be increased considerably without much alteration in the oxygen consumption. The oxygen cost of breathing has been found to range between 0.3 and 1.8 ml./l. of ventilation at minute volumes up to about 50 l./min. In other words, in the resting normal subject the respiratory apparatus only consumes about 3 to 14 ml. of oxygen/min., or less than 5 per cent of the total oxygen consumption. At levels of ventilation of about 50 l./min. the ventilatory apparatus utilizes a greater proportion of the total oxygen consumption; and at still higher ventilations, the oxygen cost per unit of ventilation becomes progressively greater and may become a significant proportion of the total metabolism. In the example shown, the oxygen requirement of the respiratory apparatus in the normal subject is about 30 per cent of the total oxygen consumption when the ventilation is 70 l./min.

In the patient with emphysema the oxygen cost of breathing at rest is about 4 to 10 times that of the normal. Even at low ventilations, then, the oxygen consumption of the respiratory apparatus may amount to as much as 25 per cent of the total oxygen consumption in patients with emphysema. Similarly, the oxygen cost of breathing in the obese subject is about 4 times the normal, and in patients with congestive heart failure it is about twice that of the normal.

Figure 28 also illustrates that in patients with respiratory insufficiency the disproportionate increase in oxygen consumption with increases in ventilation occurs at a much lower ventilation than it does in normal subjects. In the patient with emphysema even a slight increase in ventilation increases the oxygen consumption precipitously; the respiratory apparatus consumes an exceedingly high proportion of the oxygen consumption. In the example shown the respiratory apparatus requires more than 30 per cent of the oxygen consumed at a ventilation of only 20 l./min. The increased oxygen requirements of the respiratory apparatus in these conditions may not cause disability at rest but may be an important cause of decreased effort tolerance.

OXYGEN COST OF BREATHING AND EXERCISE

During exercise the minute ventilation and the oxygen consumption rise. During mild to moderate exercise the ventilation usually bears an approximately linear relationship to the total oxygen consumption. However, as the severity of the exercise increases and the oxygen consumption reaches 50 to 75 per cent of the maximum possible, the ventilation rises out of proportion to the oxygen consumption. In other words, during mild exercise the ventilatory equivalent for oxygen remains relatively constant, but when the exercise becomes severe the ventilatory equivalent rises.

It has been suggested that exercise tolerance may depend on the relationship between the total oxygen uptake and the oxygen consumption of the respiratory apparatus during the exercise. Thus, if the proportion of the total oxygen uptake being utilized by the respiratory apparatus during exercise is high, the amount of oxygen available to the nonrespiratory tissues will be reduced. Therefore, a stage may be reached when the total amount of oxygen being consumed during exercise is insufficient to meet the needs of both the respiratory muscles and the other exercising muscles. As a result, either the exercising muscles or the respiratory muscles, or both, must go into more oxygen debt, and exercise tolerance may be limited.

Figure 29 shows the relationship between ventilation and oxygen consumption during increasing exercise in normal subjects. The total oxygen consumption is divided into the portion required by the respiratory muscles at equivalent ventilations and that consumed by the nonrespiratory tissues. It can be seen that at low ventilations the proportion of the total oxygen consumption being utilized by the respiratory apparatus is very small (roughly 2 per cent of the total) so that 98 per cent is available for the rest of the body. As the severity of the exercise increases, the rise in ventilation is associated with a disproportionate increase in the oxygen cost of breathing so that the respiratory apparatus takes a larger and larger proportion of the total oxygen uptake. In the normal subject the oxygen cost of the respiratory apparatus never reaches the stage at which breathing costs so much that there is not sufficient oxygen available to meet the

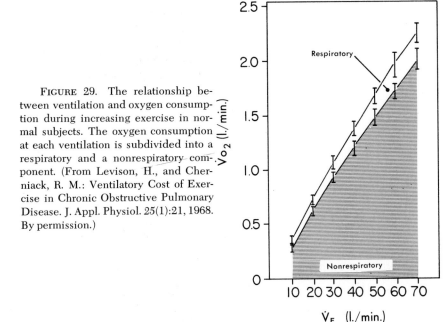

FIGURE 29. The relationship between ventilation and oxygen consumption during increasing exercise in normal subjects. The oxygen consumption at each ventilation is subdivided into a respiratory and a nonrespiratory component. (From Levison, H., and Cherniack, R. M.: Ventilatory Cost of Exercise in Chronic Obstructive Pulmonary Disease. J. Appl. Physiol. 25(1):21, 1968. By permission.)

needs of both the respiratory muscles and the other exercising muscles.

In patients with cardiopulmonary disease in which the oxygen cost of breathing is high, however, the likelihood of such a circumstance arising is much greater. The relationship between ventilation and the oxygen consumption and its components during exercise in patients with emphysema are presented in Figure 30. It can be seen that the total oxygen consumption at any ventilation is lower in patients with emphysema than it is in normal subjects. Furthermore, at each level of ventilation, the amount of oxygen consumed by the respiratory muscles is higher and the oxygen available for non-

FIGURE 30. The relationship between ventilation and oxygen consumption during increasing exercise in patients with emphysema. The oxygen consumption at each ventilation is subdivided into a respiratory and a nonrespiratory component. (From Levison, H., and Cherniack, R. M.: Ventilatory Cost of Exercise in Chronic Obstructive Pulmonary Disease. J. Appl. Physiol. 25(1):21, 1968. By permission.)

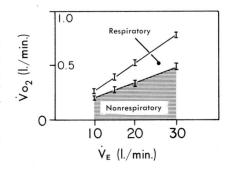

respiratory work is less in patients than in normal subjects. The mean oxygen cost of breathing, which in this case was 6.3 ml./l. of ventilation at rest, increased to 9.3 ml./l. of ventilation, even at low levels of exercise and ventilation. The high requirements of the respiratory apparatus may therefore play a major role in limiting exercise tolerance in patients with respiratory disease.

EFFICIENCY OF THE RESPIRATORY MUSCLES

In order to calculate the efficiency of the respiratory muscles, one must know the total mechanical work of breathing and the oxygen consumption of the respiratory muscles at a given ventilation. The formula for estimating this is

$$\text{Efficiency (per cent)} = \frac{\text{Mechanical work (kg.m.)}}{\text{Oxygen cost (kg.m.)}} \times 100$$

The total mechanical work of breathing performed on the lungs can be approximately determined by using the esophageal pressure as an index of the intrathoracic pressure. The total work performed in moving the lung, chest wall and abdominal contents, however, cannot be measured directly in the spontaneously breathing subject. On the other hand, the efficiency with which an added respiratory work load is handled may be calculated by measuring the extra oxygen which is consumed while the subject breathes through a known inspiratory resistance. By this method, the efficiency of the respiratory muscles in normal subjects has been found to vary between 5 and 10 per cent. The mechanical efficiency of the respiratory muscles is therefore low, even in the normal person, and it is much lower than that reported for other forms of muscular work. It has been suggested that the efficiency of the respiratory muscles in patients with emphysema is reduced to between 1 and 3 per cent. The mechanism of reduction in efficiency of the respiratory muscles in emphysema has not been elucidated, but a similar reduction in efficiency can be induced by breathing through increased resistance. It is possible that this is due to the alteration in functional residual capacity in this condition, the mechanical advantage of the respiratory muscles being reduced in the inspiratory position.

Chapter 2

The Pulmonary Circulation

The transport of oxygen and carbon dioxide between the lungs and the tissue cells depends on the convective movement of blood in the circulatory system (see Fig. 1). In this chapter the main emphasis will be on special features of the pulmonary circulation, and it will be assumed that the reader has a general understanding of the principles of hemodynamics.

The pulmonary circulation resembles the systemic circulation in several ways: it has a pump, the right ventricle; a distributing system, the pulmonary arteries and arterioles; an exchange system, the pulmonary capillaries; and a collecting system, the pulmonary venules and veins. However, the pulmonary circulation differs from the systemic circulation in that it is characterized by a low pressure within its vessels. Since the lung receives all of the right ventricular output, it is evident that the low pressure in the pulmonary vessels must reflect either a relatively low resistance to flow in the pulmonary vasculature or an increased distensibility of the vessels. In fact, both factors are operative, since the pulmonary vessels are shorter, thinner, more distensible and contain less smooth muscle than systemic blood vessels.

Because of the low pressure in the pulmonary circuit, relatively small changes in extravascular pressure produce greater effects on the dimensions of pulmonary vessels than on systemic vessels. Furthermore, whereas systemic capillaries are surrounded by tissue and tissue fluid, the pulmonary capillaries are surrounded by a fluid of much lower density—the air in the alveoli. These two factors are responsible for the marked effects on pulmonary blood flow resulting from gravity or from the changes in transpulmonary pressure produced by spontaneous or artificial ventilation.

FUNCTIONS OF THE PULMONARY CIRCULATION

GAS EXCHANGE

The main function of the pulmonary circulation is to conduct mixed venous blood through the alveolar capillaries so that a proper amount of oxygen can be added and a proper amount of carbon dioxide is eliminated.

RESERVOIR FOR LEFT VENTRICLE

The pulmonary vessels contain about 900 ml. of blood, of which more than half is in readily distensible veins. Since these are an extension of the left atrium, they constitute a blood reservoir, which supplies blood to fill the left ventricle and maintain its output, even when the right ventricular pump falls behind for a few beats. Thus, the left ventricular stroke volume (output per beat) has been shown to remain unchanged for several beats, even when the pulmonary artery is completely blocked by a balloon. The larger the left atrium and the more distended the pulmonary veins, the more capacious will be the reservoir.

PROTECTIVE FUNCTION

The pulmonary vessels act as a filter to trap and prevent emboli from reaching and blocking systemic arteries, arterioles or capillaries. Because the lungs can perform their gas exchange function with fewer than half of their conducting and exchange vessels, the body can tolerate block of some pulmonary vessels far better than it can tolerate block of coronary or cerebral vessels. The pulmonary vascular bed is the site of rapid inactivation of certain endogenous substances, such as the prostaglandins, and is the site of rapid activation of angiotensin.

NUTRITION

The lungs have an additional arterial blood supply through the bronchial vessels of the systemic circulation. Although anatomists have long believed that these vessels do not supply the alveolar ducts and alveoli, physiologists believe they do, because a lung does not die when its pulmonary artery is ligated. However, recent studies of animals after unilateral pulmonary artery occlusion demonstrated that many alveoli become hemorrhagic and collapse within 1 to 3 days, although they recover later and appear almost normal after some months. The marked early changes were previously either overlooked or attributed to postoperative complications. Blood flow through the alveolar capillaries is therefore essential for the nutrition of the alveoli and alveolar ducts. Normally this blood comes through the pulmonary circulation. In its absence, the bronchial arteries can provide an adequate blood supply to these capillaries through new or expanded channels, but this requires several weeks to develop.

PRESSURE, FLOW AND RESISTANCE
IN THE PULMONARY CIRCULATION

PULMONARY PRESSURE

There are three types of pressure used in studies of pulmonary hemodynamics: absolute intravascular pressure, transmural pressure and the driving pressure.

ABSOLUTE INTRAVASCULAR PRESSURE

The absolute intravascular pressure is the actual blood pressure in the lumen of a blood vessel at any point expressed in relation to atmospheric pressure. The pressure is not the same in similar vessels in all parts of the pulmonary circulation because of the influence of gravity. In a man of ordinary height the distance between the top (apex) and bottom (base) of the lung is about 30 cm. If the main pulmonary trunk is midway between the apex and base when a man sits or stands, there is a column of blood 15 cm. high between the pulmonary trunk and arterioles in the apex and a similar column of blood between it and arterioles in the base. A column of blood 15 cm. high is equivalent to a column of mercury 11 mm. high. If the pressure in the main pulmonary artery is 22/9 mm. Hg, there is an adequate pressure to produce apical flow during systole when apical pressure would be $22 - 11 = 11$ mm. Hg but not during diastole when it would be $9 - 11 = -2$ mm. Hg. The blood pressure at the base would be $(22 + 11)/ (9 + 11)$, or 33/20. This increase in absolute pressure and in transmural pressure in the dependent vessels also distends them, according to their compliance, and decreases the resistance to flow through them. The effects of gravity are less when man lies on his side because the lungs are not so wide as they are long, and they are still less when he lies prone or supine.

TRANSMURAL PRESSURE

Transmural pressure is the difference between the pressure in the lumen of a vessel and that of the tissue around it. A greater pressure in the lumen tends to distend the vessel, just as the transpulmonary pressure distends the lungs. A greater pressure in the tissue tends to compress or collapse the vessels. The pressure around the pulmonary arteries and veins is the intrathoracic pressure. The pressure around the smaller intrapulmonary vessels (arterioles, capillaries and venules) is difficult to measure because it is neither the air pressure in the alveoli nor the intrapleural pressure, but some pressure in between.

For some purposes it is convenient to divide small pulmonary vessels into two functional groups: those which behave as if they are exposed to an extravascular pressure, which reflects the pleural pressure; and those which behave as if they are exposed to an extravascular pressure, which reflects the alveolar pressure. The former may be termed extra-alveolar vessels, and the latter designated as alveolar vessels. However, the pressure at the immediate outer surface of these vessels may differ in absolute value from the pleural or alveolar pressure. For example, it is thought by some that the alveolar pressure is not transmitted in full to the capillary surface because some of it is dissipated across the air-liquid interface.

DRIVING PRESSURE

The difference between pressures at one point in a vessel and at another point downstream is the driving pressure. It is the pressure that overcomes frictional resistance and is responsible for blood flow between these two points. The driving pressure for the total pulmonary circulation is the difference between the pressure at the beginning of the pulmonary circulation (the pulmonary artery) and that at the other end (the left atrium). The intravascular pressures in the pulmonary circulation as well as the systemic circulation are shown in Figure 31. It is possible to place catheters in the main pulmonary artery, the right and left pulmonary artery branches, the pulmonary veins and the left atrium and to measure pressure at these specific points. It is not possible to measure intracapillary pressure directly, and there are no precise values for this pressure. Since blood flows from the pulmonary arterioles directly to the capillaries and to the pulmonary venules, the capillary pressure must be less than the arteriolar pressure and higher than the venular pressure.

In a normal man, the mean pulmonary artery pressure is about 14 mm. Hg, the pulmonary capillary pressure is about 6 mm. Hg and the left atrial pressure is approximately 5 mm. Hg. The total driving pressure is therefore $14 - 5$, or 9, mm. Hg. However, in a patient with obstruction to flow at the mitral valve and an increase in all the pulmonary vascular pressures, the mean pulmonary artery pressure may rise to 30 mm. Hg, the capillary pressure to 23 mm. Hg and the left atrial pressure to 21 mm. Hg. The total driving pressure remains the same ($30 - 21 = 9$ mm. Hg), but the capillary pressure is considerably elevated (23 instead of 6), and this is close to the colloidal osmotic pressure of the plasma proteins.

In a patient with primary pulmonary hypertension due to arteriosclerosis of the pulmonary vessels, the mean pulmonary artery pressure may be 90 mm. Hg (nearly equal to the mean systemic arterial pressure), but pulmonary capillary pressure and left atrial pressure may be normal. Since the capillary pressure is normal,

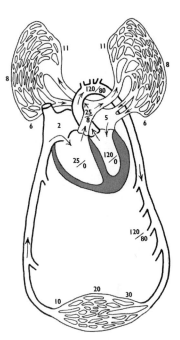

FIGURE 31. Blood pressures in the pulmonary and systemic circulations.

there is no danger of pulmonary edema, but the total driving pressure is very high (90 − 5 = 85 mm.Hg) because of resistance to flow through the arterioles. This imposes a very heavy work load on the right ventricle and can lead to right ventricular strain, hypertrophy and possibly failure. An increased right ventricular pressure does not mean that the right ventricle must fail any more than left ventricular failure necessarily follows systemic arterial hypertension; but failure is more likely than if the pressure remained normal.

It is important to recognize that the pressure may be extremely high in the pulmonary artery and normal in the pulmonary capillaries. Knowledge of the pulmonary artery pressure provides no information about the pulmonary capillary pressure; under the above circumstances there may be severe right ventricular strain and failure, but there will not be any tendency for transudation of fluid across the pulmonary capillary bed. On the other hand, an increase in capillary pressure of only 20 to 25 mm.Hg, which would not usually impose severe strain on the right ventricle if it occurred only between the right ventricle and the pulmonary capillary, may cause fulminating pulmonary edema and death.

VOLUME OF PULMONARY BLOOD FLOW

Blood flow may be measured by many techniques. One is the direct Fick method, which requires measurement of the O_2 uptake/

min. and the O_2 concentration in the arterial and mixed venous blood using the following equation:

$$\text{Blood flow (l./min.)} = \frac{O_2 \text{ uptake (ml./min.)}}{a - \bar{v} \text{ difference for } O_2 \text{ (ml./l.)}}$$

Other methods of measuring pulmonary blood flow use dye dilution or a body plethysmograph. The plethysmograph method is of special interest because it measures instantaneous flow through the pulmonary capillaries. With this method it has been shown that pulmonary capillary blood flow is pulsatile. This is because, in the pulmonary circulation, the arteriolar resistance is normally low and the pulmonary arterial pulse is transmitted to the capillary blood. This provides more time for gas exchange as long as the right ventricular stroke volume is less than the volume of the capillary bed. If the stroke volume exceeds the capillary volume, some blood may rush through the capillaries and have less time for gas exchange.

OVERALL RESISTANCE TO FLOW

Just as with airway resistance, vascular resistance is calculated from an equation similar to Ohm's law for electrical circuits relating resistance and current flow to electromotive force.

In any vascular system

$$\text{Resistance (R)} = \frac{\text{Driving pressure } (\Delta P)}{\text{Blood flow (Q)}}$$

In conventional physical terms pressure is measured in dynes/cm.^{2} (force/unit area), blood flow is measured as cm.^{3}/sec. and pressure/flow, or resistance, becomes (dynes/cm.^{2})/(cm.^{3}/sec.), or (dynes $\times$ sec.)/cm.^{5}, or dynes $\times$ sec. $\times$ cm.$^{-5}$ This calculation tends to be cumbersome; therefore, blood pressure is usually expressed in mm. Hg and flow in l./min.; the resistance unit is then mm. Hg/l./min. In the pulmonary circulation with a driving pressure of 9 mm. Hg at a flow of 6 l./min., the resistance is 9/6 or 1.5 mm. Hg/l./min. (1/10 that in the systemic circulation).

In the normal pulmonary circulation, most of the resistance to flow occurs in the arterioles and the capillaries; the venous system offers little resistance to flow, and the pressure difference between the end of the capillaries and the left atrium is believed to be less than 1 mm. Hg.

The effects of an increased pulmonary vascular resistance depend in part on the type of vessel involved. If the increased resistance is in the venules or veins, then the transmural pulmonary capillary pressure rises, and pulmonary edema may result; if it is in the arteries or arterioles, the pulmonary artery pressure will rise, but the pulmonary capillary pressure does not rise. In any location, an increase in pulmonary vascular resistance is followed by an increased right ventricular pressure and right ventricular strain.

DISTENSIBILITY AND COLLAPSIBILITY

The compliance (capacitance, volume distensibility) of the pulmonary vascular bed is far greater than that of the systemic vascular bed. Unlike analogous systemic vessels, the pulmonary arteries are more distensible than the pulmonary veins, and the large arteries are more compliant than the small ones. The pulmonary capillary bed as a whole exhibits a good deal of overall volume distensibility, and individual capillaries vary widely in the amount of blood they contain. Nevertheless, most physiologists believe that healthy capillaries, once fully open, strongly resist passive distension, even by very high internal pressures. The resistance to flow through a capillary bed can be lowered if previously closed capillary channels open; resistance to flow through any individual capillary can decrease if it changes from a flattened to a round shape and has a greater cross-sectional area. Closed capillaries may open because previously closed arterioles open or because the intracapillary pressure rises above the "extravascular pressure." Presumably, capillaries do not dilate actively, but disease or change in their chemical environment may permit them to dilate. For instance, in patients with mitral stenosis the capillaries may be so wide that 3 or 4 red blood cells can flow through abreast, whereas in normal capillaries, red blood cells file through one by one or may even have to squeeze through.

The high compliance of pulmonary vessels allows the volume of blood in the lungs to change over fairly wide limits with relatively little change in pressure. This is an advantage in that any transient discrepancies in the volume output of the right and left ventricles can be accommodated by the pulmonary blood reservoir. Normally about 10 per cent of the total circulating blood volume is in the lungs. The distribution of blood between the pulmonary and systemic vascular beds varies with posture, with the state of contraction of pulmonary in relation to systemic vascular smooth muscle, and with any factor which tends to influence the difference between intra-abdominal and intrathoracic pressures.

During a normal inspiration the fall in pleural pressure distends the intrathoracic portions of the venae cavae and right atrium. The resulting increased flow into the heart increases the right ventricular stroke volume. The left ventricular stroke volume also increases, but to a smaller extent, so that the pulmonary blood volume increases during inspiration. By contrast, during artificial ventilation, the application of intermittent positive pressure at the airway raises the mean intrathoracic pressure, and this impedes the venous return to the heart, thereby resulting in a decrease in pulmonary blood volume.

About 30 per cent of the total pulmonary blood volume is in the arteries, about 10 per cent is in the capillaries, and about 60 per cent is in the veins. Normally the pulmonary capillary bed contains only about 75 to 100 ml. of blood, but this is contained in a multitude of capillaries whose surface area has been estimated at 70 m.² The amount of blood in the pulmonary capillaries increases as much as three- to fourfold during exercise. There is also an increase in pulmonary capillary blood volume when pulmonary congestion is present as a result of an increased pulmonary venous pressure.

CAPILLARY EXCHANGE IN THE LUNG

The pulmonary blood-gas barrier (alveolocapillary membrane) is freely permeable to oxygen, carbon dioxide, anesthetic gases and inert gases as well as water, alcohols and hydrocarbons, but it is quite impermeable to ions, urea, glucose and to macromolecules. It has been postulated that the selective permeability is due to the effects of these solutes on the structure of water, which is the major constituent of the barrier. Since the permeability of the blood-gas barrier for water is high, it exchanges freely between the intravascular and extravascular compartment. It is generally believed that fluid leaves and re-enters pulmonary capillaries in a manner analogous to systemic capillaries and that fluid movements are subject to a similar balance of hydrostatic and osmotic forces.

Water introduced into the alveoli passes rapidly into the pulmonary capillary blood. This is because the pulmonary capillary pressure of a healthy man (6 to 8 mm. Hg), which tends to filter fluid from the blood into the alveoli, is always far below the colloid osmotic pressure of the plasma proteins (25 to 30 mm. Hg), which tends to pull fluid from the alveoli into the blood. Thus, the low capillary pressure provides a mechanism for preventing transudation of fluid from the blood to the alveoli and for speeding absorption of any fluid in the alveoli into the blood. However, rapid absorption of fluid can be a hazard. For example, the rapid absorption of large quantities of water that sometimes occurs in freshwater drowning causes hemolysis of red blood cells, large increases in plasma volume and overload of the heart. In addition, aerosols of drugs such as isoproterenol or procaine, intended only for the airways, will enter the blood almost as rapidly as if they were injected intravenously if they reach the alveolar surface.

Pulmonary edema develops as a result of either a change in the permeability of the pulmonary capillaries, as is seen to be the case with various chemical irritants, such as phosgene, or an imbalance of the pressure determining fluid exchange across the capillary walls. The pulmonary venous pressure must rise above 20 mm. Hg before pulmonary edema becomes apparent. When the intracapillary pressure is high, red blood cells may be extravasated as a result of rupture of capillaries. The extravascular water content of the lung is also increased by a fall in the colloid pressure of the plasma. When fluid is extravasated at very rapid rates, the ability of the lymphatics to drain the fluid is exceeded, and large amounts of fluid may accumulate in the lung.

LYMPHATICS IN THE LUNG

Although the total cardiac output traverses both the systemic and pulmonary circuits, the lymph flow from the lungs is estimated to be less than one-tenth of the flow from the rest of the body. The low net filtration of fluid from pulmonary capillaries is ascribed to the fact that the capillary pressure is low and that adjacent endothelial cells of the capillaries are closely bonded together and sit on a continuous basement membrane. Some protein does manage to escape into the lymphatics from the capillaries but again this is only one-tenth of the amount which leaks through the systemic capillaries. It is important to emphasize that estimates of lymph flow from the lungs are likely to be overestimates, since they are made by collecting lymph from the right lymphatic duct, which drains the lymphatics from the bronchi and from the pleural, pericardial and peritoneal cavities in addition to the lungs.

THE BRONCHIAL CIRCULATION

In man, the bronchial arteries usually arise from either the proximal portion of the thoracic aorta or one of the first two intercostal arteries. Each lung possesses at least one bronchial artery. These vessels follow the course of the bronchial tree into the lung parenchyma, where they branch elaborately and rejoin to form plexuses around the bronchi and in the bronchial submucosa. The bronchial arteries supply the lower part of the trachea, the bronchi as far as the respiratory bronchioles, and the visceral pleura. By means of anastomoses with numerous other vessels, they also supply the vasa vasorum of the pulmonary artery and vein, the vagi and the mediastinal structures, particularly the pericardium and the tracheobronchial lymph nodes.

In the normal person, blood brought to the lungs via the bronchial arteries may follow one of two courses during its return to the heart. In the proximal part of the major bronchi, some of this blood is carried via the bronchial veins into the azygos veins and then to the right atrium. More distally, the venous drainage enters into the pulmonary veins. The pulmonary veins therefore normally carry small amounts of poorly oxygenated blood. About 1 per cent of the cardiac output passes through the bronchial circulation into the pulmonary veins. The amount contributed via the bronchial arteries and pulmonary veins constitutes about one-quarter of the physiological right-to-left shunt seen in normal persons.

DISTRIBUTION OF BLOOD FLOW

The behavior of the blood flow in any particular part of the lung depends on the relationship of the intraluminal pressures (arterial, capillary, venous) and the state of contraction of smooth muscle existing in that region. Since the lung has an appreciable height in erect man in relation to generally low pressure in pulmonary vessels, it is apparent that the vessels near the top of the lung must have a lower pressure than those at the bottom of the lung. Similarly, the venous pressure is different at different levels of the lung. Thus, it can be predicted that blood flow should vary in different parts of the lung. The first direct confirmation of this prediction was provided when radioactive tracers, which could be detected with sensors placed on the surface of the chest, became available. The most commonly used tracers are of two types: radioactive gases and particles labeled with radioactive isotopes. An example of the gas is radioactive xenon, a gas which because of its low solubility is evolved into the alveolar gas almost immediately after entry into the pulmonary circulation. Following its intravenous injection, it becomes distributed in the alveolar gas in different parts of the lung in amounts proportional to their blood flow. An example of the particles which are used is macro-aggregated albumin labeled with radioactive iodine. Following intravenous injection the albumin particles become lodged in small pulmonary vessels in different parts of the lung in a pattern determined by their blood flow.

Typical patterns of distribution of pulmonary blood flow are shown in Figure 32. The blood flow is less at the apex than at the base of the upright lung (sitting or standing) owing to the effect of

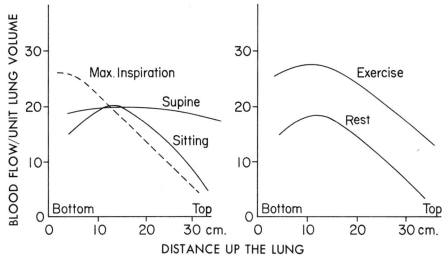

FIGURE 32. The effect of posture, lung inflation and exercise on regional pulmonary blood flow.

gravity. Blood flow does not increase uniformly with increasing distance down the lung but falls off again near the bottom. This has been explained on the basis that alveoli at the bottom of the lung, being relatively less inflated than those at the top, exert less of a distending force on the extra-alveolar vessels, which are therefore narrower and offer greater resistance so that flow decreases. When the normal subject lies down, the apical basal blood flow differences are largely abolished, since the two parts of the lung are nearly at the same hydrostatic level. If the subject lies on his side, the dependent lung is better perfused than the contralateral lung.

A maximal inspiration increases the gradient of blood flow, probably because the alveoli at the bottom of the lung expand more during the large inspiration than do those at the top, thereby distending the extra-alveolar vessels with a resultant fall in resistance so that blood flow at the bottom of the lung increases.

Figure 32 also demonstrates the effect of exercise on the distribution of blood flow in the lung. It can be seen that blood flow at the top of the lung increases relatively more than it does at the base during exercise, although the perfusion gradient (flow per unit vertical distance) may be nearly the same during exercise as it is at rest.

The use of fairly simple mechanical models provides considerable insight into the factors determining the distribution of pulmonary blood flow. For example, small pulmonary vessels behave like collapsible tubes passing through a compression chamber such as that shown in Figure 33. The pressure surrounding the collapsible

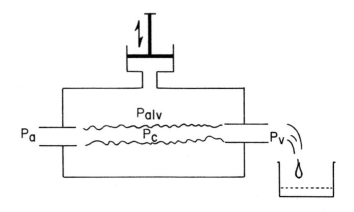

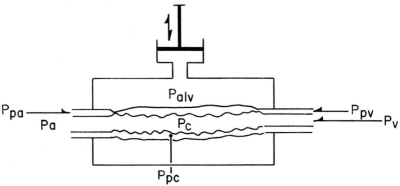

FIGURE 33.   The upper model represents a small pulmonary vessel ("capillary")
as a collapsible tube which is exposed to a variable extramural pressure analogous
to alveolar pressure (P_{alv}). When the outflow pressure or "venous" pressure (P_v) is
lower than P_{alv} it does not influence flow through the vessel. Flow will be determined
by the dimension of the collapsible vessel and the inflow or "arterial" pressure (P_a).
The dimension of the vessel is determined by its transmural pressure, i.e., the difference between its intra- and extraluminal pressures ($P_{alv} - P_c$). Only when P_v exceeds
P_{alv} is it reflected "back," hence constituting an effective "back pressure" which influences flow.
     The lower model has additional elements representing extramural forces acting
on the "extra-alveolar" and "intra-alveolar" portions of the vessel. These include
periarterial (P_{pa}) and perivenous (P_{pv}) forces, such as interstitial pressure and smooth
muscle tone. Pericapillary forces (P_{pc}) may include those related to the surface tension
of the alveolar lining layer.

tube (P_{alv}) may be varied at will. Let the inflow pressure be P_a, the
outflow pressure P_v and the pressure within the collapsible tube be
P_c. Also shown in the lower half of the diagram are the perivascular
pressures. For flow to occur through this system, the inflow pressure
(P_a) must exceed all of the pressures downstream. Flow will not
occur if the intraluminal pressure (P_c) is raised by an increase in outflow pressure (P_v) or if the collapsible tube is pinched off by an increase in the extravascular pressure (P_{alv}).

Consideration of this system demonstrates that the patency of the collapsible tube is determined by P_{alv} as long as P_{alv} exceeds P_v and by P_v when P_v exceeds P_{alv}. In other words, for a given value of P_a the tube will be narrowed, resistance will increase, and flow will decrease as P_{alv} is raised. As long as P_v is lower than P_{alv} it will have no influence on the dimension of the tube, its resistance or the flow through it. This arrangement has been described as resembling that in a *waterfall* in which the flow over the fall is independent of the height of the fall. If, however, P_v is elevated so that it exceeds P_{alv}, it will constitute an effective "back pressure," determining blood flow.

Since the lung has an appreciable height between apex and base in erect man, its vascular bed can not be represented by a single collapsible tube but instead should be represented by a number of collapsible tubes arranged vertically or in parallel fashion, as shown in Figure 34. The inflow reservoir which is kept filled to a height of 23 cm. H₂O above the "artery" at the lowest part of the lung represents the pulmonary artery pressure (P_{PA}). The outflow reservoir overflows when the water level in it is higher than 11 cm. above the "vein" in the lowest part of the lung. The height of fluid in this reservoir is analogous to the left atrial pressure. A number of horizontal vascular channels link the inflow and outflow reservoirs.

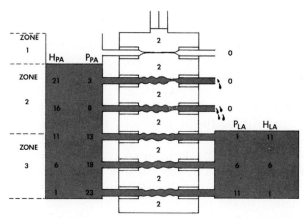

FIGURE 34.   A model which represents the pulmonary vascular bed. H_{PA} is height of inflow reservoir. P_{PA} represents pulmonary artery pressure. H_{LA} represents height of outflow reservoir. P_{LA} is left atrial pressure. Alveolar pressure (P_{alv}) equals 2 centimeters of water throughout the system.

In zone 1, P_{alv} exceeds P_{PA} so there is no flow.

In zone 2, P_{PA} exceeds P_{alv} so that flow varies with height, being greater near the bottom than at the top of the zone.

In zone 3, P_{PA} exceeds P_{alv} but P_{alv} is less than P_{LA}. Since P_{PA} and P_{LA} increase by equal amounts throughout this zone, flow through each channel in this zone is the same and does not vary with height.

These horizontal channels each consist of a rigid metal inflow tube (artery) joined to cellophane tubing (alveolar capillary), which collapses when the surrounding or outside pressure exceeds the inside pressure and is rigid when filled. The other end of the cellophane tube is joined to an outflow tube representing the pulmonary vein. Since the density of air is negligible compared with that of blood, P_{alv} is constant for all channels, and in this model, it is shown as 2 cm. H_2O. The perfusing pressure, however, depends on the height of the channel.

In the upper part of the model lung (zone 1) alveolar pressure (P_{alv}), which is $+ 2$ cm. H_2O, exceeds P_{PA}, which is 0. There is, therefore, no flow in zone 1.

In zone 2, P_{PA} for each channel exceeds P_{alv} so that in this zone the pressure gradient responsible for flow in any channel is the inflow pressure at the height of the vascular channel minus the alveolar pressure ($P_{PA} - P_{alv}$). Flow therefore varies with height, being greater nearer the bottom than at the top of the zone.

In zone 3, P_{PA} exceeds P_{alv} for every channel but P_{alv} is less than the outflow pressure (P_{LA}). The pressure gradient that determines flow through a channel in this zone is therefore the inflow pressure for that channel (P_{PA}) minus the corresponding outflow pressure (P_{LA}). In this zone the driving pressure for each channel is the same, since P_{PA} and P_{LA} increase equally with distance down this zone. Similarly, the flow through each channel in this zone is the same and does not vary with height as in zone 2.

In reality, the inflow and outflow tubes in the lung are distensible rather than rigid. Since the alveolar pressure exceeds the pulmonary capillary pressure in zone 1, there is, as in the model, no flow in this zone. In zone 2, blood flow in each channel, as in the rigid tube model, will vary, depending on the relation of the height of each channel to the height of the perfusion reservoir. In this case, however, the flow will not only be determined by the collapsible capillary, but it will also be a function of the transmural pressure acting on the inflow and outflow tubes, which are distensible and variable in size. The same reasoning applies to zone 3. Where there was no variation of flow with height in the lung in the rigid tube model, the flow will vary, depending on the local resistance as determined by the local transmural pressure and distensibility of the vessels.

REGULATION OF THE PULMONARY CIRCULATION

The right ventricle behaves very much like the left ventricle. Its beat is slowed by parasympathetic stimulation and accelerated by sympathetic stimulation. It obeys Starling's law of the heart and responds to increased diastolic stretch with increased force of contraction and with increased stroke volume. It responds to the same chemicals and drugs (acetylcholine, norepinephrine, isoproterenol, digitalis) that affect the left ventricle.

The main question is: do the pulmonary vessels respond to the same stimuli and in the same way as systemic vessels? Until recently there was some doubt about the presence of significant vasomotor control of the pulmonary vessels. Histologists saw very little smooth muscle in pulmonary arterioles; physiologists found only small changes after injection of drugs that caused vasoconstriction elsewhere; and teleologists reasoned that there was no need for regulation because all the cardiac output must flow through the lungs, and one resistance (a low one) would permit the right ventricle to pump it through with minimal work. It is now known that there is enough smooth muscle in pulmonary arterioles to alter resistance (not much is needed in a low-pressure system) and that it can hypertrophy remarkably in pathologic conditions, such as mitral stenosis. The hypertrophy is most marked in the lower lobes where vascular pressures are highest because of the force of gravity. It is also known that electrical or reflex stimulation of the sympathetic nerves to the lung causes vasoconstriction and that drugs can cause vasoconstriction and vasodilation.

ACTIVE CHANGES IN PULMONARY VASCULAR RESISTANCE

Active changes in the pulmonary vascular resistance result from neural or chemical influences.

NEURAL INFLUENCES

The pulmonary vessels are well supplied with both sympathetic and parasympathetic nerve fibers. Animal experiments have provided evidence that the pulmonary vascular resistance decreases following stimulation of systemic baroreceptors, and stimulation of the aortic body chemoreceptor results in an increase in pulmonary vascular resistance.

Under normal conditions, pulmonary vasomotor tone appears to contribute little to the total resistance of the pulmonary vessels, which appear to respond mainly in a passive manner to changes in transmural pressure.

CHEMICAL INFLUENCES

The pulmonary blood vessels constrict in response to hypoxia. The vasoconstriction probably involves both pre- and postcapillary vessels and is not mediated by neural reflex mechanisms involving the central nervous system, since it also occurs in the isolated lung. Isolated pulmonary vascular smooth muscle does not contract in response to hypoxia unless remnants of lung parenchyma are attached to it. This suggests that hypoxia acts by causing the lung parenchyma to release a substance which induces vasoconstriction. In certain species it would appear that histamine may be the responsible agent.

The pulmonary blood vessels exhibit a variable response to a high PCO_2 (hypercapnia). When vasoconstriction occurs it is probably the result of an increased H^+ concentration, although some observers claim that the effect of molecular CO_2 per se is to dilate vessels. Hypercapnia associated with a low pH of the blood (acidemia), but not hypercapnia associated with a normal pH, results in vasoconstriction. Acidemia of metabolic origin also results in pulmonary vasoconstriction. The presence of acidemia of both respiratory or metabolic origin potentiates the vasoconstrictor response to hypoxia.

The pulmonary vessels constrict in response to certain agents, such as histamine, epinephrine, norepinephrine, serotonin, *E. coli* endotoxin and alloxan. The direct effects of these vasoactive substances may be masked by passive changes in transmural pressure which occur as a result of the effect of these agents on the heart and systemic vessels. Furthermore, the vasoconstriction induced by agents such as epinephrine may be offset by their effects on airway smooth muscle. For example, bronchodilatation may increase the ventilation of a portion of lung, thereby raising the partial pressure of oxygen and lowering the partial pressure of carbon dioxide, and, in addition, may increase alveolar volume. These effects would offset the increase in vascular resistance produced by epinephrine.

Isoproterenol and acetylcholine dilate constricted pulmonary arterioles. Acetylcholine is occasionally injected into the pulmonary circulation in order to determine whether the vascular resistance decreases, and if it does, it is concluded that the increased resistance was due, at least partly, to vasoconstriction rather than to atherosclerosis or other organic obstruction. Similarly, the inhalation of oxygen leads to vasodilation and a fall in pulmonary vascular resistance when anoxic vasoconstriction is present.

PATHOLOGICAL CHANGES IN PULMONARY
VASCULAR RESISTANCE

The pulmonary vascular resistance may increase in many pathological conditions, in which the increased resistance may be in the artery, arterioles, capillaries, venules or veins. Among the causes of an increased pulmonary vascular resistance are intraluminal obstruction due to thrombi or emboli (blood clots, parasites, fat cells, air, tumor cells, white blood cells or platelets); disease of the vascular wall, such as sclerosis, endarteritis, polyarteritis or scleroderma; destructive or obliterative diseases, such as emphysema and interstitial pulmonary fibrosis; or compression of vessels by masses of infiltrative lesions. The causes of an increased pulmonary vascular resistance are discussed in greater detail in Chapter 15.

Chapter 3

Oxygen and Carbon Dioxide Exchanges Between Gas and Blood

PROPERTIES OF GASES

Before we discuss gas exchange in the lungs, an explanation of certain physical properties of gases is essential. If a volume of gas is placed in a container, the gas expands until it fills the container because its molecules diffuse very rapidly throughout it. The gas exerts a pressure which is dependent on the amount of bombardment of the walls of the containing vessel by its molecules. According to *Boyle's law,* the pressure of the gas will rise if the volume of the container is reduced because the molecules of gas are closer together and increase their bombardment of the walls of the container. Similarly, according to *Gay-Lussac's law,* the pressure of a gas is proportionate to its temperature, provided the volume is kept constant. The pressure rises when the temperature of the gas is elevated, because the speed of molecular movement increases, causing greater bombardment of the molecules on the boundaries of the confining space. If a mixture of two or more gases is confined within the same space, each gas behaves independently, as if it alone were in that space. The molecules of each gas are uniformly distributed throughout the space, and the pressure of each gas depends on its own concentration, regardless of the concentration of the other gases.

The pressure which any gas exerts, whether alone or mixed with other gases, is called the *partial pressure,* or the *tension,* of that gas. It is indicated by the letter "P" preceding the symbol for the gas. For example, the partial pressure of oxygen is denoted by PO_2 and that of carbon dioxide by PCO_2. The total pressure exerted by a mixture of gases is the arithmetic sum of the partial pressures of all the different gases which make up the mixture. The total pressure of air at sea level, which is 760 mm. Hg, is the sum of the partial pressures of

70

the oxygen, carbon dioxide, nitrogen and the inert gases, such as argon and neon, which it contains. Since there is 20.94 per cent oxygen, 0.04 per cent carbon dioxide and 79 per cent nitrogen in ambient air, their partial pressures are 159, 0.3 and 600 mm. Hg, respectively. The remainder of the atmospheric pressure is due to the traces of inert gases which are present. When air enters the lungs it becomes diluted by, and saturated with, water vapor. At body temperature (37° C.) this exerts a partial pressure of 47 mm. Hg. Since the total gas pressure remains at 760 mm. Hg, the partial pressures of O_2, CO_2 and N_2 in saturated air become 149, 2 and 563 mm. Hg, respectively.

When the partial pressure of a gas is different in two parts of a system, a concentration gradient exists between the two parts. The gas diffuses readily between the two parts of the system, but the number of gas molecules diffusing from the region of high concentration to the region of low concentration is much larger than the amount diffusing in the reverse direction. If the system is left undisturbed, the diffusion of the gas continues until its partial pressure is the same in both parts of the system. The rate at which the gas diffuses depends upon the diffusing properties of the gas involved and the steepness of the concentration gradient.

If one exposes a liquid free of gas to air, gases will diffuse from the air phase to the liquid phase until the partial pressure of each of the various gases is the same in the two phases. The volume of gas which must be transferred from the air phase to the liquid phase before a partial pressure equilibrium is achieved is ordinarily related to the solubility of the gases in the liquid phase. Using various levels of Po_2 in the gas phase, it can be demonstrated that the volume of O_2 dissolved in the plasma is linearly related to the Po_2. For example, if 1 liter of blood plasma is exposed to a continuous stream of water-saturated gas having a Po_2 of 100 mm. Hg, oxygen will be taken up by the plasma until the plasma Po_2 is also 100 mm. Hg, and the total amount transferred will be approximately 3 ml. (the solubility of O_2 in plasma = .003 ml./mm. Hg/100 ml. plasma).

It is important to note that even at a Po_2 as high as that in alveolar air (149 mm. Hg) only 4.5 ml. of O_2 would be dissolved in 1 liter of plasma.

Of the total amount of oxygen and carbon dioxide in the blood, less than 5 per cent is present in simple solution. Reversible chemical reactions are responsible for the transport of the remainder of the two gases, and in both cases, hemoglobin plays a major role. The exchange of oxygen and carbon dioxide between the systemic capillaries and the tissues is illustrated in Figure 35, and the exchange which takes place at the alveolocapillary membrane is illustrated in Figure 36.

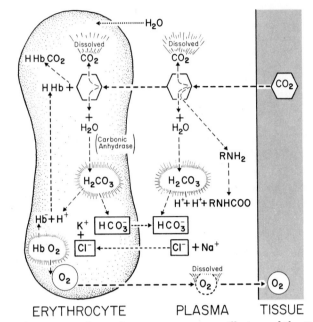

FIGURE 35.   Gas exchange between systemic capillaries and the tissues.

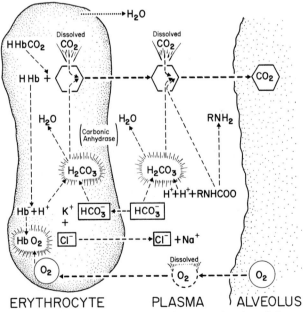

FIGURE 36.   Gas exchange between the pulmonary alveoli and the capillaries.

OXYGEN IN BLOOD

Since the partial pressure of oxygen is high in the alveoli and low in the mixed venous blood, oxygen diffuses from the alveoli into the pulmonary capillary blood. It is carried in the blood in two ways: as dissolved oxygen in physical solution in the plasma and combined with the hemoglobin in the erythrocytes. The amount of oxygen which is dissolved and the amount which is combined with hemoglobin both depend upon the partial pressure of oxygen in the arterial blood.

OXYGEN IN PHYSICAL SOLUTION

As was pointed out previously, the amount of oxygen which dissolves in a given volume of plasma is directly proportional to its partial pressure in the gaseous phase which, in turn, is in equilibrium with the oxygen tension in the plasma. Since the partial pressure of oxygen in the arterial blood in normal persons is approximately 100 mm. Hg, the amount of oxygen in physical solution in the plasma is about 3.0 ml./liter of plasma. In the venous blood, in which the partial pressure of oxygen is about 40 mm. Hg, there is 1.2 ml./liter of plasma. Thus, the oxygen in solution in the plasma diminishes by only 1.8 ml./liter as the blood passes through the tissues. Since the oxygen requirement of resting man is about 250 ml./min., the cardiac output would have to be 140 l./min. at rest and 800 l./min. during moderately strenuous exercise if plasma were the only transporting medium for oxygen. Fortunately, the gas transport medium is whole blood and not just plasma.

OXYGEN COMBINED WITH HEMOGLOBIN

Most of the oxygen in the blood is carried in the erythrocytes in combination with hemoglobin as oxyhemoglobin (HbO_2). Hemoglobin which is not combined with oxygen is called reduced hemoglobin (Hb).

One gram of hemoglobin is capable of combining chemically with 1.34 ml. of oxygen. In a normal man who has a hemoglobin content of 15 grams/100 ml., the blood is therefore capable of carrying 20.10 vol. per cent of oxygen as oxyhemoglobin, in addition to the comparatively small amount dissolved in the plasma. Although hemoglobin is capable of combining with this amount of oxygen, it does not normally do so. The extent to which hemoglobin combines with oxygen is usually expressed as the percentage saturation and is illustrated in the following formula:

$$\text{per cent saturation} = \frac{\text{oxygen content (HbO}_2)}{\text{oxygen capacity (HbO}_2 + \text{Hb)}} \times 100$$

The oxygen saturation of the arterial blood in a normal person breathing room air is about 97 per cent. The saturation of hemoglobin depends upon the partial pressure of the oxygen in the plasma. When the oxygen tension is high, most or all of the hemoglobin combines with oxygen; when the oxygen tension is low, as in respiratory disease, only a small amount of the hemoglobin combines with oxygen.

Unlike the amount of dissolved oxygen in the plasma, which is directly proportional to the partial pressure of oxygen, the amount of oxyhemoglobin formed in the red blood cell is not linearly related to the tension. The relationship between the partial pressure of oxygen and the saturation of hemoglobin is expressed by the *oxyhemoglobin dissociation curve*, which is illustrated in Figure 37. The characteristic **S** shape of this curve means that the hemoglobin clings to oxygen over a fairly wide range of oxygen tension at the upper end of the scale and gives up oxygen readily at lower oxygen tensions. The converse is also true, in that hemoglobin takes up oxygen very readily at the lower oxygen tensions but not at the upper end of the scale. It can be seen from Figure 37 that if the concentration of oxygen in the alveoli were less than 1 per cent, little oxygen would be absorbed by the hemoglobin in the red blood cells. If the concentra-

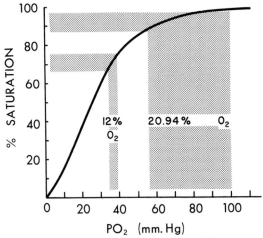

FIGURE 37.   The oxyhemoglobin dissociation curve. When an individual breathes room air at sea level (20.94 per cent O_2) the values for P_{O_2} and saturation are located on the flat part of the curve where large changes in tension are associated with small changes in saturation. In the hypoxic individual or in someone breathing air which contains only 12 per cent O_2, values for P_{O_2} and saturation are located on the steep part of the curve where small changes in tension are associated with large changes in saturation.

tion were increased to 9 per cent, which is equivalent to a partial pressure of about 60 mm. Hg, a large amount would be absorbed by the hemoglobin, and it would become 90 per cent saturated. If the oxygen concentration in the alveoli were elevated still more, the amount of oxyhemoglobin would increase further but only by a small amount. In other words, a change in the alveolar oxygen concentration from 9 to 15 per cent, so that the partial pressure rises to 100 mm. Hg, only raises the oxyhemoglobin saturation to 97 per cent. It is obvious, as well, that even if the alveolar oxygen tension were raised well above 100 mm. Hg, there would be only a slight further increase in oxyhemoglobin content.

Oxygen is brought to the tissues by the arterial blood. The oxygen which is directly available to the tissues is that in physical solution in the plasma. As it is taken up by the tissue cells, the partial pressure of the oxygen in the plasma falls so that the oxyhemoglobin begins to dissociate. In this way, oxygen is liberated from the red blood cells into the plasma and is then made available to the tissues. The oxyhemoglobin dissociation curve illustrates that the hemoglobin relinquishes oxygen readily when the oxygen tension drops below 60 mm. Hg. Since the oxygen tension of the tissue cells is low (less than 10 mm. Hg), the oxygen diffuses rapidly from the blood into the tissue cells. An average of approximately 50 ml. of oxygen/liter of blood is given up by the blood to the tissues of the body. Even after the tissues have received all their requirements, the venous blood is still 70 to 75 per cent saturated with oxygen under ordinary circumstances. Part of this remainder represents a reserve that can be drawn on by the tissues with only a slight further reduction in the partial pressure of oxygen.

The amount of oxygen which is given off by the blood to a particular tissue depends not only on the oxygen tension of that tissue but also on the partial pressure of carbon dioxide, the pH and the temperature of the blood. Figure 38 shows that the oxyhemoglobin dissociation curve moves to the right whenever there is a rise in the carbon dioxide tension, the hydrogen ion concentration or the temperature. It is believed that changes in carbon dioxide tension influence the dissociation curve because of the concomitant pH changes.

The influence of these factors on the dissociation of oxyhemoglobin means that, at a given partial pressure of oxygen, the oxyhemoglobin gives up more oxygen under conditions in which there is an elevated carbon dioxide tension, a lowered pH or an elevated temperature. These effects are extremely important because they act as a safeguard for the welfare of the tissues. A decrease in the oxygen tension in the tissue capillary blood, such as occurs when the activity of the tissues is increased or when the blood flow is decreased, is accompanied by a rise in carbon dioxide tension and hydrogen ion

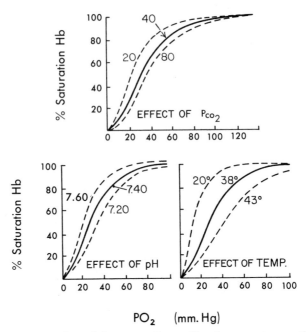

FIGURE 38.   The effect of changes in P_{CO_2}, pH and temperature on the oxyhemo-globin dissociation curve.

concentration, which in turn assists in the unloading of oxygen from the blood to the tissues. Conversely, the fall in blood carbon dioxide tension as the blood passes through the lungs causes the dissociation curve to shift to the left so that the hemoglobin is capable of taking on an additional quantity of oxygen. The effect of temperature is easily demonstrable in situations in which there is undue cooling of a tissue. When the hands are extremely chilled, for example, they may be red, not only because the tissues utilize less oxygen, but also because the oxyhemoglobin has been unable to dissociate.

The oxyhemoglobin dissociation curve of fetal blood lies to the left of the adult curve. On the other hand, if fetal hemoglobin in solution is examined, its dissociation curve is similar to that of adult hemoglobin, suggesting that the intracellular environment of fetal hemoglobin is responsible for its shifted oxyhemoglobin dissociation curve. Minor abnormalities in oxyhemoglobin dissociation have been found in a variety of metabolic or endocrine disorders in adult animals and in man; these also seem to be related to changes in the intracellular environment of hemoglobin rather than to changes in the hemoglobin itself. Recently, considerable attention has been directed at the possible role of 2,3,-diphosphoglycerate (DPG), which is nearly equimolar with hemoglobin in human red blood cells, in accounting for the shift in the oxyhemoglobin dissociation curve seen in disease, because it lowers the affinity of hemoglobin for oxygen.

Carbon monoxide competes with oxygen for binding with the iron in hemoglobin, and because its affinity for hemoglobin is about 250 times greater than that of oxygen, it is firmly bound. Not only does it compete with oxygen, but it increases the affinity of unbound iron atoms for oxygen. Thus, the oxygen capacity of the hemoglobin is reduced by carbon monoxide, and the oxygen which is carried by the hemoglobin is firmly bound and not readily given up to the tissues. When methemoglobin is formed as a result of oxidation of an iron atom to the ferric state, the oxyhemoglobin dissociation curve is altered in a manner similar to the effects of carbon monoxide.

HYPOXIA

The term "hypoxemia" means that there is a diminution in the oxygen content of the arterial blood, but it does not differentiate between a diminution due to a reduced partial pressure of oxygen, a diminution due to a lowered oxygen carrying capacity of the hemoglobin, or a diminution due to both. The term "hypoxia" means that there is a decrease in the amount of oxygen available to the tissues, regardless of the cause or the location. Hypoxia may be present even though both the arterial oxygen tension and content are normal. It has been classified into four main types: hypoxic, anemic, circulatory and histotoxic.

HYPOXIC HYPOXIA

In hypoxic hypoxia the tissues are supplied by blood in which the oxygen tension is lower than normal; that is, the hemoglobin is incompletely saturated with oxygen. This condition occurs in patients who are suffering from respiratory or cardiac diseases, in which there is an abnormality in gas exchange. As will be described later, the abnormality may be due to alveolar hypoventilation, altered ventilation-perfusion ratios, a diffusion defect, true venous admixture or a combination of these disturbances. This type of hypoxia is also present when the concentration of oxygen in the inspired air is lower than normal, e.g., at a high altitude.

ANEMIC HYPOXIA

In anemic hypoxia the tissues are supplied by arterial blood in which the oxygen tension is normal and the hemoglobin is almost completely saturated with oxygen. Since the hemoglobin content is low, however, both the oxygen content and the oxygen capacity of the blood are lower than normal. As a result, the tissues may not receive sufficient oxygen. This variety of hypoxia may be encountered in all of the anemic states as well as in certain conditions in which toxic substances combine with hemoglobin, such as carbon monoxide poisoning and methemoglobinemia. This combination prevents the uptake of oxygen by the hemoglobin so that the oxygen content is low.

CIRCULATORY HYPOXIA

This condition may be encountered in cases of generalized circulatory insufficiency, such as shock or congestive heart failure, or when there is a localized obstruction to arterial blood flow. Similarly, a localized venous occlusion produces local hypoxia because it impedes the flow of blood into and out of the capillaries. It may also develop when the tissue utilization of oxygen increases to an extent which is greater than the available supply of oxygen, as in violent exercise or in thyrotoxicosis. The blood which arrives at the tissues may have a normal oxygen tension and content, but the quantity of blood, and therefore the oxygen supply to the particular organ, may be too small for its metabolic demands.

HISTOTOXIC HYPOXIA

Some toxic substances, such as cyanide, interfere with the ability of the tissues to utilize the oxygen. Under such circumstances, the tissues may become exceedingly hypoxic, even though the partial pressure and content of oxygen in the arterial blood are normal.

CARBON DIOXIDE IN THE BLOOD

The carbon dioxide produced in the tissues diffuses into the systemic capillaries and is eliminated at the pulmonary capillaries.

TRANSPORT AS DISSOLVED CARBON DIOXIDE

Some of the carbon dioxide is transported between the systemic and pulmonary capillaries in a physically dissolved form in both plasma and erythrocytes. In the plasma, some of this dissolved carbon dioxide reacts with water to produce carbonic acid. This hydration of carbon dioxide takes place according to the equation

$$CO_2 + H_2O \leftrightarrows H_2CO_3$$

The equilibrium of this reaction in the plasma is far to the left so that the concentration of dissolved carbon dioxide is about 1000 times greater than the concentration of carbonic acid. The amount of dissolved carbon dioxide depends on its solubility coefficient, its partial pressure and the temperature. At body temperature, 0.067 vol. per cent or 0.0301 mM./l. of carbon dioxide is dissolved in plasma for every mm. Hg partial pressure of carbon dioxide. In the arterial blood, in which the carbon dioxide tension is normally about 40 mm. Hg, there is approximately 1.2 mM./l. of dissolved carbon dioxide, and in the venous blood, in which the tension is about 46 mm. Hg, there is 1.38 mM./l. of dissolved carbon dioxide. However, this is an increase of only 0.4 vol. per cent, or 0.18 mM./l., and the blood transports considerably more carbon dioxide than this. About 4 vol. per cent or 2 mM./l. of carbon dioxide enters the systemic capillary blood as it passes through the tissues. Most of this is carried as bicarbonate.

TRANSPORT AS BOUND CARBON DIOXIDE

When carbonic acid is formed, it ionizes according to the equation

$$H_2CO_3 \rightleftharpoons H^+ + HCO_3^-$$

Since only a minute amount of H_2CO_3 is formed in the plasma, only a small amount of bicarbonate is formed. On the other hand, the plasma bicarbonate content increases considerably when the blood traverses the tissue capillaries because the red blood cells are capable of promoting the formation of bicarbonate from CO_2. They do so for three reasons:

First, they contain an enzyme called *carbonic anhydrase* which catalyzes the hydration of the CO_2 diffusing from tissues through the plasma into the red blood cells to form carbonic acid at a rapid rate.

$$CO_2 + H_2O \underset{\text{carbonic anhydrase}}{\rightleftharpoons} H_2CO_3 \rightleftharpoons HCO_3^- + H^+$$

Second, the hemoglobin in the red blood cell provides basic groups which neutralize the H^+ ions formed by the dissociation of H_2CO_3, thereby promoting the formation of HCO_3^-

$$Hb^- + H^+ + HCO_3^- \rightleftharpoons HHb + HCO_3^-$$

The efficacy of hemoglobin as a buffer is enhanced by deoxygenation, since reduced hemoglobin is a better H^+ ion acceptor than oxyhemoglobin.

The formation of HCO_3^- in the red blood cells results in a concentration gradient between the cells and the plasma, and HCO_3^- diffuses quickly out of the cells. Since the red blood cell membrane is relatively impermeable to cations, electrical neutrality is preserved by an influx of Cl^- ions into the red blood cells which is equivalent to the efflux of HCO_3^- ions. This phenomenon is called the "*chloride shift.*" The hydration of CO_2 and the dissociation of carbonic acid result in an increase in the osmolarity of the red blood cell and, as a result, water enters the cells and increases their volume.

Finally, red blood cells further promote carbon dioxide transport because hemoglobin provides many more amino groups for the formation of carbamino compounds than do the proteins of the plasma according to this reaction:

$$Hb—N\begin{matrix} H \\ \\ H \end{matrix} + CO_2 \rightleftarrows Hb—N\begin{matrix} H \\ \\ COO^- \end{matrix} + H^+$$

Carbamino CO_2 accounts for about one-quarter of the arteriovenous CO_2 difference.

As is shown in Figure 36, the reverse of the processes which have been described takes place in the lungs. Because the partial pressure of carbon dioxide is 46 mm. Hg in the mixed venous blood and only about 40 mm. Hg in the alveoli, the blood gives up its excess carbon dioxide to the alveoli. Because of the high solubility of this gas in an aqueous media, its diffusion is rapid, and equilibrium between the carbon dioxide tensions of the pulmonary capillary blood and the alveolar air is established promptly. About 30 per cent of all the carbon dioxide which is exchanged is given up from combination with hemoglobin as carbamino-carbon dioxide when oxygen, whose partial pressure in the alveoli is about 100 mm. Hg, passes through the plasma into the red blood cells and oxygenates the hemoglobin to approximately 97 per cent of its capacity.

In contrast to what takes place in the tissues, the amount of diffusible anions decreases and the number of nondiffusible anions in the red blood cells increases so that the equilibrium for anions between the red blood cells and the plasma is once again altered. Consequently, the diffusible anions are redistributed, and some Cl^- leaves the red blood cell and HCO_3^- enters it. On entering the red blood cells, the HCO_3^- combines with H^+ to form H_2CO_3, and this in turn is dehydrated to carbon dioxide and water; the carbon dioxide then passes through the plasma into the alveoli. At the same time, the osmotic equilibrium between the red blood cells and the plasma is once again maintained by the movement of water out of the red blood cells into the plasma.

All of the reactions which have been described, with one exception, are very rapid. The exception is the dissociation of carbonic acid into carbon dioxide and water and the reverse form of this reaction. This is a slow process, and if the elimination of carbon dioxide were to depend on it alone, only 10 per cent of the available carbon dioxide would be removed from the blood during its passage through the pulmonary capillaries. As pointed out earlier, the red blood cells contain a high concentration of *carbonic anhydrase* which accelerates the reversible reaction of the formation of carbonic acid from CO_2 and water. The rate at which all the reactions involving carbon dioxide proceed has no effect on the equilibrium which is finally reached. However, the rate of the circulation of the blood sets a definite limit within which these reactions must take place. An erythrocyte is present in the lungs for a period of less than a second, and it is during this brief time that the reactions which liberate the carbon dioxide from the mixed venous blood into the alveolar air must take place. The reverse chloride shift is important in this regard, for without it, it would be impossible for the bicarbonate to enter the red blood cells from the plasma, where it is rapidly dehydrated to carbon dioxide by the carbonic anhydrase.

The capacity of the blood to carry carbon dioxide is expressed in the *CO_2 dissociation curve* which is illustrated in Figure 39. Unlike the oxyhemoglobin dissociation curve, the CO_2 dissociation

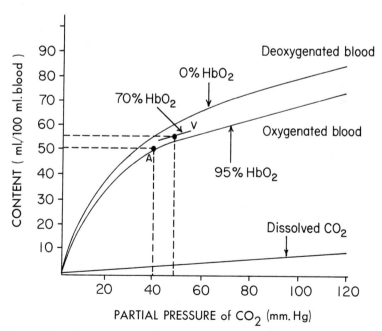

FIGURE 39. The in vitro CO_2 dissociation curve. The upper two curves show total CO_2 content in deoxygenated and oxygenated blood. The arterial point (*A*) and the venous point (*V*) indicate typical values obtained in normal resting man.

curve is nearly linear in the physiological range of PCO_2, especially when the effect of oxygenation of hemoglobin is taken into account.

DIFFUSION OF GAS IN THE LUNG

When blood is exposed to air, the rate at which the gas will equilibrate between the blood and air phases depends on four factors. The rate of diffusion of a gas across the blood-gas barrier is directly proportional to the solubility of the gas in the barrier between the two phases, the partial pressure difference between air and the blood, and the surface area available for diffusion, and it is inversely proportional to the square root of the molecular weight of the gas. Carbon dioxide diffuses 20 times more rapidly between air and blood than does oxygen, because even though it is a larger molecule than oxygen, its solubility is 25 times as great.

When gases diffuse between the air and the blood in the lungs certain complicating features are encountered. For example, an O_2 molecule in an alveolus is separated from an iron atom in a hemoglobin molecule in a red blood cell by the alveolar epithelium, basement membranes, the capillary endothelium, plasma and the intracellular fluid. These components form the blood-gas barrier to diffusion. The difference in partial pressures across this alveolocapillary barrier is greatest at the point where the venous blood enters the capillary and least at the point where the blood leaves the capillary. The size of the partial pressure gradient along the alveolocapillary barrier is dependent on the slope of the dissociation curve for each gas. This is illustrated in Figure 40, which shows the changes in the partial pressures of oxygen and carbon dioxide in the blood as it passes along the lung capillary, a process which has been estimated to take approximately 0.75 second at rest.

As demonstrated earlier, the slope of the oxyhemoglobin dissociation curve is steep at low levels of oxygenation and relatively flat at high levels. The exchange of oxygen from the alveolus to the capillary, therefore, takes place first in the steep portion and then in the flat part of the dissociation curve. Since the initial pressure gradient for oxygen is very large, oxygen moves rapidly from the alveoli to the capillaries, and about 95 per cent of the diffusion of oxygen takes place before the blood has passed halfway along the capillary. The equilibration of the partial pressure of oxygen on either side of the barrier takes place during the remaining half of the transit time in the capillaries. Very little gradient exists normally at the end of the capillary so that the partial pressure of oxygen in the pulmonary vein is almost equal to that in the alveolus.

The carbon dioxide dissociation curve is steep at all levels, and

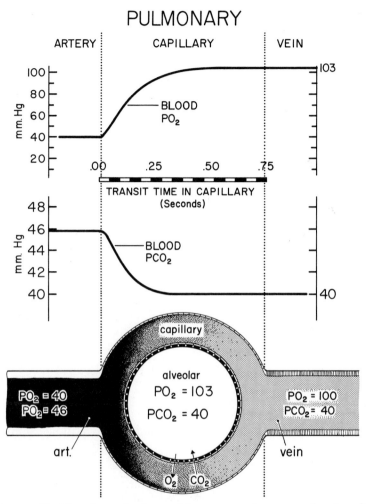

FIGURE 40. The change in the partial pressures of oxygen and carbon dioxide as blood passes along the pulmonary capillary.

it was formerly believed that the equilibration of carbon dioxide between the alveolus and the capillary takes place in about 0.072 second. However, since the evolution of CO_2 into alveolar gas is partly dependent on the oxygenation of the hemoglobin, total equilibration of carbon dioxide cannot occur more rapidly than oxygenation. It is likely that no significant difference in partial pressure of carbon dioxide between gas and blood ever develops because an overall resistance to diffusion which is great enough to cause a significant carbon dioxide gradient would be associated with such a fantastic partial pressure difference for oxygen that survival would be impossible.

Oxygen and carbon monoxide, which have a great affinity for hemoglobin, have proved to be most satisfactory for the qualitative estimation of the diffusing capacity of the lungs. In order to calculate the diffusing capacity of the lungs for a specific gas, it is necessary to know the amount of gas which is diffusing across the blood-gas barrier per minute as well as the mean gradient of its partial pressures between the alveolus and the pulmonary capillary. This is indicated in the following formulae:

$$D_{O_2} = \frac{\dot{V}_{O_2}}{P_{A_{O_2}} - P_{C_{O_2}}}$$

and

$$D_{CO} = \frac{\dot{V}_{CO}}{P_{A_{CO}} - P_{C_{CO}}}$$

where D is the diffusing capacity of the particular gas, oxygen or carbon monoxide, in ml./mm. Hg/min.; $\dot{V}$ is the volume of the gas which is diffusing per minute; and $P_A - P_C$ is the mean partial pressure gradient of that particular gas between the alveolus and the capillary.

THE VOLUME OF THE DIFFUSING GAS

The amount of oxygen or carbon monoxide which diffuses across the blood-gas barrier in 1 minute can be determined by estimating the difference between the amount of gas which is inhaled and the amount which is exhaled. The formula for the calculation of the oxygen consumption is

$$\dot{V}_{O_2} = \dot{V}_I (F_{I_{O_2}}) - \dot{V}_E (F_{E_{O_2}})$$

where $\dot{V}_{O_2}$ is the oxygen consumption per minute, $\dot{V}_I$ the inspired volume/min., $\dot{V}_E$ the expired volume/min., and F the concentration of the particular gas in the inspired air (I) and the expired air (E).

Similarly, the amount of carbon monoxide which diffuses across the blood-gas barrier is calculated from knowledge of the volume of gas which is breathed and the concentrations of carbon monoxide in the inspired and expired air. The formula is therefore similar to the one above, except that carbon monoxide is substituted for oxygen.

$$\dot{V}_{CO} = \dot{V}_I (F_{I_{co}}) - \dot{V}_E (F_{E_{co}})$$

THE MEAN ALVEOLOCAPILLARY PARTIAL PRESSURE GRADIENT

The mean partial pressure gradient is a single figure which expresses the integral with respect to time of a changing gradient between the alveolus and the pulmonary capillary. The partial pressure gradient which exists varies along the course of the pulmonary capillary and diminishes from the point at which the venous blood arrives at the alveolus to that point along the course of the capillary where the partial pressures of the gas phase and the blood phase approach equilibrium, as is shown in Figure 41. The figure also shows the mean pulmonary capillary oxygen tension, with respect to time, determined by means of identifying the value of PO_2 at which the shaded areas designated X and Y are equal. It is this mean gradient which is used in order to calculate the diffusing capacity of the lungs for oxygen.

Because of its remarkable affinity for hemoglobin, it is much easier to measure the mean gradient for carbon monoxide. Measurable quantities of carbon monoxide can diffuse into the pulmonary capillary blood without producing a significant partial pressure in the plasma. In practice, therefore, the partial pressure of carbon monoxide in the pulmonary capillary blood is considered to be zero so that the mean partial pressure gradient between the alveolus and

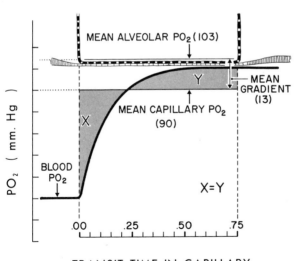

TRANSIT TIME IN CAPILLARY

(seconds)

FIGURE 41. The change in the partial pressure of oxygen as blood passes along the pulmonary capillary. The mean alveolocapillary gradient is also shown.

the capillary is equal to the mean alveolar carbon monoxide tension. This is not quite true, however, since it has been shown that the speed of the reaction between carbon monoxide and hemoglobin is slow and therefore interposes a significant resistance to the transfer of the gas from the alveolus to the hemoglobin molecule. Although there is little evidence to support this, the same can be presumed to be true for oxygen. This suggests that measurements of the diffusing capacity of the lung are affected not only by the resistance of the blood-gas barrier but also by chemical reactions within the red blood cell.

The resistance to the diffusion of carbon monoxide may be expressed as the reciprocal of the diffusing capacity:

$$1/D_{L_{CO}} = \frac{\text{partial pressure gradient}}{\text{CO uptake}}$$

and is made up of a membrane component $1/D_M$ and a blood component $1/D_B$.

$$\text{Thus, } \frac{1}{D_{L_{CO}}} = \frac{1}{D_M} + \frac{1}{D_B}$$

D_B represents the volume of CO which is taken up by blood in the pulmonary capillaries for each mm. Hg partial pressure. It is often expressed as $V_c \times \theta$, where V_c is the volume of blood in the pulmonary capillaries, and θ is the volume of CO which 1 ml. of blood will take up for each mm. Hg partial pressure.

$$\text{Thus, } \frac{1}{D_{L_{CO}}} = \frac{1}{D_M} + \frac{1}{V_c \times \theta}$$

The amount of CO taken up by the blood, i.e., the value of θ for carbon monoxide, diminishes in the presence of increased oxygen levels because of the competition between oxygen and carbon monoxide for Hb. This explains why $D_{L_{CO}}$ decreases when the concentration of inspired oxygen is increased. By determining $D_{L_{CO}}$ at several levels of inspired P_{O_2} a relationship such as that shown in Figure 42 may be derived. From an analysis of the slope of such a relationship it is possible to estimate the volume of blood in the pulmonary capillaries and, from the intercept, the size of the membrane component of the diffusion resistance can be derived.

Contrary to general opinion, an impaired diffusion of oxygen from the alveolar air to the pulmonary capillary blood, as shown in Figure 43, is seldom the primary cause of a low arterial oxygen saturation. With the exception of a relatively rare group of cases which have a specific type of alveolar pathology, arterial hypoxia in pul-

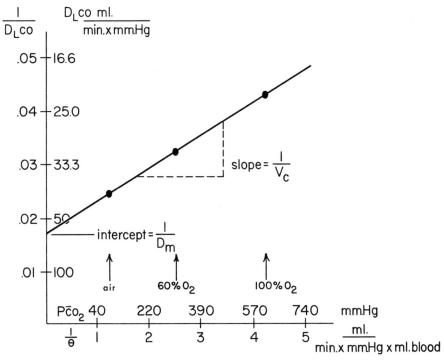

FIGURE 42. The diffusing capacity of the lungs for carbon monoxide ($D_{L_{CO}}$) measured at three levels of inspired oxygen concentration. A linear relationship is obtained when the reciprocal of the diffusing capacity is plotted against the mean capillary PO_2 ($P\bar{c}_{O_2}$) or the reciprocal of the reaction coefficient $\left(\dfrac{1}{\theta}\right)$.

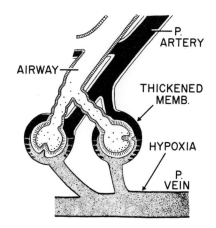

FIGURE 43. Effect of a diffusion defect on gas exchange. Note that the blood leaving the alveoli (the end-capillary blood) has not come into equilibrium with alveolar gas.

monary disease usually results from either an inadequate alveolar
ventilation or a poor correlation between ventilation and perfusion.
Thus, the finding of a low diffusing capacity may merely reflect these
abnormalities of gas exchange, rather than a diffusion defect.

ALVEOLAR VENTILATION

We have considered the two main processes subserving gas exchange: namely, the convective movement of air and blood, which
is an active process; and the passive equilibration of air and blood
by diffusion. Let us now consider the relationship of these two processes. Convective movement results mainly from expansion of the
terminal airways down to the level of alveolar ducts. Diffusion occurs
from the alveolar duct through the alveolar spaces and the blood-gas
barrier.

Practically speaking, the all-important portion of the air that is
inspired is that which is concerned in the exchange of gases with
the blood. Gas exchange occurs only in the alveoli and not in those
parts of the respiratory system which serve as the conducting airway.
Thus, some of the air that is inspired is wasted in that it does not
take part in gas exchange.

As the air is inspired into the lungs and is carried toward the
alveolar spaces, it becomes saturated with water, which evaporates
from the surfaces of the tissues. Water vapor is similar to any other
gas, in that it exerts a partial pressure and behaves independently
from the other gases in a mixture. On the other hand, since it is in
equilibrium with the liquid phase, it behaves differently from other
gases in one respect: its partial pressure depends almost completely
on the temperature and is almost independent of the barometric
pressure. At normal body temperature, the partial pressure of water
vapor is 47 mm. Hg.

The total pressure of the gases in the alveolar air corresponds
to that of the ambient barometric pressure. Owing to the presence of
water vapor, the total pressure of dry alveolar gas is equal to that of
the barometric pressure minus 47 mm. Hg. Whenever alveolar air
or expired air is analyzed, it is reported in terms of the dry gas. In
other words, in order to determine the partial pressure of an alveolar
gas, we must multiply its fractional concentration by the barometric
pressure minus 47.

Thus, $P_A = F_A \times$ (barometric pressure $- 47$)

where P represents the partial pressure and F the fractional concentration of the
alveolar gas, A.

Since the concentration of oxygen in the alveolar air is approximately 14 per cent, that of carbon dioxide approximately 6 per cent and that of nitrogen approximately 80 per cent, their respective partial pressures are approximately 103, 40 and 570 mm. Hg.

The alveolar gas can be viewed as an equilibration chamber; its composition represents a balance between two tendencies. On the one hand, the venous blood which returns to the lung and courses through it tends to lower the P_{O_2} and raise the P_{CO_2} of the alveolar gas. On the other hand, the alveolar ventilation adds fresh air to the alveolar gas, thereby tending to raise its P_{O_2} and to lower its P_{CO_2}. An important concept, to be developed later, is that it is not the absolute value of either ventilation or perfusion that determines the alveolar gas partial pressure but rather the balance between them. In normal persons the balance between ventilation and perfusion is such that the average alveolar P_{O_2} is 100 mm. Hg, the average alveolar P_{CO_2} is 40 mm. Hg, and the blood leaving the lungs has levels of P_{O_2} and P_{CO_2} which are nearly the same as those in the alveolar gas.

It must be pointed out that although the respiratory gases in the alveoli are commonly thought of as having specific concentrations, these concentrations are in fact, changing from moment to moment and, in addition, are different in various parts of the lung. The moment-to-moment changes in alveolar gas concentration are related to the different phases of the respiratory cycle; whereas, the differences in various parts of the lung are related to variations in the ventilation-perfusion ratios of the different alveoli. Any stated value for alveolar gas concentration is some sort of average figure, therefore, and cannot describe the actual situation in all parts of the lung.

Normally the air which enters the alveoli takes part in gas exchange with the mixed venous blood in the pulmonary capillaries. In this way, the gas tensions of the blood in the pulmonary veins become approximately equilibrated with the gas tensions of the alveolar air, and "arterialized" blood leaves the alveolus (Fig. 44). In normal resting man the partial pressures of oxygen and carbon dioxide of the blood coming to the pulmonary capillaries are 40 and 46 mm. Hg, respectively, and as pointed out above, those of the blood leaving the alveoli and entering the pulmonary veins are 100 and 40 mm. Hg, respectively.

DEAD SPACE

The mouth, nose, pharynx, larynx, trachea, bronchi and the bronchioles are collectively called the *anatomic dead space.* Functionally, however, the dead space is a physiologic concept, not an anatomic one, and it may be defined as that volume of the inspired

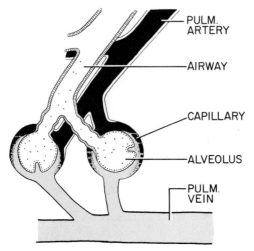

FIGURE 44. "Ideal" gas exchange. In this situation not only has blood traversing the two lung units come into complete diffusion equilibrium with the alveolar gas, but each unit contributes to the mixed alveolar gas the same proportion of gas that it contributes to the mixed arterial blood.

gas which does not take part in gas exchange and is therefore "wasted." The *physiologic dead space,* therefore, includes the volume of the inspired gas which occupies the anatomic dead space and the volume of the inspired gas that ventilates alveoli which are not perfused by capillary blood flow. In effect, there really is not such a sharp division between the ventilation of the dead space and the alveoli, because if some areas of lung are overventilated, even though normally perfused, they also contribute to the wasted ventilation and hence to the calculated dead space. In addition, some diffusion of gas probably takes place from the tracheobronchial tree into the alveoli.

In healthy persons the volumes of the anatomic and the physiologic dead spaces are almost identical. The physiologic dead space, which is approximately 150 ml. in healthy young males at rest, has been shown to increase with exercise or an increase in the tidal volume. Because of the dead space, a healthy person wastes about 20 to 30 per cent and utilizes only about 70 to 80 per cent of each tidal volume for gas exchange. In patients suffering from pulmonary disease, however, there is ventilation of alveoli in which perfusion is inadequate or absent and hyperventilation of other alveoli which are normally perfused. As a result, the physiologic dead space is increased. In these patients, therefore, a considerably smaller proportion of the inspired air is available for the oxygenation of and removal of carbon dioxide from the pulmonary capillary blood.

CALCULATION OF PHYSIOLOGIC DEAD SPACE

Measurements of the physiologic dead space are based on Bohr's formula, which simply states that the expired air consists of a mixture of two components, each with a particular composition: a component from the physiologic dead space, with the same composition as the inspired air; and an alveolar component, which has given up oxygen and received carbon dioxide.

$$\text{Thus, } V_T \times F_T = (V_D \times F_D) + (V_A \times F_A) \qquad (1)$$

where V represents a gas volume and F a fractional gas concentration; the subscripts signify the specific gas volume referred to, T being tidal gas, D dead space gas, and A alveolar gas.

For instance, if a tidal volume of 600 ml. of air containing 21 per cent oxygen were inspired and the concentration of oxygen were 16 per cent and 14 per cent in the expired and alveolar air, respectively, the dead space can be calculated:

$$0.16 \ (600) = 0.21 \ D + 0.14 \ (600 - D)$$
$$D = 171 \ ml.$$

CALCULATION OF ALVEOLAR VENTILATION

The alveolar component of the tidal volume consists of the quantity of air which remains after the dead space volume has been subtracted from the tidal volume

$$V_A = V_T - V_D \qquad (2)$$

From knowledge of the frequency of respiration per minute (f) and the tidal volume (V_T), the minute ventilation ($\dot{V}_E$) can be calculated.

$$\dot{V}_E = V_T \times f \qquad (3)$$

The alveolar ventilation per minute ($\dot{V}_A$) can, therefore, be calculated from the following formula:

$$\dot{V}_A = (V_T - V_D) \times f \qquad (4)$$

The alveolar ventilation also may be calculated directly from the Bohr equation. Since the concentration of carbon dioxide in the dead space is zero, equation (1) becomes

$$\dot{V}_E F_E = \dot{V}_A F_A \qquad (5)$$

where $\dot{V}$ is the volume and F the fractional gas concentration, the subscripts E and A and the alveolar ventilation, respectively.

For instance, if the minute ventilation is 6.0 l./min. and the concentrations of carbon dioxide are 4 per cent and 6 per cent in the expired and alveolar gases, then the alveolar ventilation is

$$0.04 \ (6.0) = 0.06 \ (\dot{V}_A)$$

and

$$\dot{V}_A = 4 \ l./min.$$

Even though the minute ventilation is kept constant, the alveolar ventilation will be affected by changes in respiratory frequency. This is illustrated in Table 2, which represents a subject in whom the dead space is 150 ml. and the ventilation is 8 l./min. It can be seen that as the respiratory rate increases, the alveolar ventilation decreases. Similarly, with a constant minute ventilation the alveolar ventilation will fall if the tidal volume diminishes. Alveolar hypoventilation as a result of rapid shallow respirations is frequently found in patients who are suffering from kyphoscoliosis or severe obesity.

Table 3 demonstrates that the alveolar ventilation per minute also falls if the dead space is increased and the minute ventilation and the respiratory rate remain constant. This situation arises particularly in patients with emphysema, in whom the physiologic dead space is large. Normally, an increase in the tidal volume would compensate for this effect of an enlarged dead space, but the capacity for such an increase is frequently diminished in patients with chronic respiratory disease.

An increase in the dead space or a decrease in the tidal volume, therefore, results in the same net effect, namely, a reduction in the alveolar ventilation, with consequent effects on the arterial blood gas tensions. If an increase in the dead space and a decrease in the tidal volume should occur simultaneously, the situation would, of course, become severely aggravated.

In addition, it should be pointed out that even though the alveolar ventilation may be adequate while at rest, it is frequently inadequate during exercise in patients with respiratory disease.

TABLE 2

EFFECT OF RESPIRATORY RATE AND TIDAL VOLUME ON ALVEOLAR VENTILATION WHEN MINUTE VENTILATION AND DEAD SPACE ARE CONSTANT

$\dot{V}_E$ (l./min.)	V_D (ml.)	V_T (ml.)	f	$\dot{V}_A$ (l./min.)
8.0	150	1000	8	6.8
8.0	150	500	16	5.6
8.0	150	250	32	3.2

TABLE 3

EFFECT OF INCREASE IN DEAD SPACE ON ALVEOLAR VENTILATION WHEN MINUTE VENTILATION AND RESPIRATORY RATE ARE CONSTANT

$\dot{V}_E$ (l./min.)	V_D (ml.)	V_T (ml.)	f	$\dot{V}_A$ (l./min.)
8.0	150	500	16	5.6
8.0	200	500	16	4.8
8.0	250	500	16	4.0

ALVEOLAR VENTILATION AND CARBON DIOXIDE PRODUCTION

Since the alveolar ventilation serves to promote the exchange of oxygen and carbon dioxide between the body and the environment, the adequacy or inadequacy of a given level of alveolar ventilation must be judged in relation to the body's oxygen consumption or carbon dioxide production. In a steady state the metabolic production of CO_2 by the body is equal to the amount of CO_2 being eliminated by the alveoli; the latter is simply the difference between the volume of CO_2 entering and leaving the alveoli per unit time.

Since only negligible amounts of CO_2 enter the alveoli in the inspired air,

$$CO_2 \text{ production} = \text{alveolar ventilation} \times \text{alveolar } CO_2 \text{ concentration}$$

$$\text{or alveolar } CO_2 \text{ concentration} = \frac{CO_2 \text{ production}}{\text{alveolar ventilation}}$$

This equation can be expressed in terms of P_{CO_2} rather than CO_2 concentration as follows:

$$P_{CO_2} \text{ (mm. Hg)} = \frac{CO_2 \text{ production (ml./min.)}}{\text{alveolar ventilation (l./min.)}} \times 0.863$$

The factor 0.863 converts concentration to partial pressure and, in addition, corrects for the fact that the volume of CO_2 produced is usually expressed as the dry gas volume at a standard temperature and pressure (STPD), and ventilatory volumes are expressed as the wet gas volume at body temperature and pressure (BTPS). An analogous relationship can be derived between alveolar ventilation and the alveolar P_{O_2}.

Clearly, an increase in CO_2 production and O_2 consumption, as occurs during exercise, would result in an increase in alveolar P_{CO_2} and a decrease in alveolar P_{O_2} if alveolar ventilation were to remain unchanged. A decrease in alveolar ventilation at a given metabolic rate, as occurs in severe lung disease, will also result in an increase in alveolar P_{CO_2} and decrease in alveolar P_{O_2}. The mixed alveolar P_{CO_2} and P_{O_2} are, therefore, indicators of the adequacy of alveolar ventilation with respect to the metabolic demands of the tissue.

In practice, it is difficult to obtain a valid sample of the mixed alveolar gas, since there is reason to believe that even in normal persons alveolar gas composition may be different in various parts of the lung. However, although the arterial P_{CO_2} may differ from the P_{CO_2} of mixed alveolar gas, the difference is usually small at rest, and it is generally considered that the arterial P_{CO_2} is a measure of the "effective" alveolar P_{CO_2}. We can therefore substitute the arterial P_{CO_2} for the alveolar P_{CO_2} as an indicator of the normality or abnormality of alveolar ventilation. When alveolar ventilation is abnormally low for a given CO_2 production (hypoventilation), the arterial P_{CO_2} is high. Conversely, when the alveolar ventilation is abnormally high for a given CO_2 production (hyperventilation), the arterial P_{CO_2} is low. On the other hand, the arterial P_{O_2} is not a reliable measure of the alveolar P_{O_2} because it is influenced by factors other than alveolar ventilation to a much greater extent than is the P_{CO_2}.

ALVEOLAR VENTILATION AND THE ACIDITY
OF THE BLOOD

Normally the lungs eliminate the CO_2 equivalent of about 15,000 mEq. of carbonic acid each day, while the kidneys excrete 60 to 80 mEq. in fixed acids. Thus, the respiratory system is quantitatively most important in regulating the acid-base balance of the body. This regulation is dependent upon the relationships between alveolar ventilation and the concentrations of CO_2, bicarbonate and hydrogen ions in extracellular fluid.

Molecular CO_2 in the blood and extracellular fluid is, as we have already seen, in equilibrium with HCO_3^- by virtue of the hydration-dissociation reactions:

$$CO_2 + H_2O \underset{\text{Hydration}}{\overset{K_H}{\rightleftarrows}} H_2CO_3 \underset{\text{Dissociation}}{\overset{K_O}{\rightleftarrows}} H^+ + HCO_3^-$$

The two reactions are intimately related and are usually considered as a single reaction with the two rate constants combined as an "apparent" rate constant K_a. Furthermore, since the concentration of carbonic acid is only one-thousandth of that of molecular CO_2, the mass action form of the equation is usually written in terms of CO_2

and bicarbonate. Thus,

$$H^+ = K_a \frac{CO_2}{HCO_3^-}$$

Since the amount of dissolved CO_2 is directly related to the partial pressure of CO_2, P_{CO_2} multiplied by the solubility coefficient 0.03 may be substituted for the CO_2 concentration in the formula to give

$$H^+ = K_a \frac{0.03\ P_{CO_2}}{HCO_3^-}$$

When the hydrogen ion concentration is expressed in moles per liter, the constant K_a has a value of 8×10^{-7} in blood at body temperature. When hydrogen ion concentration is expressed in nanomoles per liter the constant becomes 800 so that

$$H^+\ (\text{nanomoles/liter}) = 800 \times \frac{0.03\ P_{CO_2}\ \text{mm. Hg}}{HCO_3^-\ \text{m moles/1.}} = \frac{24\ P_{CO_2}}{HCO_3^-}$$

The relationship between carbonic acid and the anion bicarbonate in the plasma is used clinically to establish the existence and the severity of any disturbances in the acid-base balance. In this case, the relationship is governed by the Henderson-Hasselbalch equation:

$$pH = pK_a + \log \frac{HCO_3^-}{H_2CO_3}$$

or

$$pH = pK_a + \log \frac{HCO_3^-}{0.03\ P_{CO_2}}$$

The pK_a for blood at body temperature is 6.10.

In normal arterial blood the bicarbonate concentration is approximately 24 millimoles per liter and the P_{CO_2} is 40 mm. Hg. Hydrogen ion concentration is therefore

$$24 \times \frac{40}{24} = 40 \text{ nanomoles per liter}$$

and the pH is

$$6.10 + \log \frac{24}{0.03 \times 40} = 6.10 + \log \frac{24}{1.2} \text{ or } 7.40$$

The Henderson-Hasselbalch equation illustrates that the pH of the blood plasma remains unchanged as long as there is a constant ratio between the levels of bicarbonate and dissolved carbon dioxide (or the carbon dioxide tension). As can be seen, the ratio of bicarbonate to dissolved carbon dioxide is normally maintained at 20:1. Whenever this ratio is altered by either respiratory or metabolic conditions, the pH becomes abnormal.

It can now be clearly seen that there is an important link between the alveolar ventilation and the acidity of the blood; a link which depends on the central role played by CO_2. At a given level of metabolic activity or carbon dioxide production, the hydrogen ion concentration (cH^+) is proportional to the P_{CO_2}, which in turn is inversely related to the alveolar ventilation. When the alveolar ventilation is decreased in relation to CO_2 production, CO_2 is retained excessively and the P_{CO_2} and cH^+ increase (i.e., hypercapnia and acidemia are present). When the alveolar ventilation is increased in relation to CO_2 production, CO_2 is eliminated excessively, and the P_{CO_2} and cH^+ decrease (i.e., hypocapnia and alkalemia are present).

Alveolar hypoventilation with consequent hypercapnia and acidemia has a particular clinical importance and is encountered frequently. The defect may be in the lungs, the thoracic cage or the neural regulatory mechanisms. Hypercapnia develops whenever the total ventilation falls or when the physiologic dead space increases without a proportionate rise in the minute ventilation. The arterial carbon dioxide tension also rises whenever the metabolic production of carbon dioxide rises without a proportionate increase in the alveolar ventilation. This is particularly true when the work of breathing is great, for under such circumstances, increases in ventilation may be associated with the production of more carbon dioxide than can be eliminated by the lungs.

A sudden fall in alveolar ventilation only results in a transient decrease in CO_2 elimination because, as CO_2 is retained, the alveolar P_{CO_2} rises and the amount of CO_2 eliminated over a period of time is gradually restored to its original value. A new steady state is established in which CO_2 production and elimination are again equal, but this is now at a higher level of alveolar and hence extracellular fluid CO_2. It has been calculated that in an average adult male about 35 ml. of CO_2 will be retained for each mm. Hg rise in P_{CO_2} resulting from an acute decrease in alveolar ventilation.

When the arterial carbon dioxide tension rises the amount of bicarbonate and total carbon dioxide also increases. Unfortunately, this acute increase in total carbon dioxide content is not easily recognizable, for it is still within the normal range. Because of the increase in carbon dioxide tension, the ratio between the bicarbonate and the dissolved carbon dioxide is less than 20:1. As a result, the pH falls, and the patient suffers from a condition called respiratory acidemia.

In response to hypercapnia which persists the kidney increases its H^+ ion excretion and the renal tubular cells generate bicarbonate which passes into the blood. This tends to restore the ratio P_{CO_2}/HCO_3^- and hence the cH^+ to a normal value. As pointed out earlier, an increase in CO_2 will, by virtue of its hydration to H_2CO_3 and the subsequent dissociation, directly increase the HCO_3^- concentration. However, this is a relatively small effect compared to the effect of renal retention of HCO_3^- and does little to offset the effect of an increase in CO_2 on cH^+.

Hypocapnia and alkalemia due to an increase in alveolar ventilation in relation to CO_2 production is also observed frequently. It is brought about by direct or reflex stimulation of the respiratory centers in the brain. It is encountered particularly in patients with hypoxic hypoxia due to respiratory disease. Other common causes are cerebral damage such as a cerebrovascular accident or the ingestion of a drug, such as salicylate, which is a respiratory stimulant. It is also seen occasionally in highly emotional or apprehensive persons. When the partial pressure of carbon dioxide falls the plasma bicarbonate level also falls, but the ratio of bicarbonate to dissolved carbon dioxide is still greater than 20:1, so the pH rises, resulting in a condition called *respiratory alkalemia.* If the hypocapnia persists, excess cations, and in addition bicarbonate anions, are excreted by the kidneys, while chloride is conserved. If the plasma bicarbonate level falls sufficiently, the ratio of bicarbonate to dissolved carbon dioxide may return toward its normal value so that the cH^+ may be almost normal. Since the P_{CO_2} of extracellular fluid is determined by the function of the lungs, and its bicarbonate is controlled mainly by renal function, the cH^+ of extracellular fluid has been said to depend on the ratio of lung function to renal function. Thus, the respiratory system is also involved in compensation for metabolic disturbances leading to abnormal acid-base states. These "metabolic" disturbances of acid-base balance occur when the relationship between fixed anions and fixed cations in the blood is altered. For instance, in diabetic ketosis excess H^+ ions react with bicarbonate to form carbonic acid and the bicarbonate level and the pH fall. This is called *metabolic acidemia.* The rise in cH^+ stimulates ventilation so that the arterial P_{CO_2} is secondarily lowered. In this way, the ratio of bicarbonate to dissolved carbon dioxide tends to return to normal so that the pH is nearly normal. Conversely, when excess OH^- is present in the blood, it reacts with carbonic acid so that the bicarbonate level and the pH rise, resulting in a condition called *metabolic alkalemia.* The carbon dioxide tension tends to rise secondarily because the lowered cH^+ inhibits respiration. In metabolic conditions, therefore, the respiratory system acts as the compensatory device whereby the arterial carbon dioxide tension is altered secondarily in order to restore the normal ratio of bicarbonate to dissolved carbon dioxide so that the pH may be maintained at a normal level. This is because the neural mechanisms influencing the activity of the respiratory muscles, and hence alveolar ventilation, are sensitive to changes in the acid-base state of the extracellular fluid. The factors involved in the control of breathing will be discussed later.

ALVEOLAR VENTILATION AND PERFUSION

The ratio of the alveolar ventilation to the pulmonary capillary blood flow determines the gas composition of the blood leaving the lung. This can be demonstrated mathematically. Recall that the amount of oxygen taken up from alveolar gas over a given period of time is equal to the difference between the amount inspired and the amount expired from the alveolar gas in that time or

Amount inspired − Amount expired = Oxygen uptake

$$\dot{V}_A(F_{I_{O_2}}) - \dot{V}_A(F_{A_{O_2}}) = \dot{V}_{O_2}$$

The oxygen taken up from the alveolar gas by the blood equals the difference between the amount delivered to the lung in the mixed venous blood and the amount leaving the lung in the systemic arterial blood, or

Amount in arterial blood − Amount in mixed venous blood =
Oxygen uptake

$$\dot{Q}/(C_{a_{O_2}}) - \dot{Q}\,(C_{\bar{V}_{O_2}}) = \dot{V}_{O_2}$$

The two equations representing oxygen uptake can be combined as follows:

$$\dot{V}_A\,(F_{I_{O_2}} - F_{A_{O_2}}) = \dot{Q}\,(C_{a_{O_2}} - C_{\bar{V}_{O_2}})$$

From this the relationship between alveolar ventilation and perfusion ($\dot{V}_A/\dot{Q}$) can be derived

$$\dot{V}_A/\dot{Q} = \frac{C_{a_{O_2}}' - C_{\bar{V}_{O_2}}}{F_{I_{O_2}} - F_{A_{O_2}}}$$

This equation indicates that at a fixed value of inspired oxygen concentration ($F_{I_{O_2}}$) and at a given level of mixed venous oxygen content ($C_{\bar{V}_{O_2}}$) the oxygen content of arterial blood and of the alveolar gas will be determined by the ratio of alveolar ventilation to perfusion. The absolute value of ventilation or perfusion is unimportant in this respect.

A similar expression can be derived for carbon dioxide exchange. Namely

$$\dot{V}_A/\dot{Q} = \frac{C_{\bar{V}_{CO_2}} - C_{a_{CO_2}}}{F_{A_{CO_2}}}$$

Since at any time in a steady state the $\dot{V}_A/\dot{Q}$ ratios in terms of O_2 must be identical to the $\dot{V}_A/\dot{Q}$ ratios in terms of CO_2, we may write

$$\frac{\dot{V}_A}{\dot{Q}} = \frac{C_{a_{O_2}} - C_{\bar{v}_{O_2}}}{F_{I_{O_2}} - F_{A_{O_2}}} = \frac{C_{\bar{v}_{CO_2}} - C_{a_{CO_2}}}{F_{A_{CO_2}}}$$

From this equation it can be seen that for given values of $F_{I_{O_2}}$, $C_{\bar{v}_{CO_2}}$ and $C_{\bar{v}_{O_2}}$ the values of $F_{A_{O_2}}$ and $F_{A_{CO_2}}$ and hence $P_{A_{CO_2}}$ and $P_{A_{O_2}}$ will be determined by the ratio of ventilation to perfusion. By graphical analysis it is possible to determine, for given values of $F_{I_{O_2}}$, $C_{\bar{v}_{O_2}}$ and $C_{\bar{v}_{CO_2}}$, the values of $P_{A_{CO_2}}$ and $P_{A_{O_2}}$ which would satisfy the equation at several values of $\dot{V}_A/\dot{Q}$.

This procedure results in the $O_2 - CO_2$ diagram shown in Figure 45.

As has been discussed earlier, the distribution of both the inspired gas and the pulmonary blood flow are not uniform throughout the lungs, even in a healthy person. Similarly, the relationship between the blood and gas distribution ($\dot{V}_A/\dot{Q}$ ratios) is not uniform throughout the lung (Fig. 46) so that gas concentrations must differ from region to region. Fortunately, in healthy subjects, these regional differences are not large enough to materially interfere with gas exchange, and the mixed arterial blood has nearly the same partial pressures of oxygen and carbon dioxide as that of mixed alveolar gas.

VENOUS-ADMIXTURE-LIKE PERFUSION

When there is perfusion of inadequately ventilated alveoli, as is illustrated in Figure 47, *A*, or in the extreme case, perfusion of

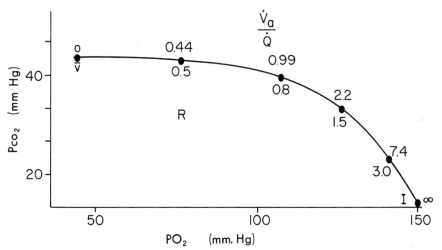

FIGURE 45. A curve may be drawn which joins the points (representing the values of P_{O_2} and P_{CO_2}) which are determined by given values for the respiratory exchange ratio (R), the ventilation perfusion ratio ($\dot{V}_A/\dot{Q}$), the composition of mixed venous blood (V) and inspired air (I).

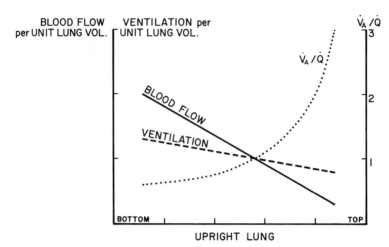

UPRIGHT LUNG

FIGURE 46.   Regional blood flow and ventilation. Both ventilation and blood flow decrease from bottom to top but the ratio between them changes so that the upper regions are overventilated in relation to their perfusion and the lower regions are relatively underventilated.

nonventilated alveoli, a low ventilation-perfusion ratio is present. Under such circumstances, a portion of the pulmonary blood is only slightly aerated, if at all. This poorly aerated blood leaves the capillary and then mixes with fully "arterialized" blood coming from the other pulmonary capillaries. This *venous-admixture-like perfusion* leads to hypoxia and slight hypercapnia in the arterial blood. Hyper-

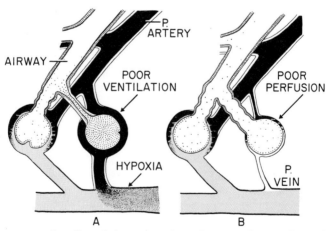

FIGURE 47.   The effect of alterations of ventilation-perfusion relationships on gas exchange. *A*, Low $\dot{V}_A/\dot{Q}$ areas contribute poorly oxygenated blood to the systemic circulation—an effect which is similar to that resulting from venous-admixture (shunt). *B*, High $\dot{V}_A/\dot{Q}$ areas contribute gas to the mixed expired air which is high in O_2 and low in CO_2 concentration—an effect which is similar to that resulting from an increase in dead space.

capnia may not develop, however, if there is sufficient hyperventilation of the remaining perfused alveoli. On the other hand, owing to the shape of the oxyhemoglobin dissociation curve, hyperventilation of these alveoli will only add a limited amount of oxygen to the blood. This means that hyperventilation cannot compensate for hypoventilation of abnormal areas of lung to correct arterial hypoxia to any significant degree.

DEAD-SPACE-LIKE VENTILATION

Whenever the ventilation of alveoli is maintained but the blood perfusion is limited (Fig. 47, *B*) or, in the extreme case, when there is no perfusion, a high ventilation-perfusion ratio is present. The gas entering these alveoli takes little part, if any, in gas exchange, and the small amount of blood flowing through these alveoli contributes relatively little to the composition of the mixed arterial blood. The gas leaving such alveoli tends to have a composition more nearly like the gas in the tracheobronchial tree, thus contributing to the physiological dead space, so that it has been called *dead-space-like ventilation.* Although a high ventilation/perfusion ratio, per se, does not result in arterial hypoxemia, the large amount of wasted ventilation means that alveolar ventilation will be low unless the total ventilation is increased. Adequate oxygenation and carbon dioxide elimination, as evidenced by the presence of normal arterial oxygen and carbon dioxide tensions, may occur in the presence of excessive dead-space-like ventilation, but only if the normally perfused alveoli are hyperventilated. Such a compensatory hyperpnea is often observed clinically.

It is important to emphasize that hypoxia develops if the ratio of the alveolar ventilation to the perfusion is not uniform throughout the lungs, even though the total alveolar ventilation and the total pulmonary blood flow are normal. As a result of variations in the ventilation-perfusion ratios throughout the lung, there is an increase in the difference between the alveolar and the arterial partial pressures of oxygen, (the alveolar-arterial or A-a difference). This is an increase in the overall difference between the mixed alveolar gas and the mixed pulmonary capillary blood. There may be no difference whatever between the partial pressures in the gas phase of a particular alveolus and that of the blood leaving it.

Disturbances in the ventilation-perfusion ratios and increased A-a differences are predominant in patients suffering from emphysema. In patients with pulmonary disease, both abnormally high and low ventilation-perfusion ratios frequently coexist. In the early stages, compensatory hyperpnea may insure an adequate effective alveolar ventilation, and the arterial carbon dioxide tension may be normal,

despite the presence of hypoxia. In the later stages, however, because of the mechanical disturbances in the lungs, the patient is
frequently unable to increase his ventilation sufficiently to provide
an adequate alveolar ventilation. Under these circumstances, the
low arterial PO_2 is associated with a high PCO_2.

TRUE VENOUS ADMIXTURE OR SHUNT

A lower than normal arterial oxygen tension may also occur when
mixed venous blood, which has not come into contact with alveoli,
enters and mixes with blood in the pulmonary vein or the systemic
circulation. This situation, which is called *true venous admixture,*
or shunt, is illustrated in Figure 48.

Even in healthy persons approximately 2.5 per cent of the total
pulmonary blood flow enters the arterialized systemic circulation
by means of the thebesian and the bronchial veins, which empty
into the left side of the heart and the pulmonary veins, respectively.
There is an increase in the amount of true venous admixture in those
congenital heart diseases in which blood is shunted from the right
side of the heart to the left side; in pulmonary arteriovenous aneurysm, in which blood is shunted from the pulmonary artery to the
pulmonary veins; and a variety of other conditions in which the lungs
may be normal. As a result, considerable arterial hypoxia is present
in such situations. However, because the lungs themselves are usually healthy, no carbon dioxide retention develops. In fact, the
hypoxia frequently leads to hyperventilation with resultant hypocapnia.

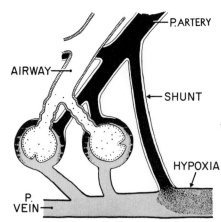

FIGURE 48. Hypoxia resulting from
true venous admixture.

Chapter 4

The Control of Breathing

It was pointed out earlier that a clear understanding of the neural control of breathing is important because some diseases and some drugs may interfere with breathing, and hence gas exchange, through their effects on the nerves and muscles of respiration. Neural mechanisms are also important in compensating for defects in gas exchange or acid-base balance resulting from the effects of disease or drugs on the lungs, kidneys or other organs. A complete description of the neural mechanisms involved in human respiration is not possible, since experiments which would provide the pertinent information cannot be carried out for technical or ethical reasons. The aim of this chapter will therefore be to briefly describe the information which has been derived from animal experiments and to emphasize its relevance to human respiration. A general scheme depicting some important neural components in the regulation of respiration is shown in Figure 49.

THE CENTRAL CONNECTIONS OF RESPIRATORY NERVES

It has become useful to refer to the central connections of respiratory nerves as the respiratory centers, but it is important to realize that this is a term of convenience and should not be taken to mean that there are clearly defined "nuclei" concerned with respiration. The nerve cells which participate in the central regulation of respiration are widely dispersed and may be found in the cerebral cortex, hypothalamus, pons and medulla.

The cortical cells are concerned with the voluntary influence on respiration and with those involuntary influences which require high levels of integration—such as talking, laughing and crying. Breathing can be altered voluntarily, as in voluntary hyperventilation or breath-holding. There are many other acts which presumably

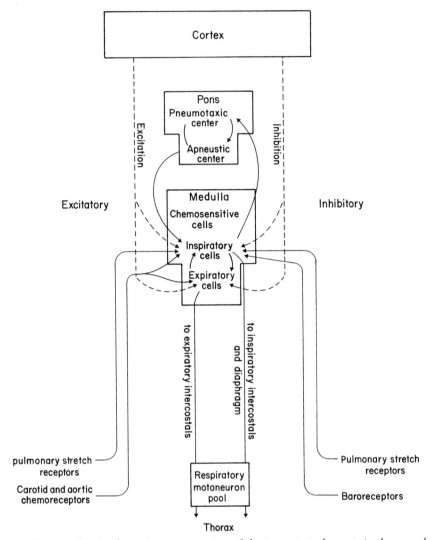

FIGURE 49.   A schematic representation of the important elements in the neural regulation of respiration. (From Mountcastle, V. B.: Medical Physiology. C. V. Mosby, St. Louis, 1968, p. 704.)

involve the higher centers, such as pain, apprehension and excitement, all of which tend to augment respiration. Furthermore, the higher centers play a role in the hyperpnea of exercise. The cerebral cortex is not essential for the mere maintenance of rhythmic respiration; this is a function which is served by neurones in the brain stem.

The nerve cells which are responsible for the maintenance of rhythmic respiration are located in the medulla. Activity of some of these cells results in inspiration; activity of others results in expiration. The two types of cells interact with each other and, in addition, are influenced by impulses coming to them from the pons, the glossopharyngeal and vagus nerves, and other locations in the brain stem such as the reticular activating system. The influence of the pons on the medullary cells includes facilitation of inspiration which, if uncontrolled, results in prolonged inspiratory spasms (*apneustic breathing*). The pneumotaxic centers, which are located in the upper third of the pons, and the vagus nerves play a role in the rhythmicity of respiration in that they periodically inhibit the inspiratory facilitation. Apneusis is thought by some to represent the effect of activity of the reticular system and by others to be the result of the activity of a discrete "apneustic center."

RESPIRATORY REFLEXES

The respiratory reflexes which have received the most attention are those in which the afferents arise in the lung, the central chemosensitive areas and the peripheral chemosensitive areas.

REFLEXES ARISING IN THE LUNG

THE INFLATION OR STRETCH REFLEX

Hering and Breuer demonstrated in 1868 that maintained distension of the lungs of anesthetized animals would decrease the frequency of respiratory effort. They showed this to be a reflex which was mediated by afferent vagal fibers. It is often called the *"Hering-Breuer reflex."* The afferent impulses travel in a particular type of vagal fiber that is temperature-sensitive. The impulses traveling in these fibers are thought to be inhibitory because inflation of the lungs leads to an increase in impulse frequency in the afferent fiber and a simultaneous decrease of electrical activity in inspiratory muscles. The receptors for this reflex are probably located in the bronchi or bronchioles.

Earlier physiologists attributed a major role in the regulation of respiration to this reflex and felt that it was responsible for terminating inspiration, exciting a tonic inhibition of the respiratory center, and perhaps also regulating the work of breathing. The reflex is well developed in animals and appears to be active in newborn babies. By contrast, it would appear to be inactive in adults, since blocking the vagi has little effect on the normal pattern of breathing, unless the tidal volume is over a liter.

HEAD'S PARADOXICAL REFLEX

Head demonstrated in 1889 that inflation of the lungs of rabbits would cause an additional reflex inspiratory effort if the Hering-

Breuer reflex inhibition of respiration were prevented by a partial vagal block. The phenomenon has been termed *"Head's paradoxical reflex"* or, more simply, the *"gasp reflex."* The receptors for this reflex lie in the lungs, and their activity appears to be augmented by progressive collapse of the lungs so that a tidal inspiration becomes sufficient to produce a "positive feedback" and a self-augmented gasp or "complementary" cycle. Newborn animals, including human neonates, also exhibit a "gasp reflex." Although this reflex disappears in the human after the first week of life, it is of physiological advantage while present in that it aids inflation of the lungs. This reflex has been shown to be vagally mediated. It is possible that this vagal mechanism may underlie the sighs or self-augmenting cycles seen in adults when there is a tendency for lung collapse.

OTHER REFLEXES ARISING IN THE LUNG

Bilateral vagotomy prevents the hyperpnea and hyperventilation which is associated with marked deflation of the lung such as may occur with a pneumothorax, vascular congestion or following the injection of serotonin. This suggests that the hyperventilation occurring under these conditions is reflex in nature. Although there is some evidence that the response is mediated by receptors in the lung which respond to deflation and to changes resulting from pulmonary embolism or congestion, the extent to which they account for the ventilatory response seen in intact animals has not been established conclusively. It has been suggested that the rapid shallow breathing in these conditions is more appropriate for the correction of potential asphyxial changes than it is for the reinflation of collapsed parts of the lung.

Tachypnea also occurs in man in association with pulmonary embolism and in situations which are associated with a raised pulmonary venous pressure. The reflex nature of the respiratory stimulation in these situations has not been proved but it is a useful working notion. Lung receptors are also thought to contribute to the unpleasant sensation of breathing CO_2 or breath-holding, since the breath-holding time is prolonged by vagal block.

REFLEXES ARISING IN THE TRACHEOBRONCHIAL TREE

In response to irritants, mechanoreceptors in the subepithelial regions of the airways give rise to hyperpnea and cough and, in addition, may produce bronchoconstriction and systemic hypertension. Similar effects may be produced by the injection of histamine or serotonin. Cough is not always a part of the response, however, and one may only observe reflex stimulation of breathing. It is obvious that the relative contribution of so-called deflation receptors and mechanoreceptors in the airways to the tachypnea seen in such complex conditions as pulmonary embolism cannot be judged with much confidence at the present time.

REFLEXES ARISING IN CENTRAL CHEMORECEPTORS

A major portion of the increase in ventilation which occurs in response to an elevation of the arterial CO_2 tension is the result of stimulation arising within the central nervous system. It is now believed that the chemosensitive areas which are responsible for the ventilatory response to CO_2 are not the classical medullary respiratory centers but rather areas which are anatomically separate. On the basis of the time course of the response to acute changes in blood P_{CO_2} or cH^+ concentration, it has also been postulated that a major part of central respiratory chemosensitivity resides in areas distinct from the "surface" receptors. In the cat, chemosensitive areas are located near the ventrolateral surface of the medulla, near the roots of the ninth and tenth cranial nerves. The connections between these areas and the respiratory neurones have not been delineated.

The direct chemical stimulus which activates the central chemosensitive areas is thought to be an increase in the H^+ ion concentration of the extracellular fluid, which is presumed to be in direct contact with these areas. The central areas which are not protected by a permeability barrier to ions will respond directly to changes in H^+ or HCO_3^- in the blood, but those areas, including the ones exposed to cerebrospinal fluid, which are protected by a barrier, will not respond readily to these ionic changes. In contrast to H^+ and HCO_3^-, CO_2 is freely diffusible and therefore is capable of increasing local cH^+ so that the areas beyond such a barrier will respond to CO_2 changes.

In view of our ignorance concerning the precise location of the central chemosensitive areas as well as their relative contribution to overall central chemosensitivity, it is probably best to refer to the "central component of chemosensitivity" rather than to "central chemoreceptors."

REFLEXES ARISING IN PERIPHERAL CHEMORECEPTORS

There are two main collections of receptor cells which lie outside the central nervous system and which respond to changes in the P_{O_2}, P_{CO_2} or cH^+ of the arterial blood. One collection of cells is located in the carotid body which lies in the bifurcation of the common carotid artery; the other collection lies above the aortic arch between the subclavian and common carotid arteries on either side and below the arch between the aorta and pulmonary artery. The impulses arising in the carotid body reach the central nervous system via the glossopharyngeal nerve, and the impulses arising in the aortic chemoreceptors are carried by the vagus nerve.

The carotid and aortic chemoreceptors are similar in that their stimulation results in an increased rate, depth and minute volume of ventilation so that alveolar ventilation is increased. They are stimulated particularly by a decrease in arterial oxygen tension but also by an increase in arterial CO_2 tension or in hydrogen ion concentration, a decrease in their blood flow relative to their metabolic needs, and an increase in blood temperature. The stimulating effect of P_{CO_2} may be due to the associated changes in cH^+ in the immediate environment of the chemosensitive elements. There may be interaction of these stimuli, so it is apparent that the degree to which the peripheral chemoreceptors respond to a given stimulus depends on the coincident levels of the other stimuli.

The cardiovascular effects of the carotid and aortic chemoreceptor reflexes differ in that the local stimulation of the carotid receptors produces bradycardia, and stimulation of the aortic receptors produces tachycardia and systemic vasoconstriction. In addition, it has been demonstrated that local stimulation of the carotid chemoreceptors produces an increase in pulmonary vascular resistance, an increase in bronchiolar tone and an increase in secretion from the adrenal cortex and medulla. Since they have not been studied, the effects of aortic chemoreflexes on pulmonary vessels, bronchi and the adrenal gland are not known.

PERIPHERAL AND CENTRAL CHEMOSENSITIVITY

Before the discovery of the peripheral chemoreceptors it was generally assumed that hypoxemia, hypercapnia and acidosis stimulated the medullary respiratory centers directly. It is now known that acute hypoxia depresses ventilation if the peripheral chemoreceptors are denervated. However, if the hypoxemia is sustained, there is a delayed increase in respiratory rate and a decrease in tidal volume which persists for some time after the hypoxemia is eliminated. The net effect of this delayed respiratory stimulation under these circumstances is an increase in total ventilation but not in alveolar ventilation. This is in contrast to the increase in alveolar ventilation which results from hypoxic stimulation of the peripheral chemoreceptors.

The respiratory effects of an increase in cH^+ on the aortic and carotid bodies are similar to those seen in response to a low P_{O_2}.

Metabolic acidosis and alkalosis stimulate and depress ventilation respectively over a range of arterial pH between 7.3 and 7.5 by a direct effect on the peripheral chemoreceptors. Below a pH of 7.3, and possibly above a pH of 7.5, it would appear that changes in cH^+ directly affect the intracranial chemoreceptors.

The hyperpnea associated with CO_2 inhalation is depressed only slightly by denervation of the aortic and carotid bodies, suggesting that the peripheral chemoreceptors contribute little to the ventilatory response to an increase in P_{CO_2}. Most of the ventilatory response to CO_2 originates from the more sensitive receptors which are located intracranially. However, if the arterial P_{CO_2} is elevated in the presence of a decreased P_{O_2}, the peripheral chemoreceptor component of the respiratory response is increased.

Since the peripheral receptors are highly perfused structures, the chemical composition of the fluid bathing the receptor cells changes abruptly whenever the composition of the blood changes. In other words, these receptors are adapted to respond to acute changes in blood composition. This is reflected in the fact that their discharge fluctuates even with normal respiration, probably as a result of oscillations of the arterial P_{O_2}, P_{CO_2} and cH^+. Conversely, the central chemosensitive areas are exposed to an environment which changes slowly because of the time required for the extracellular fluid in these areas to come into equilibrium with the blood. Thus, the ventilatory response to CO_2, as a result of stimulation of the peripheral chemoreceptors, although small, occurs within a few seconds, while the much greater central response due to stimulation of the central component of chemosensitivity may take six to ten minutes or more to be fully developed.

The central chemoreceptors have a much lower level of blood supply in relation to their metabolic rate than do the peripheral receptors. The composition of the extracellular fluid surrounding the central chemosensitive areas may therefore change markedly in response to changes in blood flow. Since carbon dioxide affects both the central receptors and the blood vessels that supply these receptors, the integrated effect of a change in CO_2 represents the resultant of these two influences. Thus, a rise in blood P_{CO_2} as a result of alveolar hypoventilation will raise the P_{CO_2} in the brain, and this will tend to stimulate an increase in ventilation. However, the increased P_{CO_2} also dilates the blood vessels in the brain so that carbon dioxide removal increases, thereby tending to lower the central P_{CO_2}. The increase in ventilation and the cerebral vasodilation which develop in response to an elevated P_{CO_2} both operate to counteract the effect of hypoventilation on the composition of the extracellular fluid in the brain.

The ventilatory response to stimulation of both central and

peripheral chemoreceptors appears to subserve the immediate regulation of cH^+ in blood and in the extracellular fluid of the brain through its effect on P_{CO_2}. Such mechanisms are necessarily imperfect, since they act only while cH^+ is abnormal. More complete but much slower compensation is brought about by changes in extracellular fluid and blood concentrations of HCO_3^-, Na^+, K^+ and H^+ resulting from active energy-dependent processes occurring in the brain and kidney. Such changes, by restoring blood and extracellular fluid cH^+ to more nearly normal values, may have the effect of "resetting" the chemoreceptors at a new level so that they may remain responsive to acute changes in P_{CO_2}.

Under ordinary circumstances, the peripheral chemoreceptors do not play a major role in the control of respiration. In contrast, impulses arising from the central chemoreceptors are sometimes essential for breathing. A reduction of arterial P_{CO_2} in anesthetized man and animals causes apnea. Also, respiratory efforts are temporarily suspended in conscious dogs when arterial CO_2 is lowered by artificial ventilation. In conscious man the results are variable, but apnea may follow voluntary hyperventilation, particularly if the peripheral chemoreceptor drive is eliminated by high levels of P_{O_2}. The stimulus for continued breathing in subjects who fail to manifest apnea presumably arises from other inputs to the respiratory center, such as those arising in the reticular activating system.

REFLEXES ARISING IN OTHER RECEPTORS

PRESSORECEPTORS

There are receptors in the adventitial coat of the aortic arch and the carotid sinus which are sensitive to alterations in the blood pressure and chiefly influence the cardiovascular system, although they also affect respiration to a lesser extent. The impulses arising from these receptors are inhibitory; a rise in the systemic blood pressure inhibits ventilation, and a fall in blood pressure leads to an increase in ventilation, presumably by reducing a pre-existing inhibitory influence. These responses are only moderate in degree, and their role in the control of respiration in man is not clear.

RECEPTORS IN MUSCLES AND JOINTS

Afferent activity from any receptor, particularly those involved in muscle activity, influences the tone or level of excitability of many, if not all, of the anterior horn cells. It would not be surprising, therefore, to find that the respiratory movements are influenced by tension and stretch receptors in the muscles and joints of the extremities, or, for that matter, anywhere in the body. The change in ventilation associated with passive movements has been attributed to some such mechanism. In addition, it is believed that receptors in the muscles, tendons and joints of the extremities reflexly contribute to the hyperpnea of exercise.

It has been suggested that "the act of breathing involves the participation of motor control mechanisms which adjust the tension developed by the inspiratory muscles so that they change in length by the amount appropriate to the tidal volume demanded, despite changes in mechanical conditions" (Campbell). The postulated neural mechanism for adjusting the tension development in the inspiratory muscles is based on an interplay between the α motorneurones which innvervate them and the γ motor system which controls the intrafusal fibers of the muscle spindles. If the shortening of the inspiratory muscle is impeded while the intrafusal muscle continues to contract, then the tension in the annulospiral receptor of the muscle spindle will rise, resulting in an increase in afferent discharge. This is relayed to the α motor neurones and results in an increase in the force of contraction of the inspiratory muscles, thereby compensating for the effect of any increase in load.

THERMORECEPTORS

Receptors sensitive to variations in blood temperature are located in the anterior hypothalamus, and others which respond to alterations in surface temperature are located in the skin. The principal thermoregulatory centers receiving impulses from these thermoreceptors are situated in the hypothalamus. These centers discharge the appropriate impulses over the somatic and visceral motor nerves to control the production and elimination of heat. It is assumed, at least in animals, that there are connections between the thermoregulatory centers and the respiratory centers. In dogs, the respiratory passages constitute a very important means of heat elimination. In these animals, stimulation of either the peripheral or the central thermoreceptors produces panting. This mechanism for temperature regulation is relatively unimportant in man, but artificial elevation of body temperature does lead to hyperventilation. During sustained fevers the pulmonary ventilation is increased by an amount which is out of proportion to the associated elevation in the metabolic rate. Since changes in cH^+ and in solubility of carbon dioxide in the body fluids are both directly affected by changes in temperature, it may be these factors which are influencing the ventilatory response associated with an increase in temperature in the human.

RESPIRATORY CHEMOSENSITIVITY IN MAN

CARBON DIOXIDE

A rise in arterial carbon dioxide tension is the most potent of all the known chemical influences on ventilation. The arterial carbon dioxide tension normally is about 40 mm. Hg, and if it is gradually raised by inhaling increasing percentages of carbon dioxide in air, the ventilation increases in a relatively linear fashion. Although the inhalation of 5 per cent carbon dioxide is readily tolerated normally, higher percentages become increasingly distressing, and the subject may become disoriented and apprehensive. In general, headache, dizziness and mental changes such as drowsiness and confusion develop at an arterial carbon dioxide tension of about 80 mm. Hg. The inhalation of about 15 per cent carbon dioxide no longer increases the ventilation, the maximal ventilation being approximately 70 to 90 l./min. This may coincide with a loss of consciousness and the onset of muscular rigidity, tremors and generalized convulsions. When 30 per cent carbon dioxide is inspired, deep anesthesia is induced. At a concentration of 40 per cent, the ventilation becomes depressed, and death may occur if this concentration is maintained for any length of time.

If the arterial P_{CO_2} drops acutely below the normal level, ventilation falls. On the other hand, if low carbon dioxide tensions are maintained for any length of time, as in a patient who is being artificially ventilated, spontaneous ventilation may not be depressed even at lower than normal levels of arterial P_{CO_2}. The adaptation to low P_{CO_2} involves a reduction in HCO_3^- concentration in the central chemosensitive areas. This restores the local H^+ concentration to normal so that these areas may discharge normally at low P_{CO_2}. If CO_2 is inhaled under these circumstances, the ventilatory response may be greater than normal. This is because any increase in P_{CO_2} in the presence of the low HCO_3^- concentration results in an exaggerated increase in cH^+ and the maintenance of a higher than normal level of ventilation. When the HCO_3^- concentration is increased to normal levels following recovery from chronic hypocapnia, the ventilatory response to CO_2 is also abnormal.

In patients with respiratory disease and chronic hypercapnia, some tolerance to the narcotic effects of carbon dioxide may develop so that mental clarity may be present at levels of arterial carbon dioxide tension which produce extreme depression in patients or experimental subjects who are acutely hypercapnic. Nevertheless, if the respiratory centers should become depressed, as in severe hypoxia, or when depressant drugs such as morphine or barbiturates have been administered, the narcotic and depressant effects of inhaled carbon dioxide may occur at a much lower concentration. In such situations, therefore, the use of carbon dioxide in an attempt to stimulate respiration may actually lead to a further depression of ventilation.

When there has been chronic carbon dioxide retention, there is an increase in the HCO_3^- concentration of the extracellular fluid in the central chemosensitive areas. This restores the local H^+ ion concentration to normal. Under these circumstances, acute changes in arterial PCO_2 may induce deleterious effects. For instance, if, in a patient with chronic carbon dioxide retention and a compensatory elevation of plasma HCO_3^-, the arterial PCO_2 is lowered rapidly by mechanical ventilation, there will be a corresponding change in PCO_2 in the central chemosensitive areas, but, because of the high HCO_3^- concentration, there will be an exaggerated fall in H^+ ion concentration and a resultant central respiratory depression. The central alkalosis may also seriously impair cerebral blood flow, for it will result in cerebral vasoconstriction and lead to or aggravate coma. Thus, as is pointed out later, restoration of the arterial PCO_2 to normal levels in patients with chronic hypercapnia should proceed slowly so that the active processes involved in reducing the HCO_3^- concentration have enough time to work.

The status of the respiratory center has been assessed clinically by measuring the ventilatory response to inhaled carbon dioxide. Thus, patients who are suffering from severe emphysema often demonstrate a lower than normal ventilatory response to the inhalation of carbon dioxide, and it is likely that chronic elevation of the arterial PCO_2 has reduced the sensitivity of the respiratory center in these patients. A similar situation is seen in normal subjects who have been exposed to an environment of 3 per cent carbon dioxide for some time. The diminished ventilatory response is probably related to an elevated buffering capacity of the blood and extracellular fluid so that a given change in PCO_2 does not produce the usual increase in cH^+ ion concentration.

Another factor which influences the ventilatory response to carbon dioxide in emphysema is the increased work of breathing. As is shown in Figure 50, the ventilatory response to carbon dioxide is improved when bronchial obstruction is reduced by the use of bronchodilating drugs in patients with emphysema. Conversely, the ventilatory response falls in normal subjects when they breathe through an artificial airway resistance. These findings indicate that the ventilatory response to carbon dioxide measures the response of the total respiratory system, not just that of the respiratory center, and that an abnormal response does not necessarily mean that the respiratory center has lost its sensitivity. The measurement that

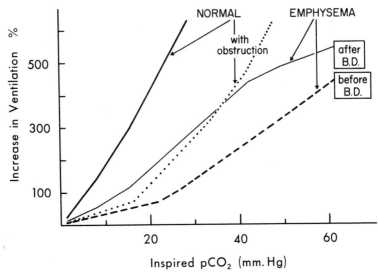

FIGURE 50.   The ventilatory response to inhaled CO_2 in normal subjects and patients with airway obstruction. The ventilatory response of the normal subject is depressed by having him breathe through an artificial airway obstruction. The patient's response is increased if airway obstruction is ameliorated by administration of a bronchodilator.

would be desirable in order to measure the sensitivity of the respiratory center is the number of impulses coming from the respiratory center, but this is obviously unobtainable. On the other hand, measurement of the response of the respiratory muscles—for example, the amount of mechanical work done during breathing—may be informative. The change in ventilatory mechanical work in response to inhaled CO_2 in normal subjects is unaltered when they breathe through an artificial airway resistance, but the change in mechanical work in response to changes in arterial P_{CO_2} in patients with emphysema and hypercapnia is lower than normal. This suggests that the sensitivity of the respiratory center may indeed be reduced in patients suffering from chronic carbon dioxide retention.

ACIDITY

The adaptation to a metabolic acidosis or an alkalosis is similar to that seen with changes in P_{CO_2}. An acute metabolic acidemia stimulates the aortic and carotid chemoreceptors and leads to an increase in ventilation and, as a result, a decrease in the arterial and brain extracellular fluid P_{CO_2}. This lowers the brain cH^+, thereby diminishing the central drive to ventilation and offsetting the full effect of the peripheral chemoreceptors. After about 24 hours, the brain cH^+ is restored to normal by a proportionate reduction in HCO_3^-. When this has taken place, ventilation is increased above normal because slight increases in PCO_2 will be associated with greater than normal changes in cH^+. If, at this stage, the blood HCO_3^- is rapidly restored to normal, the ventilation still remains elevated, because any decrease in ventilation would result in a rise in arterial and brain PCO_2 and a resultant increase in brain cH^+. This sequence of events would explain the frequently reported observation of continued hyperventilation after acute correction of diabetic or renal acidosis. Return to normal breathing depends on the restoration of brain cH^+ to normal by active transport mechanisms. Converse changes are seen with metabolic alkalosis, such as occurs with excessive vomiting.

HYPOXIA

If an exceedingly brief period of hypoxia is induced by the inhalation of two breaths of a hypoxic gas mixture, the ventilation is increased as soon as the oxygen tension falls below 90 mm. Hg. On the other hand, marked respiratory stimulation in healthy persons as a result of exposure to longer periods of hypoxia is the exception rather than the rule. There is only a mild increase in ventilation with decreasing inspired oxygen concentration until the concentration of oxygen has been reduced to about 14 per cent, after which further reductions are associated with more marked respiratory stimulation. This is equivalent to an altitude of 10,000 feet or an arterial PO_2 of approximately 60 mm. Hg. During the inhalation of 10 per cent oxygen, which lowers the arterial PO_2 to approximately 40 mm. Hg, respiration is increased by about 17 per cent. The maximal response, a ventilation of about 40 l./min., occurs during the inhalation of 4 per cent oxygen, but hypoxia of this severity can be tolerated for only a few minutes, and even then, only at the risk of acute circulatory failure, unconsciousness and convulsions.

The difference in the responses between the exceedingly brief and the "steady state" periods of hypoxia is probably due to the compensatory mechanisms which take place in the latter situation. In the steady state the initial hyperventilation is not accompanied by a corresponding increase in metabolism. The carbon dioxide tension falls in both the arterial blood and the central chemosensitive areas, resulting in a decrease in cH^+, which reflexly inhibits the respiratory center and opposes the stimulation induced by the hypoxia. On the other hand, it has been shown that if the carbon dioxide tension is kept normal or elevated, experimentally induced hypoxia leads to a marked increase in ventilation. This suggests that as long as the respiratory center is not inhibited by hypocapnia or alkalosis hypoxia is indeed a powerful stimulus to respiration.

When man ascends to high altitude, the arterial oxygen tension falls so that there is stimulation of the carotid and aortic chemoreceptors. This causes hyperventilation and a decrease in arterial and brain P_{CO_2} and in cH^+. The alkaline shift in central cH^+ diminishes the normal stimulus originating from the central chemoreceptors and partially offsets the effect of impulses originating from the peripheral chemoreceptors. After a few days at altitude, the central cH^+ becomes restored to normal, and the level of ventilation, which is now the resultant of an increased peripheral chemoreceptor activity and a normal central chemoreceptor activity, is increased. When fully adapted to altitude both the blood and the central cH^+ are normal so that the hyperventilation induced by the low P_{O_2} is unopposed by alkalosis of either the blood or the brain. This explains why chronic hypoxemia is a more potent stimulus to breathing than acute hypoxemia.

Termination of the hypoxia by returning to sea level fails to restore breathing to normal immediately. The inhalation of air at sea level removes the hypoxic stimulus to breathing so that ventilation decreases. This results in a rise in P_{CO_2} and causes an acid shift in central cH^+, which stimulates the central chemoreceptors so that ventilation is prevented from falling to normal. To compensate for the elevated P_{CO_2} the central HCO_3^- rises over a period of days (presumably by active transport mechanism) so that the cH^+, and hence ventilation, are restored to normal.

Persons born at high altitude have a diminished ventilatory drive in response to acute hypoxia which is not corrected by subsequent residence at sea level. Conversely, those who are born at sea level but later live at an altitude for prolonged periods have an intact response to acute hypoxia. These observations suggest that the acute hypoxic response is irreversibly determined early in life, but the mechanism by which this comes about is unknown.

If respiratory disease is severe, hypoxia may become an important stimulus to respiration. In these patients hypercapnia is associated with the hypoxia when the alveolar ventilation becomes inadequate in relation to the carbon dioxide production. As has been pointed out above, if the hypercapnia is severe and has been present for some time, the sensitivity of the medullary respiratory centers to P_{CO_2} may be altered, a situation which is also encountered in morphine or barbiturate intoxication. Whenever the sensitivity of the respiratory centers is diminished, the peripheral chemoreceptors may become the principal regulators of the respiratory drive, and hypoxia the primary stimulus.

RELATIONSHIP BETWEEN THE WORK AND PATTERN OF BREATHING

As described in Chapter 1, it has been postulated that the respiratory rate and depth are adjusted to the level at which the least amount of work or force will bring about the body's required alveolar ventilation. Formulae predicting the optimum respiratory frequency at a particular alveolar ventilation have been presented, and these indicate that the respiratory rate which is chosen is dependent upon the mechanical time constant of the respiratory system (i.e., the product of the compliance and the airflow resistance).

These optimum respiratory frequencies have the following basis: in order to produce a particular minute alveolar ventilation at low respiratory frequencies, large tidal volumes are necessary. However, a large tidal volume is disadvantageous because the elastic work increases as the square of the tidal volume so that the muscle force needed to overcome the elastic recoil of the lungs and the thorax is correspondingly large. To produce the same alveolar ventilation at high respiratory frequencies, dead space ventilation, and hence total ventilation, must be increased if the alveolar ventilation is to be maintained. The increased rates of airflow necessitate increased muscle force and rate of work in overcoming the flow resistance of the respiratory system. Figure 27 illustrates that the optimum frequencies fall between these two extremes.

If the mechanical impedance is increased, the respiratory muscles must overcome an additional load. An increase in elastic resistance (i.e., a reduction in compliance) and an increase in flow resistance both increase the mechanical impedance, but they have mutually opposing effects on the mechanical time constant. According to these prediction equations, the respiratory frequency should increase when the compliance is reduced and decrease when the flow resistance is increased. Indeed, it has been demonstrated that the respiratory frequency increases (and the tidal volume falls) when an external elastic resistance is added to normal subjects (Fig. 27, *B*) and that the respiratory rate falls (and the tidal volume increases) when normal subjects are obliged to breathe through an artificial resistance (Fig. 27, *C*).

Obviously, the errors involved in applying these formulae to patients with respiratory disease may be very great, for a sine wave pattern of inspiration is assumed, and the respiratory flow actually approximates a square wave in patients with bronchial obstruction. In addition, expiration is assumed to be passive in the equations, and this is seldom the case in respiratory disease. Thirdly, in a patient with respiratory disease, chemical stimuli such as PO_2, PCO_2 and pH play a large part in the control of the respiratory rate and depth.

Nevertheless, the altered respiratory patterns encountered in patients with pulmonary disease often conform with these principles. In patients with respiratory disease in whom the elastic resistance is increased one would expect the respirations to be rapid and shallow, and this is indeed what is observed. For example, in obese subjects or in patients with kyphoscoliosis in whom the compliance of the "chest wall" is low, the respiratory rate is increased and the tidal volume reduced.

In patients with bronchial obstruction, in whom the nonelastic resistance is increased, one would expect the respirations to be slow and deep. Thus, patients with chronic bronchitis and emphysema in whom the resistance to airflow is great and the compliance of the lungs essentially normal would be expected to breathe slowly and deeply. However, this is rarely the case, and these patients usually breathe rapidly and shallowly. It has been postulated that this is because these persons are breathing at a high lung volume, i.e., at the flat part of the pressure-volume curve of the lungs and chest wall, and that the resultant high elastic resistance is an important determinant of the respiratory pattern.

THE REGULATION OF VENTILATION IN RESPIRATORY DISEASE

When respiratory function is impaired, the minute ventilation may be elevated because of stimulation of either the central or peripheral chemoreceptors by abnormal blood gas tensions or other receptors in the lungs. However, it would appear that whenever the work of breathing or the effort required to do this work is increased, the activity of the respiratory centers may be modified and ventilation may be limited. This can be illustrated by healthy subjects whose ventilation is decreased when they breathe through an artificial airway obstruction. It has been suggested that the body tolerates the resultant hypercapnia instead of expending the effort that would be required to keep the arterial P_{CO_2} at a normal level. This may actually be beneficial, for it has been pointed out that a further increase in ventilation in an attempt to lower the arterial P_{CO_2} would require so much oxygen that little would be available for nonventilatory muscular work. Nevertheless, these considerations suggest that hypercapnia is not as effective a stimulus to respiration when the work of breathing is increased as when it is normal.

Aside from laboratory experimentation, it is unusual to find only a single chemical stimulus altered in patients with respiratory disease. Table 4 demonstrates that when the ventilation changes in

TABLE 4

THE ALTERATIONS IN CHEMICAL AGENTS
DURING VARIOUS CONDITIONS

CONDITION	ARTERIAL pH	ARTERIAL P_{CO_2}	ARTERIAL P_{O_2}
Inhalation of 5 per cent CO_2 in oxygen	↓	↑	↑
Inhalation of 10 per cent O_2 in nitrogen	↑	↓	↓
Voluntary hyperventilation	↑	↓	↑
Acute alveolar hypoventilation	↓	↑	↓

response to a stimulus, other respiratory stimuli are also affected, and each makes a contribution to the total respiratory response. On occasion, the major chemical agents may work together in stimulating ventilation; in other situations, some may excite and others may inhibit the respiratory centers. For instance, as has been described earlier, the stimulant effect of hypoxia may be counteracted by the depressant effect of the hypocapnia and alkalemia which develop secondarily because of the hyperventilation.

In patients with right-to-left shunts or in such conditions as pulmonary consolidation, atelectasis, congestion or fibrosis, in which there are areas with low ventilation-perfusion ratios the ventilation increases because of stimulation of the peripheral chemoreceptors in the carotid and aortic bodies. As a result of the increased ventilation, the patient may have persistent hypocapnia as well as alkalemia, both of which would tend to depress the ventilatory response to hypoxia.

PERIODIC BREATHING

Breathing is ordinarily regular. It may become irregular under conditions in which there are rapid changes in the neural drives to respiration or interference with the feedback of information from the respiratory apparatus to the "respiratory centers."

Variations in the pattern of breathing may be induced experimentally. For instance, this may occur when a subject breathes through a long dead space. The rebreathing of carbon dioxide, which accumulates in the dead space, stimulates ventilation. As a result of this increased ventilation, carbon dioxide is washed out of the dead space so that the inspired gas contains less CO_2 and now ventilation decreases. This decrease is followed by reaccumulation of CO_2 in the dead space, and once again ventilation is increased. The "hunting" process continues until the subject comes into equilibrium with the expired carbon dioxide in the dead space and has reached a "steady state." This irregular pattern of breathing is particularly evident if the subject breathes room air through the dead space. If oxygen is inhaled through the dead space, the oscillations in breathing pattern are reduced.

Alternate waxing and waning of ventilation is also produced if the circulation time to the brain is increased by lengthening the distance through which blood travels on its way to the brain from the heart. Under these conditions changes in blood gas tensions are sensed by the central chemoreceptors only after a delay. As a result, the ventilatory response lags behind the changes in arterial blood gas tensions. Thus, any tendency for CO_2 to increase will not be sensed immediately, and the PCO_2 will rise to high levels. This will lead to an increase in ventilation and a subsequent lowering of PCO_2. Because of the delay, the low PCO_2 is not detected immediately so that ventilation continues at a high level and PCO_2 continues to fall. When the blood with the very low PCO_2 finally reaches the chemoreceptors, ventilation may cease. Once again PCO_2 begins to rise, but again this is not immediately sensed, and ventilation remains depressed, allowing the PCO_2 to rise to high levels. This cyclic change in gas tensions and ventilation therefore continues to be perpetuated.

The commonest form of periodic breathing encountered clinically is known as Cheyne-Stokes respiration. As is illustrated in Figure 51, this is a series of respirations which wax and wane, each sequence of breaths being interrupted by a period of apnea. It is encountered clinically in patients with congestive heart failure, presumably because of the increased circulation time to the brain. This breathing pattern is also seen in patients who have cerebral damage due to trauma or disease or in whom the cerebrospinal fluid

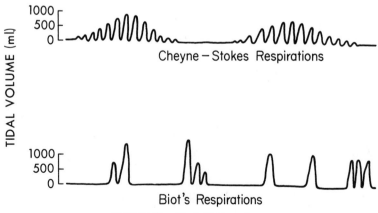

FIGURE 51.   Periodic breathing.

pressure is increased. Although the presence of this type of breathing is considered to be an ominous sign, it need not be, for it can be reversed, particularly if it is caused by congestive heart failure. In such patients, the administration of oxygen frequently abolishes the periodic breathing.

Another type of periodic breathing, known as Biot's respiration, which is also shown in Figure 51, is most frequently associated with brain damage. There may be one or more respiratory efforts of varying depth with prolonged unequal pauses in between sequences of breaths.

In view of the many interrelated factors which affect respiration and their variability, one wonders how regular breathing ever occurs. Nevertheless, periodic breathing in which the respiratory pattern is markedly irregular occurs in only a small number of clinical conditions. Irregular respirations also occur occasionally in healthy persons residing at high altitude or even at sea level during light sleep. In addition, when healthy infants are born after less than 37 weeks of gestation they frequently exhibit periodic respirations. This is not seen very often in infants after 38 weeks of gestation.

Chapter 5

Respiration Under Stress

EXERCISE AND ALTITUDE

In noting the title and first heading of this chapter, two questions may occur to the reader: What relationship does the physiology of respiration under stress have to the patient with respiratory disease? Why are exercise and altitude considered together?

There are two main answers to the first question. First, most patients with respiratory disease complain, to some extent, of limited exercise tolerance and frequently only experience symptoms on effort. Second, abnormalities in cardiorespiratory function may be undetected at rest but manifest themselves during exercise.

The answer to the second question becomes apparent when one reviews the relationships indicated in Figure 1 in the introduction of this book; this figure delineates the oxygen transport system. It is clear that both exercise and altitude constitute challenges to the oxygen transport system, in that both would be associated with a fall in tissue oxygenation in the absence of homeostatic responses. A second reason for linking exercise and altitude is that the limitations to a man's existence at an altitude include both his ability to withstand hypoxia as well as his ability to work and move about.

THE NORMAL RESPONSE TO EXERCISE

Exercise may be classified in various ways, but the two most important factors determining a person's response to work are the type of exercise being performed (i.e., large muscle groups vs. small muscle groups or weight bearing vs. movement) and the duration of the exercise. The type of exercise which will be discussed in this chapter is that which employs large muscle groups and movement, such as those involved in running, cycling and swimming.

The cardiorespiratory responses to exercise in a normal subject pedaling on a cycle ergometer for 10 minutes at each of several in-

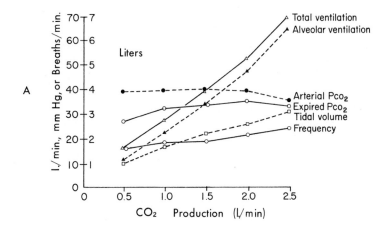

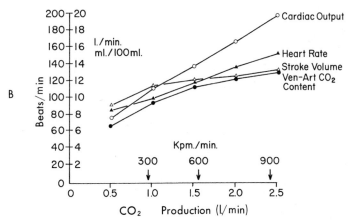

FIGURE 52. Changes in cardiorespiratory variables during exercise at three intensities on a cycle ergometer. Average values for respiratory parameters (*A*) and cardiovascular parameters (*B*) are shown. (From Campbell, E. J. M.: Exercise Tolerance. The Scientific Basis of Medicine Annual Reviews. University of London, The Athlone Press, 1967. By permission.)

tensities of exercise are shown in Figure 52, *A* and *B*. The ventilation is increased in proportion to the intensity of the work as a result of an increase in both frequency and tidal volume. The ratio of ventilation to O_2 consumption (ventilatory equivalent for O_2; ventilation coefficient) increases during particularly heavy work when a steady state cannot be maintained. At this stage, further increases in work intensity are associated with a smaller increase in O_2 consumption than occurs in light work, lactic acid accumulates in the blood, and any further increase in ventilation is mainly due to an accelerated rate of breathing.

THE HYPERPNEA OF EXERCISE

The hyperpnea of muscular exercise is associated with changes in many variables which may act as stimuli to breathing, and it is the interaction of these influences which is believed by many to account for the ventilatory response. The factors that are involved are neurogenic, proprioceptive, chemical and thermal.

The neurogenic factors which may be involved in the hyperpnea of exercise include proprioceptive influences from the limbs and impulses from higher brain centers. By studying the changes in ventilation which occur immediately on starting or at the cessation of exercise before there is time for changes in chemical stimuli to occur, the influence of nonchemical and presumably neural factors can be assessed. Such studies indicate that as much as 40 per cent of the total drive to ventilation during exercise can be related to movement-related factors. However, the interpretation of the ventilatory transients at the beginning or end of exercise is complicated by "learned" responses. Such transients may thus be influenced by cortical factors as well as by reflexes arising in the periphery.

The main chemical stimulus to ventilation during exercise is thought to be related to cH^+. Although the changes in cH^+ during moderate exercise may be relatively small, they are positively correlated with changes in ventilation. The cH^+ and ventilation are even more closely correlated during the more pronounced anaerobic metabolic acidosis of heavy exercise. These findings suggest that the hyperpnea of muscular exercise is in part due to acid-base changes, but the major locus of action of the cH^+ during exercise has yet to be established.

The role of hypoxia in the hyperpnea of exercise is difficult to establish. In healthy persons the arterial P_{O_2} is normal during exercise. It has been shown that a single breath of oxygen during exercise is sufficient to produce, within a few seconds, a 10 to 15 per cent decrease in ventilation. Although the arterial P_{O_2} is normal during exercise, this fall in ventilation following the inhalation of oxygen has nevertheless been attributed to a lessening in peripheral chemoreceptor drive. It has been suggested that the changes in cH^+ which occur during exercise increase the sensitivity of the peripheral chemoreceptors so that even normal levels of P_{O_2} are associated with an increased impulse traffic.

The influence of P_{CO_2} on ventilation during exercise is difficult to assess, since it is often normal or decreased rather than increased. It has been proposed that the P_{CO_2} may act as a fine controller of the ventilatory drive during exercise, in that when other ventilatory drives are excessive with respect to metabolic CO_2 production, the resultant low P_{CO_2} acts centrally to check the excessive ventilation.

When other drives result in a level of ventilation which is inadequate with respect to CO_2 production, the increased P_{CO_2} provides a further stimulus to ventilation.

The body temperature rises as much as $2°$ C. or more during exercise, and such a change is known to stimulate ventilation at rest. However, if one assumed the same degree of response to temperature during exercise, it would still only account for 10 to 15 per cent of the total ventilation response.

If the response to the above stimuli at rest can be extrapolated to the condition of exercise, then it would appear that the level of ventilation achieved during steady state exercise can be almost entirely accounted for by an increase in blood cH^+, by muscle movement and by the change in body temperature. The residual portion still unaccounted for may be due to the inappropriateness of such an extrapolation or to other factors which are as yet not perfectly understood.

THE CIRCULATORY RESPONSE TO EXERCISE

The circulatory response to exercise serves to provide an increased supply of oxygen to the working muscles, to remove CO_2 and acid metabolites from them and to dissipate heat. The response involves an increase in cardiac output, vascular dilatation in the working muscles, and diversion of blood flow away from the nonworking areas.

The increase in cardiac output which occurs during exercise in the erect posture is the result of both an increase in stroke volume and in heart rate. At the start of exercise the stroke volume is increased because of a shift of blood from the periphery into the thorax and an increased diastolic filling of the heart. Once exercise has begun, the stroke volume rises further with increasing work intensity because of an increase in systolic emptying that occurs as a result of an adrenergically mediated increased force of contraction, and there is a decrease in peripheral resistance. The acceleration of the heart rate at the start of exercise is vary rapid. It is associated with a decrease in the duration of diastole and has been attributed to release of vagal inhibition. With continued exercise of a given intensity the heart rate increases more slowly to a higher steady state level. This secondary increase in heart rate has been attributed to adrenergic influences; probably of a reflex nature, since at the cessation of exercise the heart rate decreases abruptly. Proprioceptor, chemoreceptor and baroreceptor reflexes may all be involved. The heart rate increases almost linearly with work intensity and reaches a maximum of 200 beats per minute in youth. This maximum declines with advancing age to values of about 160 in the seventh decade of life.

The diversion of blood flow from nonworking areas occurs because there is vasoconstriction in the splanchnic vascular beds and a fall in the vascular resistance of the working muscles. The fall in resistance occurs because of both arteriolar dilatation and a hundredfold increase in the number of open capillaries. The arteriolar dilatation occurs almost immediately when exercise begins, suggesting that a reflex inhibition of vasomotor tone may be involved. As work continues, the accumulation of vasodilator metabolites and the increased temperature also contribute to the decrease in vasomotor tone. The vasomotor responses to exercise are influenced considerably by the environmental temperature. As core temperature increases during exercise, cutaneous vasodilation occurs because of hypothalamically mediated decreases in vasomotor tone. In hot environments, the cutaneous blood flow is increased at the expense of flow to the working muscles so that work capacity is consequently reduced.

THE METABOLIC RESPONSE TO EXERCISE

The metabolic response to an exercise lasting more than a few minutes is characterized by an increased utilization of both fat and carbohydrate. With prolonged exercise in a fasting person, the ventilatory exchange ratio (R) declines toward 0.7, and plasma free fatty acid and glycerol concentrations increase, suggesting that fat mobilization and utilization are the main mechanisms for providing energy. In the presence of anaerobic metabolism, the R value rises, often to values greater than 1.0. This high ventilatory exchange ratio does not reflect the tissue respiratory quotient but rather the fact that as the lactic acid concentration increases in the blood, the amount of carbon dioxide eliminated from the lungs increases because the CO_2 released from the bicarbonate stores is eliminated together with the carbon dioxide produced by tissue metabolism. A rise in R to high levels during exercise can be used as an indirect measure of the degree of metabolic acidosis present and, by extension, as a measure of the presence of anaerobic metabolism.

For most of the activities which are undertaken in ordinary daily life the exercise period often lasts for only a few seconds or a few minutes. During such short periods, the respiratory, circulatory and metabolic changes occur very rapidly, and a steady state is not achieved. It has been clearly established that the ability to perform short bursts of exercise does not depend on the immediate ability of the circulatory and respiratory system to meet the oxygen requirements of the tissues, but rather on the ability to meet the energy costs during the recovery phase. For brief periods of exercise we "exercise now and pay later." As Campbell said: "Patients base their estimate of exercise tolerance on their experience of the difficulty they have in paying later; and they learn not to exercise too hard because the bill, when it comes, is more than they can comfortably pay."

The bill which must be paid has classically been measured in terms of that amount of oxygen consumed after the cessation of exercise which is in excess of the resting oxygen consumption. The excess oxygen consumed during recovery was termed the "oxygen debt" by A. V. Hill. The energy formed by this extra oxidation during recovery is used, in part, to replenish the high energy stores within the muscles and, in addition, to remove substances, chiefly lactic acid, which are formed in the anaerobic pathways of energy metabolism. These two energy requirements have been referred to as the alactacid and the lactacid components of the energy debt. The anaerobic mechanisms of energy release serve two functions. During maximal work they permit energy to be expended in excess of the person's ability to perform aerobic metabolism. In work of any intensity, the anaerobic reactions permit a rapid initial release of energy before oxygen utilization can proceed at the required rate. The abilities to sustain aerobic and anaerobic exercise are linked.

EXERCISE TOLERANCE AND PHYSICAL FITNESS

The ability to perform exercise depends on factors which are related to motivation as well as to the functional capacities of the oxygen transport system. In general, it is neither realistic nor useful to determine the absolute maximum amount of work that can be generated by the organism. Instead, it has been found that the aerobic working capacity (i.e., the work intensity at which the oxygen consumption reaches its maximum) is a useful determination. This measurement, which is readily determined, correlates well with the sense of well being. In addition, an increase in maximum oxygen consumption is associated with an increase in fitness resulting from training. The relationship between aerobic working capacity and the response to a submaximal exercise is not a linear one in the sense that untrained subjects cannot perform at more than 50 per cent of their maximal oxygen uptake when working continuously for an hour, whereas highly trained subjects are able to maintain a work intensity requiring 80 to 90 per cent of the maximum oxygen consumption.

The factors which force normal subjects to stop exercising during maximum effort are extremely difficult to evaluate. The subjective accounts of the "reasons" for stopping vary somewhat from one person to another for the same exercise and between different types of exercise. The physiological event which leads to the breaking point in maximal work lasting a few minutes is an inadequate supply of oxygen to the working muscles. This is not due to an inadequate level of ventilation or oxygen diffusing capacity, since alveolar Po_2 and Pco_2 and the alveolar-arterial Po_2 difference are normal. Instead, it is circulatory factors, related partly to the amount of blood flow coming to the working muscles and partly to the ability of the working muscles and their vascular beds to transfer oxygen, which normally limit exercise tolerance.

EXERCISE IN PATIENTS WITH RESPIRATORY DISEASE

It is obvious that respiratory disease may impair exercise tolerance by a variety of mechanisms. In patients with severe disturbances in gas exchange, the impairment may result because of an inadequate oxygenation of the blood or because an excessive proportion of the oxygen consumption is expended in overcoming the resistances to ventilation. Limitation of the ventilatory response to exercise in relation to the rates of CO_2 production and oxygen consumption is reflected in an increased alveolar and arterial Pco_2 and a decreased alveolar and arterial Po_2. Severe mismatching of ventilation and perfusion or a failure of the diffusing capacity for oxygen to increase in proportion to the oxygen consumption during the exercise results in an increase of the alveolar-arterial oxygen tension difference. In patients with cor pulmonale the oxygen transport may also be impaired because of a restricted cardiac output, and this will be reflected in a lower than normal mixed venous oxygen content. The application of exercise tests to the assessment of patients with respiratory disease is considered further in Chapter 7.

While ventilatory impairment clearly limits exercise ability, limitation of exercise tolerance because of this factor is relatively uncommon compared to the more frequently encountered limitation due to invalidism or physical unfitness. Despite marked disturbances in respiratory function, considerable improvement in exercise tolerance may be achieved when such patients undertake a program of exercise training. The training effect is often not due to improved ventilatory function but rather to improved circulatory function — in particular, to an increase in the proportion of the cardiac output which is being diverted to the working muscles.

THE NORMAL RESPONSE TO LIFE AT ALTITUDE

The response to altitude is, in essence, the response to hypoxia. This has already been considered, in part, in Chapter 4. The respiratory adaptations to altitude include hypoxic stimulation of chemo-reflexes, which is sustained, and an initial decrease in blood and central cH^+ due to hypocapnia, which is gradually offset by active processes which lower the bicarbonate concentrations. Although the ventilatory response to altitude hypoxia is the major adaptation of the respiratory system, it has also been observed that the residual volume, functional residual capacity and vital capacity are increased in natives at high altitude. The increased gas reservoir in the lungs is advantageous in that short periods of breath-holding or hypoven-tilation will not result in as great a drop in alveolar PO_2 as might occur with small lung volumes. The diffusing capacity for oxygen is also said to be increased in those who have become acclimatized to alti-tude, and this may be important in their performance of exercise.

In acutely acclimatized persons, the hemoglobin dissociation curves are normal when the acid-base changes are taken into account; whereas in natives at altitude, the dissociation curve is shifted to the right, indicating a diminished affinity for oxygen. Nevertheless, the increase in circulating hemoglobin due to the hypoxic stimula-tion of erythropoiesis results in an arterial oxygen content which may be near values found at sea level, even though the arterial PO_2 is reduced. In addition, the transfer of oxygen to the tissues occurs along the steep portion of the hemoglobin dissociation curves. These two facts mean that the required amount of oxygen can be unloaded to the tissues at altitude without leading to a decrease in capillary PO_2 which is so great that the oxidative potential of the tissue is im-paired.

In contrast to the respiratory responses which persist, circula-tory adaptations in the oxygen transport system, such as tachycardia and increased cardiac output, are transient. The ventilation and oxygen consumption are linearly related to work intensity during exercise at altitude. At 20,500 ft., on Mt. Everest, where the inspired PO_2 of 73 mm. Hg is about half that at sea level, the maximum oxygen consumption of climbers was about half of the maximum value at sea level. Both the maximum voluntary ventilation and the maximum ventilation achieved during exercise were increased by about 30 per cent at this altitude, presumably because of the reduced density of the atmospheric air.

ARTIFICIAL ATMOSPHERES

The effects of exposure to excessive concentrations of carbon dioxide and carbon monoxide have been considered previously. These gases may accumulate in closed system environments, and the nature of their toxicity has been well established. As man's range of activities has broadened to encompass aerospace and undersea environments, knowledge of the effects of excessive pressures of oxygen and inert gases have permitted him to create suitable artificial atmospheres to meet the demands of these environments.

HYPEROXIA

Excessive pressures of oxygen may result in deranged function in two general ways: by replacement of the inert gas, nitrogen; and by direct chemical toxicity. Because of nitrogen, the gas volume reservoir in the lungs and other gas-containing spaces in the body is maintained. When communication with the external environment is blocked, absorption of oxygen and carbon dioxide occurs rapidly, but nitrogen is absorbed slowly because it is poorly soluble in body fluids. If the oxygen concentration of the inspired gas is increased at the expense of nitrogen, the development of airway obstruction can lead to rapid collapse of the lung.

The direct chemical toxicity of oxygen is manifested mainly in the lungs and the central nervous system. The pulmonary effects include bronchial irritation, cough and a fall in vital capacity after 24 hours of exposure to 80 per cent oxygen. Higher concentrations and longer exposures may lead to bronchopneumonia, pleural effusion and impairment in the mechanical properties of the lung and gas exchange.

Pressures of oxygen in excess of 2 atmospheres produce CNS toxicity. This places a depth of 30 feet as the practical limit for the use of pure oxygen in diving. If a gas mixture containing 10 per cent oxygen in helium is inhaled rather than pure oxygen, the equivalent depth limit is increased to 600 feet. The manifestations of CNS toxicity are neuromuscular irritability progressing to generalized convulsions. The appearance and severity of CNS effects depend on the oxygen pressure, the duration of exposure and the activity of the subject. The CNS effects are aggravated by increased CO_2 concentrations.

Hyperoxia also leads to contraction of the visual fields in adults, but the most serious ophthalmic effects occur in premature infants who develop severe vascular changes leading to blindness if they are given high concentrations of oxygen to breathe. The use and abuse of increased pressures of oxygen in the treatment of anoxic states is considered in more detail later.

INERT GASES

In the case of inert gases, the effects of excessive pressures are both direct and indirect. The direct effects are those which mainly involve the excitable tissues, narcosis being the most dramatic manifestation in humans. The threshold for narcosis decreases with increasing molecular weight, being lowest for radon, highest for helium and intermediate for nitrogen.

The indirect effects of inert gases are those related to rapid decompression of the body; they may occur following compression of divers, caisson workers and subjects in pressure chambers. When compression occurs with a person breathing a gas mixture containing an inert gas such as nitrogen, the partial pressure of nitrogen increases and additional nitrogen becomes dissolved in body fluids. If decompression occurs rapidly nitrogen may come out of solution to form bubbles of gas in the tissues and in small vessels where they may obstruct blood flow. The symptoms produced are called *decompression sickness,* or *"bends,"* and include joint pains, paralysis, sensory loss, paraplegia and dyspnea. The symptom pattern depends on the sites at which the bubbles are formed or trapped.

Chapter 6

Special Aspects Related to the Newborn Infant

The dramatic events at the time of birth continue to intrigue the physician as well as the layman. Within a few moments, the lung must replace the placenta as the organ of gas exchange, and thereafter it must continue to function efficiently for many decades. This sudden adaptation to extrauterine life also requires rapid circulatory adjustments. In order to understand this vital event a knowledge of some aspects of lung development is necessary.

THE FETAL LUNG

By the sixteenth week of gestation, the bronchial tree has 20 generations of branches. Thereafter, the respiratory bronchioles and the alveolar ducts continue to increase in number until adulthood when there are 23 generations of airway branching. In contrast to the early development of airways, alveoli do not begin to form until the fetus is about 24 weeks old. Initially the alveoli are lined by cuboidal epithelium, but as term approaches (40 weeks), the epithelium becomes flattened. The pulmonary capillary network develops from the pulmonary mesenchyme at 20 weeks and by 28 weeks has proliferated in proximity to the developing airway. The fetus is not viable before the twenty-eighth week of gestation because the pulmonary bed is unable to accommodate the entire cardiac output, and the pulmonary capillaries are separated from alveoli by mesenchymal tissue so that adequate pulmonary gas exchange is not possible.

The internal surface of the airways is lined by cells at all phases of lung development. Ciliated cells, goblet cells and brush cells are found in the trachea and bronchi by the fifteenth week of gestation. Ciliated cells are also found in the bronchioles, but the goblet cells are replaced by columnar cells with small apical secretory droplets. The lining cells of the most terminal air spaces are particularly specific to the lung and are the last to appear in lung development. Two types of alveolar cells are present—the Type I cell has a thin attenuated cytoplasm, and the Type II cell has a bulky cytoplasm containing many mitochondria, osmophilic inclusions and other organelles. The appearance of surfactant is coincident with the proliferation of Type II cells, which is evidence in favor of the idea that the Type II cell is responsible for surfactant production.

The fetal lung is not in a collapsed state in utero but instead is distended with a volume of liquid which is nearly equal to the FRC of the lung in the newborn infant. The liquid originates in the lung itself and represents an ultrafiltrate of plasma with a protein content of 0.3 gm./100 ml. There is evidence that active sodium transport occurs, and it has been suggested that the lung liquid may be formed against a considerable osmotic gradient. At one time it was thought that intrauterine respiratory movements were necessary for normal lung development and that the liquid within the lung represented aspirated amniotic fluid. This is now known not to be true, since it has been demonstrated that the fetal lung will develop normally and become distended with liquid despite ligation of the trachea in utero. Although it is known that the fetus will gasp occasionally and inhale some amniotic fluid, a rhythmic respiratory pattern is not established before birth.

PULMONARY VASCULAR RESISTANCE IN THE FETAL LUNG

The mean pressure in the pulmonary artery of the fetus is a few millimeters of mercury above the aortic pressure (about 60 mm. Hg) so that the blood flows from right to left through the ductus arteriosus. The pulmonary vascular resistance in the fetal lung is high for several reasons. The vessels in the lung, which is at a relatively low volume, are tortuous and kinked; the smooth muscle mass in the pulmonary arterioles is relatively large, and there is tonic pulmonary vasoconstriction in response to the low Po_2 (30 mm. Hg) of the intrauterine environment; the presence of pulmonary fluid in the fetal lung exerts a pressure of about 10 cm. H_2O.

PERINATAL CIRCULATION

Before birth the placenta acts as the respiratory, digestive and renal organ of the fetus. The fetal circulation is adapted to serve these functions of the placenta, and when the fetus and placenta

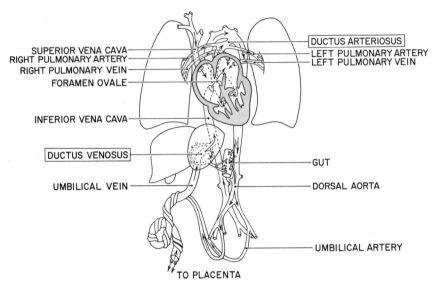

FIGURE 53.   The fetal circulation. Note the extracardiac channels through which blood is shunted. (From Avery, M. E.: The Lung and Its Disorders in the Newborn Infant, 2nd ed. W. B. Saunders Co., Philadelphia, 1964, p. 32. By permission.)

are separated at birth, rapid and dramatic circulatory changes must occur in order that adequate gas exchange can proceed in the lungs.

Figure 53 illustrates that there are two important extracardiac channels through which blood is shunted in the fetus. The first is the ductus venosus through which oxygenated blood from the placenta bypasses the portal system and enters the inferior vena cava. About 50 per cent of the inferior vena caval flow is diverted through the foramen ovale to the left side of the heart. There it mixes with the small proportion of the cardiac output which passes through the lungs. This blood, which has a relatively high oxygen content, perfuses the brain. The second extracardiac shunt is the ductus arteriosus. Through this channel, poorly oxygenated blood which is pumped out of the right ventricle (a mixture of the inferior and superior vena caval return to the heart) bypasses the lungs and enters the descending aorta. The umbilical arteries therefore deliver poorly oxygenated, hypercapnic blood to the placenta.

Because the right and left sides of the heart both contribute blood to the systemic circulation, the measurement of separate ventricular output has little meaning in the fetus. Cardiac output is therefore expressed as the combined right and left ventricular outputs and is approximately 300 ml./kg. The distribution of the combined ventricular output is related to the relative distribution of vascular resistance in the various beds.

*RESPONSE OF FETAL AND NEONATAL
PULMONARY CIRCULATION TO GASES
AND DRUGS*

The fetal and neonatal pulmonary circulation appears to be exquisitely sensitive to vasoconstrictor agents such as hypoxemia, acidosis, epinephrine, norepinephrine and serotonin. These agents produce a prompt and marked increase in pulmonary vascular resistance. The response to vasodilator agents depends on the level of the pulmonary vascular resistance. In the fetal lung, with its high pulmonary vascular resistance, acetylcholine, histamine, isoproterenol and bradykinin produce a marked fall in pulmonary vascular resistance, but in neonatal animals with a low pulmonary vascular resistance these agents have little effect. The qualitative responses are similar in the fetal, neonatal and adult pulmonary circulations, but the quantitative effects of vasoactive stimuli differs in the three groups.

THE INITIATION OF RESPIRATION AT BIRTH

In utero, the fetus exists in an environment which isolates it from tactile, thermal, visual and other stimuli. At birth the newborn infant is suddenly bombarded by the sensory stimuli of a new environment. In addition, the process of birth produces impairment of placental gas exchange, with resultant fetal hypoxemia and hypercapnia, which stimulate both central and peripheral chemoreceptors. It is the combination of these chemical and nonchemical stimuli which result in the initiation of respiration within moments of birth.

The initial inflation of the lung may be aided by Head's paradoxical reflex, or "gasp reflex," which is mediated by the vagus nerve (see Chapter 4). This reflex is present in the human neonate but disappears a few weeks after birth. It is believed that during the first inspiration the large airways are distended and that this stretch triggers a reflex augmentation of the first inspiration. This first inspiration after birth requires the application of a high transpulmonary pressure in order to overcome the viscosity of the liquid in the airways as well as the forces of surface tension and the elastic recoil of the lungs. The fetal lung contains a volume of liquid which is about 100 times more viscous than air and, as pointed out earlier, it may amount to about 40 per cent of the total lung capacity. Although this liquid within the lung increases the viscous forces which must be overcome, it also acts to distend the small airways and to keep the radius of curvature of the air-liquid interface relatively large. This, as indicated by the Laplace formula (see Chapter 1), reduces the surface forces resisting inflation.

Since the lung must function efficiently as an organ of gas exchange within a few moments after birth, the lung liquid must be cleared rapidly. About one-third of the lung liquid is squeezed from the thorax and out of the oropharynx as the infant passes through the birth canal. Of the remaining two-thirds of the lung liquid, about one-half is absorbed into the capillaries and the remainder into the pulmonary lymphatics. Thus, within a few moments after the onset of respiration the FRC has almost reached a normal value, and the internal surface area of the lungs is sufficient for adequate gas exchange.

The introduction of air into the airless lung does not result in uniform expansion because the airway resistance varies throughout the lung and depends on the size of the airways. Thus, expansion of the lung is asynchronous; groups of alveoli become fully distended, and other areas of the lung remain atelectatic. After a short period of time, however, practically all air spaces have been inflated to some extent. The aspiration of meconium, blood or mucus may result in airway obstruction and lead to complications. In order to overcome the bronchial obstruction it is necessary to develop a high and prolonged transpulmonary pressure which may result in overdistention and rupture of patent alveoli. Indeed, the highest incidence of spontaneous pneumothorax in the neonatal period occurs in those infants who demonstrate evidence of aspiration of foreign material.

Figure 54 illustrates transpulmonary pressures which were recorded from a human infant during the first 3 breaths after birth. Note that air does not begin to enter the lung until a transpulmonary pressure of -40 cm. H_2O is reached and that a peak transpulmonary pressure of -60 cm. H_2O is present transiently. Transpulmonary pressures of -80 cm. H_2O may be produced during the first few breaths and occasionally peak transpulmonary pressures of as much as -100 cm. H_2O are found. At the end of the first expiration the lungs contain a small volume of air and subsequent inspirations require transpulmonary pressures of decreasing magnitude. During the first few expirations the pleural pressure may be positive because expiration is made against a partially closed glottis. Retention of air in the lungs after expiration depends on the presence of pulmonary surfactant, which lowers the surface tension in the terminal lung units, thereby allowing alveoli to remain open at a low transpulmonary pressure.

CHANGE IN PULMONARY VASCULAR RESISTANCE AT BIRTH

The expansion of the lung with air at birth produces a drastic and immediate fall in the pulmonary vascular resistance and, in ad-

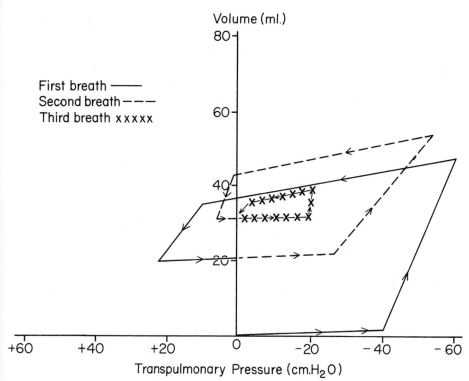

Volume (ml.)

First breath ——
Second breath — — —
Third breath x x x x x

Transpulmonary Pressure (cm.H_2O)

FIGURE 54. Transpulmonary pressures developed in the newborn human infant during the first three breaths after birth. (Modified from Avery, M. E.: The Lung and Its Disorders in the Newborn Infant. 2nd ed. W. B. Saunders Co., Philadelphia, 1964, p. 29. By permission.)

dition, a local increase in Po_2 and decrease in Pco_2 and cH^+. However, the pulmonary vascular resistance remains higher in the neonate than in the adult, and the pulmonary arterial pressure is about 40 mm. Hg after birth. With time, the pulmonary vascular resistance gradually decreases, the pulmonary artery pressure falling to normal adult levels at about 1 to 2 weeks after birth.

CLOSURE OF THE FORAMEN OVALE AND DUCTUS ARTERIOSUS AT BIRTH

At birth, *functional closure* of the foramen ovale occurs because with cessation of the umbilical circulation there is a fall of flow in the inferior vena cava and a concomitant fall in the right atrial pressure. The left atrial pressure rises because of the increased pulmonary blood flow. *Anatomical closure* of the foramen ovale may not occur for some time and indeed in 25 per cent of adults remains "probe patent."

Closure of the ductus arteriosus at birth is thought to be related to constriction, which is brought about by an increase in arterial

PO$_2$. Recently it has been demonstrated that bradykinin (a vasoactive polypeptide) is released from the lung during its initial inflation. This substance is capable of producing profound vasoconstriction of the ductus arteriosus and the umbilical artery in the presence of an arterial PO$_2$ above 40 mm. Hg. In full-term human infants a small bidirectional ductal shunt may be present until about 6 hours of age, and then a small left-to-right shunt is present up to about 15 hours of age.

POSTNATAL GROWTH AND FUNCTION OF THE LUNG

A comparison of the infant and adult measurements of pulmonary anatomy and function is shown in Table 5. The number of airways down to the level of terminal bronchioles does not increase after birth, but with lung growth, the airways elongate and the number of alveoli increases some tenfold, reaching adult values by about 8 years of age. Although the surface area of the infant lung is equal to that of the adult, when compared on the basis of body surface area or body weight, the oxygen requirements of the infant are nearly twice that of the adult. Thus, the pulmonary reserve of the infant is considerably less than that of the adult.

TABLE 5

COMPARISON OF INFANTS AND ADULT MEASUREMENTS OF PULMONARY ANATOMY AND FUNCTION

	INFANT	ADULT
Body weight (kg.)	3	70
Lung weight (gm.)	50	800
Lung surface area (sq.m.)	2.8	75
Alveolar diameter	150	300
Number of alveoli	24×10^6	296×10^6
Number of airways	1.5×10^6	14×10^6
Respiratory frequency (per min.)	36	14
Calories/kg./hr.	2.0	1.0
$\dot{V}_{O_2}$ (ml./kg./min., STPD)	7	3
$\dot{V}_{CO_2}$ (ml./kg./min., STPD)	6	3
$\dot{V}_E$ (ml./min.)	525	6000
f	35	12
V_T (ml.)	15	500
$\dot{V}_A$ (ml./kg.)	120	60
$\dot{V}_D$ (ml.)	5	150
$\dot{V}_{O_2}/\dot{V}_A$	.06	.06
FRC (ml.)	70	3000

Studies of the chemical control of respiration in newborn infants have indicated that there is a very active ventilatory response to hypoxia and hypercapnia. No major differences have been found in the ventilatory control mechanisms between infants and adults.

Because of the asphyxial insult which occurs at the time of birth, most newborn infants have a combined metabolic and respiratory acidosis. However, by 12 hours of age, the arterial pH returns to normal values as the arterial PCO_2 falls. It is of interest that in children up to 2 years of age the serum bicarbonate is slightly lower and the arterial PCO_2 is about 5 mm. Hg lower than in normal adults. The arterial pH, however, is in the normal adult range of 7.35 to 7.45. The arterial PO_2 averages only 70 mm. Hg at 24 hours of age in healthy newborn infants, but it increases to adult values within the next 48 hours. These low values in the first 24 hours represent the persistence of fetal circulatory pathways, and the considerable right-to-left shunting which occurs through the foramen ovale and the ductus arteriosus.

Chapter 7

The Application of Pulmonary Physiology to Clinical Pulmonary Function Testing

There are a variety of tests which may be used to detect disturbed respiratory function, and used judiciously, they are an essential component of the clinical evaluation of a patient with respiratory complaints. These tests of function enable the physician to follow the progress of the disease and also, because of his knowledge of the disturbances in pulmonary function, to prescribe proper therapy and to assess its effects objectively. In a case of pulmonary disability in which surgery, particularly removal of lung tissue, is planned, such tests help to assess the patient's ability to tolerate anesthetics, narcotics or the removal of lung tissue and serve as a guide to the preparation and the postoperative care of the patient. Since only one aspect of pulmonary function may be altered by some diseases, these studies occasionally assist in establishing the correct diagnosis of the respiratory condition.

The degree of sophistication and complexity of the pulmonary function tests which are used varies widely, depending on local circumstances. In this chapter we will confine the discussion to those tests which are simplest, most widely used and most helpful. They fall into two general groups: tests relating to the ventilatory function of the lungs and chest wall, and those relating to gas exchange. In clinical practice, limited studies of respiratory function, such as ventilatory function studies, usually suffice. In those cases that warrant it, the functional assessment of a patient with respiratory disease should also include tests of gas exchange at rest and during exercise.

VENTILATORY FUNCTION

The ventilatory function of the respiratory system may be altered by changes in either the elastic or the nonelastic properties of the

140

lungs and the chest wall. As was described in Chapter 1, the elastic resistance (compliance) of the lungs and the chest wall, either together or separately, can be determined by measuring the distending pressure and the resultant change in lung volume at a time when airflow has ceased.

Measurement of the static pressure-volume relationships of the lung over the total vital capacity provides an indication of its retractive force at each level of lung volume. It is also possible to measure the elastic resistance or compliance of the lungs during breathing (dynamic compliance). However, since the pressure-volume relationship over the entire range of the lung volume is not linear, the lung compliance value varies with lung volume even in a given subject. Thus, it is important when measuring dynamic compliance to relate the compliance to the lung volume at which it is determined. To correct for differences in size between persons, compliance is also expressed with reference to the lung volume at which it is measured, and in this case is called "specific compliance."

The nonelastic resistance of the lungs during breathing is assessed by measuring simultaneously the pressure within the lung and the rate of airflow at the mouth. As discussed in Chapter 1, this can be determined in a body plethysmograph or by simultaneous measurement of the airflow, volume and transpulmonary pressure. The reciprocal of the resistance to airflow (conductance) varies directly with the lung volume at which it is measured (i.e., the conductance is greatest at high lung volume where the bronchi are widest). Thus, conductance should also be expressed with reference to the lung volume at which it is measured; it is then called the "specific conductance."

In practice, measurements of static lung volumes are utilized to reflect the elastic properties of the respiratory system; the nonelastic properties are reflected in measurements of the speed with which lung volumes may be changed (dynamic lung volumes).

STATIC LUNG VOLUMES

The subdivisions of the lung volumes have been described in Chapter 1. The static lung volumes can be measured by means of the body plethysmographic technique or, except for the residual volume, by means of a simple spirometer. The residual volume can be measured by dilution techniques employing either helium or nitrogen as the reference gas. In practice, one usually measures the FRC, the residual volume being obtained by subtraction of the expiratory reserve volume from the functional residual capacity. The total lung capacity is calculated by addition of either the vital capacity and the residual volume or the functional residual capacity and the inspiratory capacity. As indicated in Chapter 1, the size of the lung volumes varies with the age and size of the subject.

A reduction in lung volume suggests the presence of a restrictive disorder because of either a reduced distensibility of the lungs, as in pulmonary fibrosis, or a reduced distensibility of the chest wall, as in kyphoscoliosis. An increase in lung volume indicates that the lungs are hyperinflated, because of obstruction of the airways, as in asthma, or a loss of lung elasticity, as in emphysema. It has been suggested that a residual volume which is greater than 30 per cent of the total lung capacity is indicative of hyperinflation, but it is important to remember that the residual volume normally increases with age; in an elderly healthy person the residual volume may be as much as 50 per cent of the total lung capacity. It is also important to remember that although hyperinflation is present in emphysema, not all patients exhibiting hyperinflated lungs have emphysema.

Determination of the vital capacity, which also varies normally according to age, body size and sex, provides an index of the distensibility of the lungs and thoracic cage. Figure 55 illustrates that the vital capacity is well correlated with measurements of the compliance of the lung and thorax. Thus, the vital capacity is reduced in any condition in which the compliance of the lung is decreased, such as pulmonary fibrosis or congestion, or in which the compliance of the chest wall is decreased, such as obesity or kyphoscoliosis. In addition,

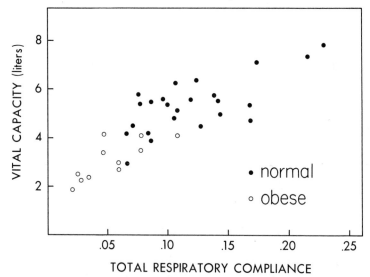

FIGURE 55.   The relationship between vital capacity and the compliance of the lung and thorax in normal and obese subjects. (From Naimark, A., and Cherniack, R. M.: The compliance of the respiratory system and its components in health and obesity. J. Appl. Physiol. *15*:377, 1960. By permission.)

since the vital capacity is determined by having the subject make a forceful maximal expiration after a maximal inspiration, it will be reduced if the respiratory muscles are weakened or paralyzed by neuromuscular disease.

A patient may be suffering from severe pulmonary disability and yet have a vital capacity well within the normal range, because the volume of the vital capacity is primarily related to the distensibility of the respiratory system. This situation is frequently encountered in patients in whom the nonelastic resistance is increased because of severe airway obstruction. Conversely, since measurement of the vital capacity depends on the effort exerted by the patient, a low vital capacity may not indicate respiratory impairment. Clearly, it is essential that the test be repeated several times in order to ensure that the maximal value has been obtained, and the examiner must be *convinced* that the maximum has been obtained.

Like values of compliance, the value of the vital capacity must be related to lung volume in order for it to be interpreted correctly. Figure 56 illustrates that the vital capacity may be reduced in patients with either pulmonary fibrosis or with airway obstruction. In fibrosis the reduced vital capacity is associated with a small lung volume. In airway obstruction the low vital capacity is associated with a large lung volume.

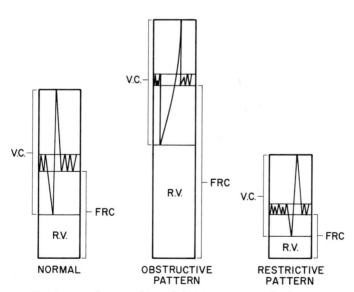

FIGURE 56.   Lung volume and its subdivisions in normal subjects, patients with airway obstruction and patients with restricted movement of the lung or thorax.

DYNAMIC LUNG VOLUMES

Considerable information about the nonelastic resistance may be obtained from tests based on determining the rate at which air flows out of the lungs during a forced expiration. A simple test, which can be employed at the bedside, is one which determines the patient's ability to blow out the flame of a match held four to six inches away from his wide-open mouth. A more objective assessment is obtained by analysis of a forced expiratory vital capacity maneuver (FEV).

The analysis of the forced vital capacity can be carried out in several ways (Fig. 57). The commonest is to calculate the volume of air expelled during a particular period of time, i.e., in the first half second ($FEV_{0.5}$), the first three-quarters of a second ($FEV_{0.75}$) or the first second ($FEV_{1.0}$). Other commonly used calculations are the peak expiratory flow rate (PEFR) or estimations of the rate of airflow while a particular volume of air is expired. The maximal midexpiratory flow rate, or MMF (the mean rate of airflow during the middle half of the forced expired vital capacity) and the maximal expiratory flow rate or MEFR (the length of time taken to expire 1.0 liter after the first 200 ml. have been expired) are examples of this technique.

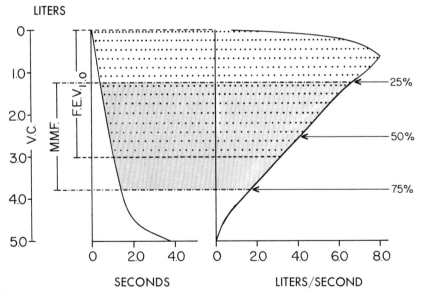

FIGURE 57.   The forced vital capacity maneuver. The timed vital capacity is shown on the left and the relationship between volume and flow is shown on the right. The maximal flow rates when 25 per cent, 50 per cent, and 75 per cent of the vital capacity have been expired are indicated by the arrows.

Not all of these analyses are equally informative, however, and most investigators prefer to use the $FEV_{1.0}$ or the MMF as indices of expiratory resistance to airflow. This choice is determined by the fact that at high lung volumes maximal flow is subject to wide variability and is very dependent on patient effort, but over the lower two-thirds of the lung volume maximal effort is not necessary to produce maximum flow. It will be recalled that Figure 19 in Chapter 1 indicated that the maximal inspiratory flow rate depends primarily on the force developed at every lung inflation. However, the maximal expiratory flow rate continues to increase with increasing pressure only when the expiration is carried out at lung volumes near full inflation. At lesser degrees of lung inflation (less than 65 per cent of the TLC) airflow only increases as effort (pressure) increases up to a certain point. After that, increased effort fails to elicit an increase in flow and may actually be associated with a slight decrease in flow.

Thus, it is apparent that any assessment of flow resistance which is based predominantly on analysis of the expiratory rate of airflow at high degrees of lung inflation, such as $FEV_{0.5}$, PEFR or MEFR, may be unreliable because the value obtained may be related more to patient cooperation and effort than to alterations in pulmonary mechanics. Conversely, when the flow rate is measured over a larger range of lung volume (e.g., $FEV_{1.0}$), or the measurement of flow rate ignores the first portion of the expiration during which flow is primarily effort dependent (e.g., the MMF), the values obtained may provide better indices of alterations in the mechanical resistances.

In emphysema and other obstructive airway diseases, these indices of airflow resistance are sharply reduced. On the other hand, in patients with a reduced compliance but no associated airway obstruction, as in diffuse pulmonary fibrosis, these indices of airflow resistance are usually normal.

Patients with chronic bronchial obstruction also suffer from considerable obstruction to airflow during inspiration. Analysis of flow rates during an inspiratory vital capacity may be made in the same manner as the forced expiratory vital capacity, but as stated previously, the measurement of flow resistance during a forced inspiration is less informative because it may be related more to the degree of effort than to changes in the mechanical properties of the lung.

It must be pointed out that measurements of airflow resistance or tests of expiratory flow which are used as indices of expiratory airflow resistance reflect mainly the resistance in the large airways and are relatively insensitive to changes in the peripheral portions of the airways. Since the small airways (less than 2 mm. in diameter) contribute less than 20 per cent of the total airway resistance, even a marked increase in peripheral airway resistance might not be reflected in the commonly employed indices of airway resistance. Thus, routine tests of dynamic lung volumes or nonelastic resistance may yield normal results in patients with predominantly "small airways" disease. However, as pointed out in Chapter 1, obstruction of small airways will alter the distribution of mechanical time constants in the lung and therefore will influence the distribution of inspired gas, particularly when the respiratory frequency is increased. A fall in dynamic lung compliance with increasing respiratory frequency is indicative of an uneven distribution of time constants throughout the lungs and therefore, in the absence of evidence of large airway disease, may be a reflection of small airway disease.

OVERALL VENTILATORY FUNCTION

The overall effect of an alteration in the elastic or nonelastic properties of the lungs is an increase in the amount of work required to overcome the mechanical resistances of the lungs. As indicated previously, this can be calculated from simultaneous measurements of the pleural pressure and the volume of air displaced during breathing. However, the work required to overcome the resistance of the chest wall cannot be measured directly.

A simple test which provides an index of the overall effects of altered mechanical properties of the lungs and chest wall is the maximum breathing capacity (MBC). The patient is instructed to breathe as hard and as fast as he can for 12 or 15 seconds, and the minute ventilation is determined. Since the rate of airflow is markedly increased during the performance of the maximal breathing capacity, this test is particularly affected by alterations in the nonelastic resistance and, to a much lesser extent, by changes in the elastic resistance. Since a maximal ventilation can be attained only by voluntary effort, the subject must be encouraged constantly during the performance of the test, and the examiner must be convinced that the patient has made a maximal effort before he interprets a low value as being abnormal. There is no apparent correlation between the maximal breathing capacity and the vital capacity. However, the relationship between the maximal breathing capacity and calculations of expiratory flow resistance, based on assessment of the forced vital capacity, is moderately close.

Another overall effect of altered mechanical properties is an abnormal distribution of air within the lung. The manner in which inspired air is distributed to the alveoli is affected by the equality of the time constants of the peripheral lung units. When two or more parallel units of lung are subjected to the same inflation or deflation pressure they fill or empty at a rate which is determined by their respective time constants. If the time constants of the units are equal, they will fill or empty uniformly, and conversely, if the time constants are unequal, there will be nonuniform filling or emptying. As was demonstrated in Figure 22, when there is no localized disease the tidal volume is distributed equally to different areas of lung. In normal subjects, tests of gas distribution indicate that inspired gas is distributed equally and suggest that the distribution of time constants is relatively uniform throughout the lung. When localized disease, such as an airway obstruction, is present, however, the time constants are unequally distributed in the lung so that the air tends to move into areas of the lung which offer the least resistance, and the inspired air is distributed unequally.

From the above, it will be clear that the assessment of the distribution of gas in the lung provides qualitative information about the degree of nonuniformity of the time constants in the lungs. Several tests of gas distribution are in use. In one, the rate at which the lungs and a spirometer reach equilibrium with respect to a foreign gas, such as helium or hydrogen, is determined. In another, the rate of dilution of nitrogen ("nitrogen washout") within the lung during the inhalation of either oxygen or a helium-oxygen mixture is estimated. The percentage of N_2 remaining at the end of a period (e.g., 7 minutes) provides an index of intrapulmonary mixing. In a "single breath" technique, the changes in expired nitrogen concentration during a forced expiration following a vital capacity inhalation of pure oxygen are recorded. As has been demonstrated in Figure 25 in Chapter 1, inequalities of time constants between lung units leading to unequal distribution of inspired air will be reflected by a rising moment-to-moment nitrogen concentration during the ensuing expiration.

A simple analysis which may provide the best index of the overall mechanical resistances to breathing may be obtained by assessment of the flow-volume relationship (Fig. 57), particularly over the last 50 per cent of the forced expiratory vital capacity. Assessment of the flow-volume relationship during a forced vital capacity provides the most sensitive assessment of resistances in the lung, and changes in the slope of the flow-volume relationship may be reflections of the inequality of time constants in the lung; the higher slopes represent air coming from areas with a low time constant, and the remainder of the curve represents air coming from areas with a high time constant.

THE INTERPRETATION OF VENTILATORY FUNCTION TESTS

The interpretation of ventilatory function tests can be best understood if one considers them as comprising two "envelopes." This is illustrated in Figure 58, in which the "static envelope" (i.e., the

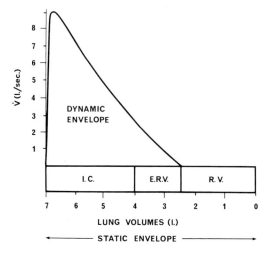

FIGURE 58. The lung volume ("static envelope") and the flow volume relationship during a forced expiratory vital capacity ("dynamic envelope") in a healthy subject.

static lung volumes) and the "dynamic envelope" (flow-volume relationship) for a normal subject are depicted.

Table 6 compares the patterns of abnormality of the standard ventilatory function tests in patients with restrictive pulmonary disease and patients with obstructive pulmonary disease. The finding of a low MMF or absolute $FEV_{1.0}$ in patients with restrictive pulmonary disease may suggest concomitant airflow obstruction. However, visualization of these measurements in the light of the two "envelopes" allows differentiation of a restrictive ventilatory pattern from an obstructive ventilatory pattern (Fig. 59).

TABLE 6

DISTURBANCES OF VENTILATORY FUNCTION IN
OBSTRUCTIVE AND RESTRICTIVE DISEASE

TEST	OBSTRUCTIVE DISEASE	RESTRICTIVE DISEASE
VC	↔ ↓	↓
$FEV_{1.0}$	↓	↔ ↓
MMF	↓	↔ ↓
MBC	↓	↔ ↓
RV	↑	↓
FRC	↑	↓
TLC	↑	↓

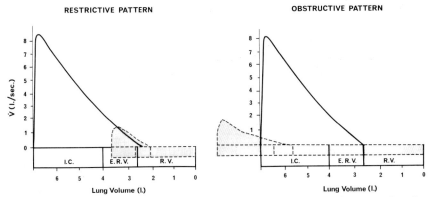

FIGURE 59.   The static and dynamic "envelopes" in restrictive disease and in obstructive disease. The solid "envelopes" represent the expected values in a healthy person of the same age and height.

In the restrictive pattern the "static envelope" is reduced in size (i.e., lung volumes are diminished). The "dynamic envelope" is also reduced in size (i.e., flow rates are low), not because of increased airflow resistance, but because of the reduced lung volume. In fact, flow rates are greater than predicted at equivalent lung volumes because of the increase in elastic recoil.

In the obstructive pattern the "static envelope" is increased in size (i.e., lung volumes are high). The "dynamic envelope" is reduced in size, but in this case the flow rates are considerably lower than predicted at an equivalent lung volume as a result of the increase in airflow resistance.

RESTRICTIVE VENTILATORY PATTERN

In the patient suffering from a restrictive disease, such as pulmonary fibrosis, the vital capacity and the total lung capacity and its subdivisions are reduced, but the maximal breathing capacity may be nearly normal. The measurement of flow rates or the MMF may be lower than predicted. However, as is indicated in Figure 59, this can be explained by the reduction in lung volume and does not reflect obstruction to airflow. In fact, the flow rates are higher than predicted at this lung volume because of the increased elastic retractive force of the lungs due to the restrictive disorder.

This type of disturbance in ventilatory function is also found when the elastic resistance of the chest cage is increased, as in obesity or kyphoscoliosis. From these measurements one may infer that the distensibility or compliance of the respiratory system is reduced and that the airway resistance is normal. Such a reduction in lung volumes is also found in patients whose respiratory muscles are unable to perform normally because of neuromuscular disease or paralysis. In this case the reduction in vital capacity and maximal breathing capacity can be attributed, in large part, to muscular paralysis rather than to reduced distensibility.

OBSTRUCTIVE VENTILATORY PATTERN

In the patient suffering from diffuse airway obstruction, the flow rates, the MMF and the maximal breathing capacity are markedly reduced, but the vital capacity may be either considerably reduced or only slightly impaired. In this case the reduction in vital capacity is due to the increase in residual volume rather than a restrictive component. The total lung capacity and the functional residual capacity are also usually greater than normal. The increased lung volume offers a functional advantage because the bronchi are wider and the lung elastic recoil is greater, and hence the resistance to airflow is easier to overcome than if the lung volume were smaller. Examination of the measurements of ventilatory function in the light of the static and dynamic "envelopes" indicates gross overdistention and flow rates which are considerably lower than would be predicted at equivalent lung volumes, a picture which is very different from that seen in the restrictive ventilatory defect.

When the analysis of the forced vital capacity and flow rates are indicative of obstruction to airflow, it is important to determine whether there is improvement after the administration of a nebulized bronchodilator. Figure 60 demonstrates the increase in vital capacity,

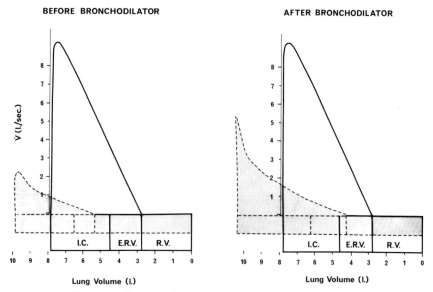

FIGURE 60. The effect of nebulized bronchodilator on "static" and "dynamic" lung envelopes in a patient with obstruction to airflow. The solid "envelopes" represent the expected values in a healthy person of the same age and height.

Note that bronchodilator resulted in little change in size of the "static envelope," although its components have altered, and that the "dynamic envelope" has increased in size, the flow rates being higher at equivalent lung volumes, indicating a reduction in airflow resistance.

and flow rates which were obtained following the inhalation of a nebulized bronchodilator in a patient suffering from diffuse bronchial obstruction. The increase in flow rate at equivalent lung volumes indicates that there has been a reduction in resistance to airflow following the inhalation of bronchodilator. The increase in vital capacity is due to a lowering of residual volume and functional residual capacity because of the reduction in resistance to airflow.

THE VENTILATORY RESPONSE TO CARBON DIOXIDE

It might be surprising to some that this section is introduced at this point, since the ventilatory response to the inhalation of either a fixed concentration of CO_2 in oxygen (e.g., 3 per cent or 5 per cent) for a period of time or a gradually increasing inspired CO_2 concentration from a spirometer containing oxygen but no CO_2 absorber, is frequently assessed to determine the status of the respiratory center sensitivity. A lower than normal ventilatory response to CO_2 has been attributed to a diminished sensitivity of the medullary respiratory center.

However, it is important to reiterate, as has been demonstrated in Figure 50, that the ventilatory response to CO_2 can be lowered in a normal subject by the introduction of an artificial airway obstruction, and that of a patient with chronic obstructive airway disease can be increased by the administration of a bronchodilating agent. Similarly, it has been demonstrated that artificially assisting ventilation increases the ventilatory response to inhaled CO_2 in normal persons. Since it is unlikely that the "respiratory center" sensitivity is changed acutely in these studies, these findings suggest that the ventilatory response to CO_2 may be an inadequate expression of respiratory center responsiveness and that mechanical factors may play a major role in limiting the ventilatory response.

The fact that the ventilatory response to inhaled CO_2 may be limited by alterations in the mechanical work of breathing is not surprising if one considers several important facts that were discussed in the earlier chapters. The arterial P_{CO_2} at any ventilation is directly related to the CO_2 production, and the oxygen cost of breathing (or CO_2 production) at any ventilation is increased when the mechanical work of breathing is high (Fig. 28). Thus, the P_{CO_2} will be higher at a particular alveolar ventilation in any person in whom the oxygen cost of breathing is high and the ventilation changes in response to P_{CO_2} changes will be lower. For the same reason the size of the physiologic dead space will influence the ventilation achieved in response to inhaled CO_2. For instance, if the dead space-tidal volume ratio is high (i.e., the alveolar ventilation/total ventilation ratio is low), then a given increase in minute ventilation and oxygen consumption will be associated with a higher PCO_2.

Thus, the PCO_2 can be expected to be higher than normal at an equivalent ventilation whenever the work of breathing is high or the proportion of the ventilation being wasted is greater than normal. Since the work of breathing and the physiologic dead space are elevated in the patient with emphysema, it is not surprising that the change in ventilation per unit change in arterial PCO_2 is lower than normal. However, it is clear that this "diminished response to CO_2" does not necessarily imply a diminished sensitivity of the respiratory centers, but rather that it may be still another reflection of ventilatory impairment.

GAS EXCHANGE

The gas exchange function of the lung is said to be normal when the blood leaving the lungs has approximately the same gas composition as the alveolar gas and the values for arterial PO_2 and PCO_2 are normal. An abnormality in gas exchange is reflected in a failure of equilibration between the partial pressure of oxygen in the alveolar gas and pulmonary capillary blood, in abnormal values for arterial PO_2 and PCO_2 or both. In many patients the abnormality in gas exchange may be slight while at rest and may become apparent only during exertion. Assessment of gas exchange should therefore be carried out both at rest and during exercise by analysis of simultaneously collected samples of arterial blood and expired air.

The arterial blood is collected anaerobically for the determination of the oxygen and carbon dioxide content of the blood as well as the PCO_2, PO_2 and pH. When an arterial puncture is difficult or undesirable, a reliable estimate of arterial PCO_2 can be obtained by having the subject rebreathe from a bag containing oxygen and a small amount of CO_2 and then monitoring the CO_2 concentration in the system. When the CO_2 in the system is equal to the mixed venous PCO_2, a transient plateau is noted. The arterial PCO_2 is then estimated by subtracting the arteriovenous PCO_2 difference of 6 mm. Hg from this value for mixed venous PCO_2.

The gas concentrations in the expired air allow the calculation of oxygen consumption and carbon dioxide production and the ventilatory gas exchange ratio (R). If the value for R is within normal limits, it can be inferred that the patient was in a steady state while the arterial blood was drawn and that any abnormalities which were found are valid reflections of a disturbance in gas exchange due to respiratory insufficiency. A low respiratory quotient suggests that the patient was hypoventilating while the blood was being drawn, and a high respiratory quotient suggests that he was hyperventilating. Under these circumstances, any abnormal values of P_{O_2} and P_{CO_2} are not an accurate reflection of the gas exchange defect which may be present.

The analysis of the gas concentrations and partial pressures in the expired air and arterial blood allows calculation of several other important parameters, such as the physiologic dead space (V_D), the dead space-tidal volume ratio (V_D/V_T) and the alveolo-arterial partial pressure difference for oxygen (A-a D_{O_2}).

PHYSIOLOGIC DEAD SPACE

As indicated in Chapter 2, part of each tidal volume is wasted (i.e., it does not take part in gas exchange), even in a healthy person. If there is a reduction in perfusion of alveoli which are well ventilated, or overventilation of alveoli which are normally perfused, much of the gas leaving these alveoli does not take part in gas exchange and its composition is close to that of the inspired air. The amount of wasted ventilation is usually determined by calculation of the physiologic dead space (Chapter 2) from the formula

$$V_D = \frac{(P_{A_{CO_2}} - P_{E_{CO_2}})}{P_{A_{CO_2}}} \times V_T$$

and

$$V_D/V_T = \frac{P_{A_{CO_2}} - P_{E_{CO_2}}}{P_{A_{CO_2}}}$$

As long as the lungs are healthy, the end-tidal P_{CO_2} is a fairly accurate reflection of the alveolar carbon dioxide tension. However, in patients with cardiorespiratory disease, it is difficult to obtain a representative alveolar sample. In practice, the arterial P_{CO_2} is used instead of the alveolar P_{CO_2} in order to calculate the physiologic dead space.

The dead space tidal volume ratio (V_D/V_T) is less than 30 per cent in normal young subjects and about 40 per cent in older subjects. A ratio greater than this suggests that there is ventilation of alveoli which have limited perfusion or, in the extreme case, alveoli which are not perfused. The gas entering these alveoli takes little part, if any, in gas exchange and is called "dead-space-like ventilation."

ALVEOLO-ARTERIAL O₂ DIFFERENCE

Unlike the arterial P_{O_2}, which may be measured directly, the true alveolar P_{O_2} cannot, and instead an "ideal" or "effective" value for alveolar P_{O_2} is calculated. This is done by considering that all perfused alveoli, with their diverse P_{CO_2} values, are a single gas exchange volume with a P_{CO_2} which is the same as the arterial P_{CO_2} and with a gas exchange ratio which is equal to that of the lungs as a whole.

Under these circumstances

$$R = \frac{P_{A_{CO_2}} - P_{I_{CO_2}}}{P_{I_{O_2}} - P_{A_{O_2}}}$$

Since $P_{I_{CO_2}}$ is virtually zero, then

$$P_{A_{O_2}} = P_{I_{O_2}} - \left(P_{A_{CO_2}} \times \frac{I}{R}\right)$$

This *effective alveolar oxygen tension* is used to estimate the difference between the alveolar and the arterial oxygen tensions (i.e., the A-a D_{O_2}). In normal persons, the A-a D_{O_2} is less than 10 mm. Hg when room air is being inhaled.

PATTERNS OF ABNORMAL GAS EXCHANGE

An abnormality of gas exchange is reflected by an increase in A-a P_{O_2} difference or a low arterial P_{O_2} with, or without, an abnormal P_{CO_2}. A low arterial P_{O_2} in patients with cardiopulmonary disease is likely to be due to alveolar hypoventilation, altered ventilation-perfusion ratios within the lung, true venous admixture, a diffusion defect or a combination of these disturbances. The salient feature of each of these disturbances is illustrated in Table 7.

ALVEOLAR HYPOVENTILATION

Although this is the most serious functional disturbance encountered in respiratory disease, it is often not recognized clinically unless it is severe. It is important to recognize that the term alveolar hypoventilation is a relative one and denotes an alveolar ventilation (no matter what the absolute value is) which is inadequate to cope with the CO_2 production. Thus, the finding of an elevated arterial P_{CO_2} in association with hypoxia is synonymous with this diagnosis. The alveolar ventilation will be inadequate in relation to the CO_2 production, and hypoxia and hypercapnia will be present whenever the work of breathing or total body metabolism is disproportionately high for a given alveolar ventilation. This situation may be present in conditions in which there is excessive dead-space-like or wasted ventilation (Table 7, *a*), as is found in emphysema, or the total venti-

TABLE 7

DISTURBANCES OF GAS EXCHANGE

	ALVEOLAR HYPO-VENTILATION		$\dot{V}_A/\dot{Q}$ ABNORMALITY		VENOUS ADMIX-TURE	DIFFU-SION DEFECT
	(a)	(b)	(c)	(d)	(e)	(f)
V_E	↔ ↑	↓	↑	↑	↑ ↔	↑
V_D	↑	↔	↑	↔	↔	↔
V_D/V_T	↑	↑	↑	↔	↔	↔
A-a PO_2 difference	↔	↔	↑	↑	↑	↑
$P_{a_{O_2}}$ (room air)	↓	↓	↔	↓	↓	↓
$P_{a_{O_2}}$ (O_2)	>500	>500	>500	>500	<500	>500
$P_{a_{CO_2}}$	↑	↑	↔ ↓	↔ ↑	↓ ↔	↓ ↔

lation is decreased (Table 7, *b*), as in barbiturate poisoning or muscular paralysis.

Adequate oxygenation and carbon dioxide elimination, as evidenced by the presence of normal arterial oxygen and carbon dioxide tensions, may still occur when there is excessive "dead-space-like ventilation" but only if the normally perfused alveoli are hyperventilated. However, if the ventilation of the perfused alveoli is inadequate to cope with the carbon dioxide production of the body, then "alveolar hypoventilation," is also present and hypoxia and carbon dioxide retention will develop. In pure alveolar hypoventilation—i.e., the only defect is an overall reduction in alveolar ventilation—the partial pressure of the gases in the alveoli and the pulmonary capillary blood come into equilibrium so that, in this situation, the A-a PO_2 difference is within normal limits.

VENTILATION-PERFUSION IMBALANCE

An A-a PO_2 difference which is greater than 10 mm. Hg indicates a defect in blood-gas equilibration between the alveoli and the pulmonary capillaries and may be due to one or more of three physiological disturbances. Nonuniformity of ventilation-perfusion ratios in the lungs accounts for the major proportion of the A-a PO_2 difference in both normal and abnormal lungs. Blood leaving the alveoli which are poorly perfused or not perfused at all (i.e., the ventilation-perfusion ratio is high) is fully oxygenated and often excessively depleted of carbon dioxide so that the arterial blood-gas tensions may be relatively normal (Table 7, *c*). However, this abnormality can be recognized by determination of the A-a PO_2 difference and the physiologic dead space; a dead space which is greater than 30 per cent of the tidal volume suggests that a greater than normal amount of nonperfused or poorly perfused alveoli are being ventilated.

When there is perfusion of inadequately ventilated alveoli, or in the extreme case, perfusion of nonventilated alveoli (i.e., the ventilation-perfusion ratio is low) a portion of the pulmonary blood is only slightly aerated, if at all. This poorly aerated blood mixes with "arterialized blood" coming from the well-ventilated and perfused alveoli; as a result, the PO_2 will be low, and the PCO_2 will be slightly elevated in the mixed arterial blood (Table 7, *d*). The arterial PCO_2 may be normal if there is sufficient hyperventilation of the well-perfused alveoli, but because of the shape of the oxyhemoglobin dissociation curve, the arterial hypoxia will not be corrected to any significant degree by the hyperventilation.

The other causes of an increased A-a PO_2 difference are shunting of nonarterialized blood past the lungs to the left side of the heart or an impairment of diffusion of oxygen from the alveoli to the capillaries. Since a failure of diffusion is rarely, if ever, a major cause of a large A-a PO_2 difference at rest in disease, the finding of a large difference is usually due to either a mismatching of ventilation and perfusion in the lung or to "true venous admixture."

TRUE VENOUS ADMIXTURE

Shunting of blood past the lungs to the left side of the heart is normally responsible for a small part of the A-a PO_2 difference. Significant degrees of oxygen unsaturation due to the admixture of unaerated blood can occur in congenital heart disease, polycythemia, liver disease and abnormal pulmonary arteriovenous communications.

A qualitative estimate of the shunt can be obtained by measuring the arterial PO_2 while the subject is breathing 100 per cent oxygen. If there is a greater than normal amount of unaerated blood being added to aerated blood, the arterial oxygen tension will not reach expected values (i.e., greater than 500 mm. Hg) when 100 per cent oxygen is being inhaled (Table 7, *e*). If one assumes a value for the arteriovenous O_2 content difference, then the amount of blood being shunted can be calculated from the following equation:

$$\text{Per cent shunt} = \frac{\text{O}_2 \text{ content difference between end pulmonary capillary and arterial blood}}{\text{O}_2 \text{ content difference between end pulmonary capillary and mixed venous blood}}$$

For instance, if the arterial PO_2 is 500 mm. Hg and PCO_2 40 mm. Hg while 100 per cent oxygen is being inhaled by a person whose hemoglobin is 20 gm./100 ml., then

Arterial O_2 content = 20 × 1.34 (O_2 carried by hemoglobin) +
500 × .003 (O_2 in solution) = <u>28.30 ml.</u>/100 ml. of blood

If the alveolar and end-capillary O_2 tensions are in equilibrium, then

end-capillary P_{O_2} = 760 (barometric pressure) −
$$47 \text{ (pressure of water vapour)} - 40 \text{ } (P_{A_{CO_2}}) = 673 \text{ mm. Hg}$$

and

end-capillary O_2 content = (20 × 1.34) +
$$(673 \times .003) = \underline{28.82} \text{ ml./100 ml. of blood}$$

If the A-V oxygen content difference is 5 ml./100 ml., then

$$\text{Per cent shunt} = \frac{28.82 - 28.30}{28.82 - 23.30} \times 100 = 9.4 \text{ per cent}$$

Though usually due to an arteriovenous aneurysm or a defect in the heart, an increase in calculated venous admixture can also occur if there is perfusion of regions of the lung which are not ventilated because of obstruction, collapse, pulmonary edema or consolidation. To determine whether an increased amount of shunting is due to true venous admixture or is the result of continued perfusion of areas of lung which are not ventilated, one can inject dye intravenously and note its appearance time in a peripheral artery. The appearance time is normal if the apparent shunting is due to perfusion of non-ventilated areas, but the dye appears earlier if a true shunt is present.

DIFFUSION ABNORMALITY

Although a diffusion defect may develop in some diseases when the alveolocapillary membrane is markedly thickened or the capillary bed considerably reduced, it is usually the associated ventilation-perfusion imbalance which accounts for the major portion of the high A-a P_{O_2} difference at rest. However, the diffusion defect may become a predominant factor, resulting in a high A-a D_{O_2} in such patients during heavy exercise or when a low concentration of oxygen is inspired. When a diffusion abnormality is present, it is often characterized by hyperventilation and a low $P_{A_{CO_2}}$ (Table 7f).

The diffusing capacity of the lungs can be assessed by using either oxygen or carbon monoxide as the reference gas. "Single-breath" and "steady-state" techniques of estimating the diffusing capacity of carbon monoxide are used most commonly because of the technical difficulties associated with the oxygen method. The "single-breath" technique is easiest to perform, but because the values are obtained under the artificial conditions of breath-holding, they may not be as relevant to the actual gas exchange conditions as "steady-state" values. On the other hand, steady-state techniques depend on an accurate estimate of alveolar carbon monoxide concentration. Use of an end-tidal sample of alveolar gas may be in error if the tidal volume is low because gas from the dead space is included in the end-tidal sample or if there is marked ventilation-perfusion imbalance. In abnormal subjects, therefore, alveolar carbon monoxide concentration is best obtained indirectly from measurements of the expired carbon monoxide concentration and the physiologic dead space.

The diffusing capacity of carbon monoxide decreases with age, probably because ventilation-perfusion mismatching increases, but possibly also because of a decrease in the vascular bed or some qualitative change in the alveolocapillary membrane. A lower than expected diffusing capacity is encountered in patients with qualitative changes in the structure of terminal lung units, as in diffuse fibrosis of the lung, or in whom a large amount of lung tissue has been destroyed by disease or removed at surgery. It is unaltered in bronchial asthma but is markedly reduced in the later stages of emphysema, probably because of gross ventilation-perfusion abnormalities and a diminution in the amount of lung surface available for diffusion.

It must be stressed that a low value for diffusing capacity does not necessarily signify a diffusion defect but may merely reflect the presence of uneven ventilation-perfusion ratios, or as pointed out above, it may be the result of an inaccurate estimate of the alveolar carbon monoxide concentration. The interpretation of a low diffusing capacity can be aided by measurement of the fractional carbon monoxide removal (i.e., the proportion of the inspired volume of carbon monoxide which is transferred across the alveolocapillary barrier). If both the diffusing capacity and the fractional removal are low, then the low value for the D_{CO} is likely not to be due to an inaccurate estimate of alveolar P_{CO} but rather is an indication of a marked abnormality in ventilation-perfusion distribution or a decrease in the effective internal surface area of the lung available for gas transfer.

PATTERNS OF ABNORMALITY DURING EXERCISE

In the patient with mild respiratory disease, abnormal gas exchange may only become evident during exercise. Since exertional symptoms are predominant in patients with cardiorespiratory disease, the assessment of gas exchange during exercise can be particularly informative. Exercise limitation may result from a variety of mechanisms, and it is essential to differentiate between nonrespiratory and respiratory causes. It is not unusual to find evidence of limited exercise tolerance due to both aspects. Table 8 indicates the changes in several gas exchange variables which can be observed during exercise in patients who are physically unfit or who have cardiovascular impairment and those who have respiratory impairment.

TABLE 8

GAS EXCHANGE ABNORMALITIES DURING EXERCISE

PARAMETER	CARDIO-VASCULAR IMPAIRMENT OR PHYSICAL UNFITNESS	VENTI-LATORY IMPAIRMENT	$\dot{V}_A/\dot{Q}$ IMBALANCE	
	(a)	(b)	(c)	(d)
$\dot{V}_E$ rise	↑ ↑ ↑	↑	↑ ↑ ↑	↑ ↑ ↑
R	↑	↓ ↔	↔	↔
V_D/V_T (%)	← ↑ ↓	↓ ↔	↓	↑
A-a PO$_2$	↑ ↔	↔	↑	↑
$P_{a_{O_2}}$	↔ ↓	↓	↓	↓
$P_{a_{CO_2}}$	↔ ↓	↑	↔ ↓	↔ ↑
pH	↓	↓	↔ ↑	↔ ↑

If the cardiovascular system is unable to cope with the increased demands of the tissues during exercise, or if the person is not physically fit, then the distribution of systemic blood flow to the exercising muscles may be inadequate so that tissue hypoxia with excessive lactate production and acidemia develop. Thus, a rise in respiratory quotient, due to accumulation of lactate, and a fall in arterial pH are useful indicators of an impaired distribution of blood flow to the exercising muscles (Table 8, *a*).

The patterns of disturbance seen during exercise in respiratory insufficiency are those related to alveolar hypoventilation, ventilation perfusion abnormality or both and occasionally a diffusion defect.

VENTILATORY ABNORMALITY

The pattern of abnormality seen when exercise is limited by an impaired ventilatory ability is illustrated in Table 8, *b*. When the work of breathing is excessive, the ventilatory response to exercise may be limited. When there is alveolar hypoventilation unassociated with other physiological disturbances the physiologic dead space-tidal volume ratio may fall or remain unchanged. The effective alveolar oxygen tension falls, but there is no failure of equilibration between the oxygen in the alveolar air and the blood perfusing the alveoli; therefore, although the arterial oxygen tension falls, the alveolo-arterial PO$_2$ difference is usually within normal limits. However, the increase in ventilation during the exercise load is inadequate to cope with the increased CO$_2$ production, and therefore, the fall in arterial PO$_2$ is associated with a rise in arterial PCO$_2$.

VENTILATION-PERFUSION ABNORMALITY

The pattern of gas exchange abnormality which is seen during exercise when there is a mismatching of blood and gas distribution is also presented in Table 8. When there is an increased A-a PO_2 difference present at rest, it may rise or fall during exercise, depending on whether or not the increase in cardiac output and ventilation result in more uniform ventilation-perfusion ratios. Although the physiologic dead space normally increases with rising tidal volumes, the V_DV_T ratio usually falls, suggesting that there is better perfusion of regions with high ventilation-perfusion ratios during exercise. In some patients, then, the arterial PO_2 and A-a PO_2 difference may improve during exercise (Table 8, *c*). However, if, despite the increased perfusion which occurs during exercise, gross mismatching of blood and gas distribution in the lungs persists or increases, then the dead space-tidal air ratio may remain unchanged or may rise, the A-a PO_2 difference may rise further and the arterial PO_2 may fall (Table 8, *d*). In patients who have obstruction of a portion of the pulmonary vascular tree, an increase in physiologic dead space and an elevated A-a PO_2 difference during exercise may be the only abnormalities demonstrated.

DIFFUSION DEFECT

A pure diffusion defect is relatively uncommon and is usually associated with ventilation-perfusion imbalance, even in diseases in which the alveolocapillary membrane is markedly thickened or in which the capillary bed is reduced. The findings during exercise are similar to those which are found when there is a $\dot{V}_A/\dot{Q}$ abnormality (Table 8, *d*).

MIXED ABNORMALITY

In many cases abnormalities in gas exchange during exercise are the result of a combination of alveolar hypoventilation and a mismatching of the distribution of blood and gas. The presence of alveolar hypoventilation will be indicated by an elevated arterial PCO_2, and the ventilation-perfusion imbalance will be indicated by the increased A-a PO_2 difference. These abnormalities may be present at rest and increase during exercise or may only become apparent during exercise.

ACID-BASE BALANCE

Assessment of the acid-base status is an essential component of the investigation of patients with respiratory disease. The current availability of relatively simple equipment for measurement of pH and P_{CO_2} has facilitated the study of acid-base balance to the extent that it should be as much a part of the assessment of a patient with metabolic or respiratory disturbances as is the hemoglobin and leukocyte count.

As has been pointed out, alterations in gas exchange leading to alveolar hyperventilation or hypoventilation affect the arterial pH and lead to consequent compensatory measures by the kidney. Similarly, metabolic disturbances leading to alterations in bicarbonate result in compensatory measures by the respiratory system.

In order to avoid confusion with respect to disturbances which result in abnormalities of acid-base balance, one should distinguish between the acid-base state of the blood and the abnormal process involved in the primary disturbance. The abnormal states of the blood are *acidemia* (in which the cH^+ is high and pH is low) and *alkalemia* (in which the cH^+ is low and pH is high). The abnormal processes leading to acid-base disturbances are *acidosis* (in which a strong acid is gained, or HCO_3^- is lost in excessive amounts) and *alkalosis* (in which a strong base is gained or a strong acid is lost). An acidosis may at first lead to acidemia, but if secondary processes have led to compensation for the primary disturbance, then the blood cH^+ may become normal. The degree of compensation may be complete or incomplete, and this is judged on the basis of whether or not the cH^+ of the blood has returned to a normal value. In the completely compensated state, the primary disturbance—i.e., the acidosis or alkalosis—will be present, but the acidemia or alkalemia will have been ameliorated.

The terms acidosis and alkalosis are further qualified according to the nature of the primary disturbance. A *respiratory acidosis* is an abnormal process in which the alveolar ventilation is inadequate in relation to the rate of metabolic CO_2 production so that hypercapnia is present. This is equivalent to the retention of the strong acid H_2CO_3. A *respiratory alkalosis* is an abnormal process in which the alveolar ventilation is excessive in relation to the metabolic CO_2 production so that hypocapnia is present. This is equivalent to a loss of strong acid. A *metabolic acidosis* is an abnormal process characterized by a primary gain of strong acid by the extracellular fluid (e.g., organic acids from metabolism or exogenous acids such as NH_4Cl or by a primary loss of HCO_3^- from the extracellular fluid through the kidney or the intestinal tract). A *metabolic alkalosis* is an abnormal process characterized by a primary gain of strong base by the extracellular fluid (as in the administration of exogenous HCO_3^-; or by a primary loss of strong acid from extracellular fluid such as loss of HCl from the stomach).

ASSESSMENT OF ACID-BASE STATUS

Determination of any two of the three variables of the Henderson-Hasselbalch equation, (pH, P_{CO_2} and CO_2 content) allows calculation of the third variable. Measurement of a single parameter, however, may be very misleading. Clearly, a low pH may reflect either a metabolic or a respiratory acidemia, and a high pH indicates a metabolic or respiratory alkalemia. A low CO_2 content may indicate either a respiratory alkalosis (low $P_{a_{CO_2}}$) or a metabolic acidosis (low HCO_3^-), and a high CO_2 content may indicate either a metabolic alkalosis (high HCO_3^-) or a compensated respiratory acidosis (high $P_{a_{CO_2}}$). Similarly, a low $P_{a_{CO_2}}$ may be present in a respiratory alkalosis or in a compensated metabolic acidosis, and a high $P_{a_{CO_2}}$ may be present in a respiratory acidosis or in a compensated metabolic alkalosis. Thus, in order to assess the acid-base status, it is essential to measure at least two of the variables.

The approach to characterization of the acid-base status varies in different laboratories. In some, the total CO_2 content of whole blood or plasma is measured in a Van Slyke apparatus and, together with the pH, is used to calculate the P_{CO_2} or bicarbonate ion concentration from the Henderson-Hasselbalch equation. In other laboratories the P_{CO_2} and pH are both measured with electrodes, and the total CO_2 content and bicarbonate concentration are determined. A third method (Astrup) consists of determining the pH of blood taken from the patient and then measuring the pH again after the blood has been equilibrated with gases containing known high and low concentrations of P_{CO_2}. The resulting relationship between pH and P_{CO_2} at these different levels allows determination of the patient's P_{CO_2} by interpolation as well as calculation of total CO_2 content and bicarbonate concentration.

Some laboratories also express the acid-base state of the patient in terms of *buffer base*. The buffer base of whole blood is the sum of the conjugate bases and includes bicarbonate and nonbicarbonate buffers. Since hemoglobin is the principal nonbicarbonate buffer, the "normal" value for buffer base varies, depending on the hemoglobin concentration. Nomograms have been constructed (Singer and Hastings) which permit calculation of whole blood buffer base if the hematocrit or hemoglobin and two of the variables in the Henderson-Hasselbalch equation are determined. The term *base excess* is used to describe the amount in mEq./liter by which the observed value for buffer base exceeds the normal value expected on the basis of the hemoglobin concentration. *Base deficit* refers to the amount by which the observed value is lower than the expected normal value.

The term base excess and base deficit are also applied to deviations from the normal value for the *"standard bicarbonate."* Standard bicarbonate is the bicarbonate concentration of whole blood sampled anaerobically and then equilibrated with a gas with a P_{CO_2} of 40 mm. Hg and a high oxygen concentration. It may also be determined by interpolation from the pH-P_{CO_2} relationship obtained by the Astrup method cited above. The normal value is 24 mEq./liter, and deviations above and below this value are termed base excess and base deficit respectively.

A base excess or a base deficit indicates only that base has been added to or lost from the extracellular fluid. The mechanism responsible for the gain or loss of base is not revealed, and a base excess may reflect either a compensated respiratory acidosis or a metabolic alkalosis. If the nature of the disturbance is known to be nonrespiratory in origin, the level of base excess or deficit may be a useful guide to therapy. It must, however, be remembered that the standard bicarbonate measured *in vitro* is not the same as the value which would be obtained if the equilibration of blood to a P_{CO_2} of 40 mm. Hg were carried out in the patient's lungs. In vitro the changes in bicarbonate content during equilibration are confined to the water of red blood cells and plasma. In vivo the changes also take place in the total interstitial fluid volume, and consequently, their effect on bicarbonate concentration—and hence on estimates of base deficit or base excess—are less. In guiding therapy it is the total amount of base excess or deficit in the extracellular fluid which must be determined, and therefore, the values obtained in a blood sample must be corrected appropriately.

Chapter 8

The Defenses of the Respiratory System

A section devoted to the basic mechanisms of respiratory disease would be incomplete without a brief consideration of some of the non gas exchange functions of the respiratory system, for these are important in the understanding of the pathogenesis of disease. The respiratory apparatus, which is designed for gas exchange with the environment, provides a major source of contact between man and his environment. In order to protect itself against many damaging agents in the environment, such as bacteria and particles or noxious gases which may pollute the atmosphere, the respiratory apparatus has elaborate defense mechanisms.

THE UPPER RESPIRATORY TRACT

The upper respiratory tract plays an important role in the defenses of the respiratory system. The ciliated epithelium in the tracheobronchial tree, the layer of mucus covering it and the alveoli are unable to function properly unless the temperature is kept close to that of the body and the air which reaches them is humidified. The upper respiratory tract protects the tracheobronchial tree and lung parenchyma by warming, humidifying and filtering the air as it is inspired through the nasal passages. No matter how cold or dry the atmospheric air may be, it normally is warmed to almost 37° C. and becomes practically saturated by the time it reaches the trachea. The nasal turbinates, which are highly vascular structures with large amounts of blood flowing through them, act as radiators of heat and warm the inspired air as it flows past them. The inspired air is moistened predominantly by the mucous glands of the nasal mucosa which normally supply about 650 ml. of water daily in order to accomplish this feat. A further slight degree of humidification is also probably carried out by the mucous glands of the trachea and bronchi. In disease or
164

in old age the nasal mucosa may not be able to deliver this much fluid; if bronchial secretions develop, they may be thick and viscid. If the inspired air enters directly into the trachea without being properly humidified and warmed by the upper respiratory tract, as may occur in patients with a tracheostomy or in those who have had an endotracheal tube instilled for some time, crusting of secretions may occur unless the inspired air is warmed and humidified artificially.

Although the upper respiratory tract is organized in such a way as to defend against the entry of foreign material into the lower respiratory tract, this defense is not totally effective. The ability of the respiratory system to defend against noxious gases is relatively poor. When aerosols or gases are inhaled, the concentration in various parts of the respiratory tree depends on respiratory dynamics, the particle size of the aerosol, and the chemical and physical characteristics of the gases. Large particles and water-soluble gases deposit mainly in the upper parts of the respiratory pathways. Smaller particles and insoluble gases settle in the deeper parts of the respiratory tree, including the alveoli, and may lead to considerable inflammation and even pulmonary edema. Fortunately, the lungs have the ability to destroy organisms or to eliminate other foreign agents.

The first line of defense against inhaled particles is at the external openings of the nasal passages, the nares, where the long hairs filter out the larger particles in the air. Because of turbulence and inertial impaction, inhaled particles larger than 10μ in diameter which escape past the external nares are largely filtered out in the nose and trapped in the mucus which coats the nasal mucous membrane.

THE SNEEZE REFLEX

Sneezing is one defense mechanism against irritant materials in the upper respiratory tract. The nervous impulses responsible for this reflex are elicited by irritation of the nasal mucous membrane and stimulation of the sensory receptors of the trigeminal nerves. The sneeze is characterized by a deep inspiration which is followed by a violent expiration with the mouth closed so that the expiratory blast is discharged through the nose.

THE LARYNX

If one inspects the glottis indirectly with a laryngeal mirror, it is seen to widen during inspiration and narrow during expiration.

Closure of the larynx protects the respiratory tract from the aspiration of foreign substances. For instance, during swallowing closure of the glottis prevents food from entering the trachea. Closure of the larynx is essential for the development of positive pressure within the thorax or abdomen, such as during a cough or defecation. Laryngospasm creating strong resistance to airflow may develop reflexly to stimuli applied to nonrespiratory organs such as the esophagus. If closure of the larynx persists for a long period, such as during severe paroxysms of coughing, deleterious effects may be produced because the greatly prolonged increase in intrathoracic pressure may interfere with the venous return to the heart and lead to circulatory collapse and syncope.

It was formerly believed that it was extremely difficult for foreign material to gain entrance into the lung. The larynx was regarded as a vigilant watchdog which went into spasm with the slightest irritation, inducing a cough which rejected the foreign material. It is now known that this process applies only to foreign material which irritates the mucous membrane of the respiratory tract. Experiments with non-irritating radiopaque oils containing iodine, such as lipiodol, have shown that foreign material can be readily aspirated into the depths of the lungs even by a normal unanesthetized person. It is evident that secretions from the upper respiratory tract can follow the same course, especially during sleep. Since the upper respiratory tract is not sterile, it is obvious that the lung may be continually contaminated by a great variety of bacteria, fungi and viruses. When one considers the complexity and tortuosity of the whole tract, which invites trapping and pocketing, it is a marvel that the lung is not a cesspool of constant suppuration. That the normal lung is not is due to the operation of very active and effective defense mechanisms which normally protect the tracheobronchial tree from aspiration of foreign substances or accumulation of secretions. Foreign material which manages to evade the defense barriers of the nasopharynx and the larynx and enter the tracheobronchial tree can be removed by other defense mechanisms. About 90 per cent of the particles between 2 and 10μ in diameter settle out on the mucociliary blanket of the tracheobronchial epithelium. The majority of the particles between 0.5 and 2 μ in diameter penetrate to the alveolar ducts and alveoli where they are deposited by gravitational forces and, to a lesser extent, by Brownian movement. The defenses likely to be involved in handling these foreign particles include the mucociliary and other defense mechanisms present in the respiratory tract which act to reduce the dose of contaminants presented to the alveoli and to remove particles trapped on their surface, the phagocytic activity of alveolar macrophages, and defenses contributed by the epithelium.

THE LOWER RESPIRATORY TRACT

MUCOCILIARY SYSTEM

The adherence and the elimination of particles which enter the respiratory tract, whether organic or inorganic, is carried out by a thin film of mucus with elastic and adhesive properties, which is constantly moving toward the epiglottis because of the whip-like activity of cilia.

RESPIRATORY EPITHELIUM

Ciliated columnar epithelium lines the rigid and noncollapsible areas of the respiratory tract, such as the nose, the paranasal sinuses, the trachea and the larger bronchi. It has been estimated that approximately 250 fine hair-like projections about 0.5 microns in length and 0.25 microns in diameter arise from the surface of each epithelial cell. In nonrigid areas, such as the oropharynx, the terminal and respiratory bronchioles, the epithelium is cuboidal and not ciliated. Secretions are carried away from these areas by the squeezing action of the surrounding muscle fibers.

Goblet cells, which are plump elongated cells, are situated either singly or in groups between the ciliated epithelial cells. They are abundant in the proximal part of the tracheobronchial tree, particularly at the bifurcations of the larger bronchi, and are more sparse peripherally. It has been shown that acetylcholine serves as the chemical mediator in the nervous control of the goblet cells.

Mucous glands are only found in airways which contain cartilage and are more numerous in the larger bronchi where the cartilage plates are more numerous. They are innervated by the cholinergic division of the autonomic nervous system; stimulation of the vagus nerve results in an outpouring of secretion.

RESPIRATORY MUCUS

A thin, transparent film of mucus covers the epithelial lining of the upper and lower respiratory tract. While it has not been possible to actually measure the amount of mucus secreted by the tracheobronchial tree under normal conditions, it has been estimated that 100 ml. of mucus is produced in the tracheobronchial tree of a healthy person every 24 hours. It contains approximately 95 per cent water, and the remainder is a mixture of mucoproteins, mucopolysaccharides and some lipid. This mixed secretion is derived from three sources: the watery serous component is derived from the capillaries and seeps out between the epithelial cells in the walls of the respiratory tract; the remainder is secreted from the goblet cells and the mucus glands in the walls of the respiratory tract. Because of its viscosity, elasticity and particularly its adhesiveness, it is able to trap, transport and eliminate foreign substances in the inspired air.

CILIA

The cilia beat in a constant, rhythmic manner at a rate of approximately 1000 to 1500 times each minute. The ciliary beat consists of a rapid forward motion, which results in the cilium becoming almost upright, and a slower recoil back to its original position, which is curved and leaning backward. The rapid forward motion is about three times as fast as the slower backward recoil, and this causes the mucus to flow toward the glottis at the rate of approximately 10 to 20 mm./minute. This would constitute approximately a mile/week. In the upper respiratory tract, mucus is propelled from the nose and sinuses to the pharynx, and in the tracheobronchial tree, mucus is propelled upward toward the glottis.

Ciliary activity carries particles and macrophages on the mucous lining layer of the respiratory epithelium to larger bronchi where the cough reflex is important in their clearance. Ciliary activity is influenced by numerous agents; it is stimulated by acetycholine, inorganic ions, weak acids and low concentrations of local anesthetics and is inhibited by low humidity, alcohol, cigarette smoke or other noxious gases.

THE COUGH REFLEX

Cough is a violent expiratory blast which takes place against a partially closed glottis. It differs from a sneeze in that it is less explosive and is perhaps easier to control voluntarily. It helps to protect the tracheobronchial tree from the entry of foreign substances or the accumulation of bronchopulmonary secretions.

A cough is induced by an irritation of the afferent fibers of the pharyngeal distribution of the glossopharyngeal nerve as well as the sensory endings of the vagus nerve in the larynx, trachea and larger bronchi. The smaller bronchioles are relatively insensitive to irritants; it has been shown that if a radiopaque solution is inserted into a bronchopleural fistula, a cough reflex is not elicited until the fluid reaches the larger bronchi. Cough may also be stimulated by impulses which arise from nerve endings located in the mucous membrane of the pharynx, the esophagus and the pleural surfaces as well as the external auditory canal. The impulses are transmitted to the "cough center" in the medulla, which sends impulses to the muscular systems of the chest and the larynx, and a cough results. The stimuli may be inflammatory, such as an infection; mechanical, such as smoke, dust or foreign bodies; chemical, such as irritating gases; or thermal, such as cold air. Thermal stimulation, however, generally occurs only if the tracheobronchial tree has already been affected by other irritants.

The act of coughing, which is illustrated in Figure 61, comprises four separate and distinct phases. The first phase, the initial irritation, induces the second phase, which is a deep inspiration. The third and fourth components comprise the expiratory act. During the short third stage, the glottis is quickly and tightly closed while the expiratory intercostal and the abdominal muscles contract forcibly so that the intrathoracic and intra-abdominal pressures rise; this may be called the "compressive phase." After the intrathoracic pressure has reached a very high level, the glottis suddenly opens slightly. Since the intra-abdominal pressure is now higher than the intrathoracic pressure, the diaphragm is pushed up, producing a violent, explosive movement of air from the lower to the upper respiratory tract. This fourth stage is the "expulsive phase." As soon as the glottis opens, the soft palate rises and closes off the nasopharynx. Consequently, any foreign material expelled from the respiratory tract by the force of the cough enters the mouth and may be expectorated.

Through the use of radiopaque oils, it has been demonstrated that the intrathoracic airways are compressed concurrently with the onset of the expiratory blast of air. Because of this narrowing, the airflow velocity becomes exceedingly great and jet-like, and any foreign material is expelled in a manner similar to that of a bullet from the barrel of a pistol. In addition, it has been shown that the bronchi, which vary in size in an undulatory manner during normal breathing, may actually develop peristaltic expulsive waves originating in the finger bronchi and traveling upward during a cough. The

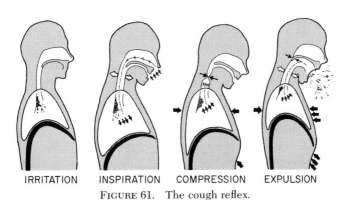

IRRITATION   INSPIRATION   COMPRESSION   EXPULSION
FIGURE 61.   The cough reflex.

bronchial undulations of normal breathing and the peristaltic waves of a cough are probably additional protective mechanisms by which foreign material is moved from the lower respiratory tract to higher levels.

In the smaller bronchioles and in the lung parenchyma, the air blast of the expulsive phase is so feeble that there may be little effect on any foreign material lying in these areas. Instead, this must be moved upward into the larger bronchi by the continuous action of the cilia. In addition, the foreign material may be forced into the larger bronchi by the normal undulating peristalsis of the bronchial tree as well as by the squeeze of the chest which occurs during the expulsive phase of a cough. Expulsion of this material may then be completed by the expiratory blast of a succeeding cough.

The diaphragm also plays an active role in coughing. During the initial deep inspiration, it contracts and descends. It remains fixed in this low position as long as the glottis is closed because the elevations of both the intrapulmonary and the intra-abdominal pressures are approximately equal. When the glottis opens during the expulsive phase, the intrapulmonary pressure falls, and the diaphragm sharply ascends because of the greatly increased intra-abdominal pressure produced by the violently contracting abdominal muscles. It is likely that the diaphragm rises passively during this phase of the cough, but it is also possible that the diaphragm regulates the expulsive force of the cough by controlling the upward push of the abdominal viscera.

THE ALVEOLAR SURFACE

Particles deposited distal to the ciliated columnar epithelium (i.e., in the terminal and respiratory bronchioles) are cleared much more slowly; their clearance depends on the rate of phagocytosis by alveolar or interstitial macrophages as well as the rate of fluid transport from alveoli to the mucociliary blanket.

While the function of the alveolar surface is to facilitate diffusion between external and internal environments, its anatomical structure is organized along the same lines as other exposed surfaces: its connective tissue resembles that of other surfaces, its blood supply is rich and its epithelium is unique.

The continuous alveolar epithelial layers are constituted of pulmonary surface epithelial cells (type I pneumonocytes) and great alveolar cells (type II pneumonocytes). "Free cells," which are large mononuclear ameboid phagocytes called alveolar macrophages, rest on this lining. Under some conditions—for example, following pulmonary edema or pulmonary infection — the pool of free cells may be enriched by other cell types derived from the blood.

Within the alveolar epithelium, secretory activity is carried out principally by the great alveolar cell (type II pneumonocyte), which is distributed with fair uniformity over the alveolar surface. The presumptive secretory product of these cells, the multilamellar bodies (or cytosomes), are products of a lysosomal system modified in this cell to favor secretion. The secretion is rich in phospholipid but probably contains protein as well; the link between it and pulmonary surfactant remains circumstantial but very strong. In addition to stabilizing the alveolar surface against collapse (see Chapter 1), it is possible that this secretion has other qualities of possible value in the lungs' defenses.

Alveolar macrophages constitute a unique feature of alveolar defense because the cells regularly scavenge the surface of the epithelium. The defensive capacity of alveolar macrophages, like that of other phagocytes, principally resides in their ability to digest harmful objects. Although large numbers of infectious particles are continuously deposited in the lung, the alveolar surface is usually sterile. It is in the phagocytic and lytic potential of the alveolar macrophages that most of the known bactericidal properties of the lungs reside. Like other phagocytes, alveolar macrophages are rich in lysosomes. These lysosomes attach themselves to the phagocytic membrane surrounding the ingested bacteria. Then the lytic enzymes kill and digest the bacteria. It has been shown that the bactericidal activity of the lungs is reduced by ethanol intoxication, hypoxia, cigarette smoke, acute starvation and corticosteroid injection. Other factors such as nitrogen dioxide and ozone are also reported to disturb macrophage function.

The lung free cells also participate in the clearance of nonliving insoluble dust and debris from the nonciliated portions of the lung. Particles remaining on the surface of the alveoli, either within free alveolar macrophages or on the fluid surface, are removed to the ciliated part of the lung. The speed of removal is determined by the macrophage migration and by the mouthward flow of alveolar capillary transudate mixed with alveolar cell secretions. The biologic half-time for removal of insoluble particles from the alveolar surface to the ciliated surface is about 24 hours.

Not all deposited particles remain on the internal surface of the lungs. Phagocytosis plays an important role in the prevention of the entry of particles into the fixed tissue of the lung, but some do enter the alveolar lining and become sequestered in the interstitial tissue or enter the lymphatics. The biological half-life of these particles can be weeks to years. The release of particles that are within cells in the alveolar wall into the alveolar space depends on the turnover time of the cells and their rate of desquamation into the alveolar spaces.

When airborne biological agents such as viruses, fungi or bacteria are inhaled, they become subject to the same mechanical clearance mechanisms as other particles. However, the ability of the biological organisms to cause a significant effect is generally not the contact time but the occurrence of multiplication. The defense against biological agents involves a second line of defense—namely, the "biocidal mechanisms"—which operates through the same media as the mechanical defense mechanism, i.e., through the mucus and phagocytic cells of the alveoli. The mucus contains biocidal agents such as immunoglobulins and lysosomes, and the phagocytic cells exert biocidal activity by killing or inhibiting multiplication of the microbes.

SECRETORY IMMUNOGLOBULINS

Respiratory secretions contain four classes of immunoglobulins: IgA, IgG, IgM and IgE. Most of these immunoglobulins are synthesized locally by the plasma cells in the submucosa of the respiratory tract; only a small portion normally is derived from serum by transudation. The contribution from serum immunoglobulins increases markedly during an inflammatory process when there is a profuse outpouring of vascular fluid. The first three classes play an important role as the body's first line of defense against invading microorganisms, and they may also help regulate the normal microorganisms which reside in the mucous membranes. IgE is the mediator of immediate hypersensitivity reaction.

Secretory IgA is the predominant immunoglobulin in respiratory secretions. It is made up of two molecules of serum IgA and small glycoprotein component, the *secretory piece*, which is linked to the serum IgA molecules by covalent disulfide bonds. The other classes of immunoglobulins present in respiratory secretions do not appear to contain secretory piece. The function of the secretory piece is not well understood, but there is some evidence that it facilitates the capability of the secretory IgA molecule to function as an antibody in secretions because of its resistance to degradation by proteolytic enzymes.

Secretory IgA has been shown to possess virus neutralizing activity but, because it is unable to fix complement, its role in protecting against bacterial infections is unclear at present. IgG and IgM, on the other hand, have both antiviral and antibacterial activities and are capable of complement fixation, thus facilitating the opsonization and phagocytosis of bacteria. Protection of the host against reinfection and mucosal colonization of noninvasive viruses appears to be better correlated with the level of secretory immunoglobulins rather than serum antibodies. Because secretory immunoglobulins are produced largely at the mucosal level, the secretory antibody response is of a greater magnitude when a viral vaccine such as influenza vaccine is applied locally to the respiratory mucosa than it is if a vaccine is administered parenterally. Certain persons suffering from a deficiency of secretory IgA, such as occurs in ataxia telangiectasia, are prone to develop recurrent sinopulmonary infections.

METABOLISM OF THE LUNG

In addition to an elaborate defense mechanism, the lung has other nongas exchange functions. The lung is a site of active metabolism, and it has been estimated that it normally utilizes as much as 10 per cent of the total oxygen consumed, and even more with pulmonary disorders such as cancer and tuberculosis. This high level of oxygen consumption is not surprising because of the presence of cellular elements, such as the type II cell, responsible for surfactant biosynthesis which possess high metabolic activity. In addition, alveolar macrophages which have been estimated to number 600,000,000 have a respiratory rate which is approximately ten times that of the polymorphonuclear leukocyte and three times that of the monocyte.

Another important function of the lung is its ability to influence the circulating level of certain vasoactive substances. It is capable of inactivating circulating bradykinin, prostaglandins, serotonin and histamine but has little effect on epinephrine. The lung also contains an enzyme which is responsible for converting the relatively inactive polypeptide, angiotensin I, to the potent vasoconstrictor, angiotensin II.

SUMMARY

Most of the important patterns of disease affecting the respiratory system are the result of inhaled biological agents such as viruses or bacteria, irritants or allergens which have bypassed the defenses of the respiratory apparatus. Consideration of the role of the non gas exchange functions of the lung in combating disease has only recently been receiving attention but is of obvious importance in the pathophysiology of pulmonary disease and in the production of signs and symptoms.

Section Two

THE MANIFESTATIONS OF RESPIRATORY DISEASE

Chapter 9

The Manifestations of Pulmonary Disease

When the defenses of the respiratory tract are strained or overcome or disturbances in function occur, symptoms and signs develop. In general, one can say that symptoms are what the patient feels, and signs are what the examiner discovers during the course of the physical examination. It is not always possible, however, to make a sharp distinction between symptoms and physical signs, for some manifestations such as dyspnea, cough and cyanosis may be both subjective and objective. There are certain primary symptoms and signs which develop as a result of altered function of the respiratory system.

PRIMARY MANIFESTATIONS

SYMPTOMS

The primary, or cardinal, symptoms of respiratory disease are excessive nasal secretions, cough, expectoration of sputum or blood, breathlessness, wheezing and chest pain.

EXCESSIVE NASAL SECRETIONS

Nasal secretions are normally swept backward to the pharynx by ciliary action, and one is usually unaware of this. Infection of the upper respiratory tract, irritants or allergens which induce an allergic response characteristically produce obstruction of the nasal passages, congestion of the nasal mucosa, an outpouring of mucus and frequent sneezing. In allergic states the mucosa appears pale and boggy, and the discharge is thin and watery. If there is infection, the nasal mucosa is hyperemic, and the discharge is usually purulent. If the paranasal sinuses are involved, pain may be felt over the corresponding areas of the face and scalp. Excessive nasal secretions may occur premenstrually, during pregnancy and in male patients who are being treated with estrogen for carcinoma of the prostate gland.

If excessive secretions accumulate, they may be felt in the back of the throat (postnasal drip), and they may induce coughing or frequent throat clearing, or "hawking." Persons who are exposed to dry air in artificially heated environments commonly have excessive postnasal secretions. A postnasal discharge is also a complaint of patients who have nasal obstruction due to a deviated septum or infection and patients who are exposed to the chronic irritation of smoke, dust or fumes. Excessive upper respiratory tract infections may lead to other manifestations of respiratory disease, particularly if the defense mechanisms of the lower respiratory tract become ineffective.

COUGH

No one goes through life without an occasional cough, and almost everyone develops a cough at some time each winter. Many adults cough a few times on first arising in the morning because of secretions in the posterior pharynx and the trachea. A cough may simply be habitual, or it may signify the presence of a serious pulmonary disease and, therefore, always deserves a thorough investigation. It is important to remember that, although the cough reflex is usually initiated in the tracheobronchial tree, the primary cause of the cough may be nonpulmonary. For example, left ventricular failure, which causes pulmonary congestion, is often associated with a cough.

Although the cough reflex, which has been described in Section One, is a defense of the tracheobronchial tree, certain of its inherent features may have detrimental effects. The deep inspiration which precedes the expiratory blast may occasionally drag secretions deeper into the peripheral portions of the lungs, or purulent secretions in one portion of a lung may be splattered throughout the lungs during the expulsive phase and then inhaled into new areas.

The Cough Syndrome. Some patients may develop lightheadedness or may even faint during a coughing spell. This is because the prolonged elevation of intrapulmonary pressure which occurs during the compressive phase of a cough interferes with the venous return to the thorax and results in a fall in the cardiac output and cerebral ischemia. When lightheadedness results from a coughing spell, it is known as "cough syndrome," and when fainting occurs it is called "cough syncope."

EXPECTORATION OF SPUTUM

Healthy persons do not ordinarily expectorate sputum, except on exposure to excessive external irritants. On the other hand, since sputum, which is brought into the pharynx by ciliary activity or a cough may be swallowed, one should not assume that there are no abnormal secretions just because no sputum is expectorated.

Whenever a patient produces sputum, it is of the greatest importance to determine its source, color, volume and consistency. If most of the sputum is cleared from the throat by "hawking" rather than by coughing, it is likely that the secretions originate in the nasal passages or the paranasal sinuses rather than in the bronchial tree. Very profuse, purulent sputum suggests the presence of gross pulmonary suppuration. If a large volume of sputum is suddenly expectorated after a short illness, a lung abscess is almost certainly present. If it has gradually increased in amount over a period of years, chronic bronchitis or bronchiectasis is the likely diagnosis.

The color of the sputum is important. Yellow sputum indicates an infection; green sputum, which is due to the presence of verdoperoxidase which has been liberated from polymorphonuclear leukocytes in the sputum, is indicative of stagnant pus in dilated bronchi (i.e., bronchiectasis), a lung abscess or an infected paranasal sinus. Many patients often say that the sputum is green early in the morning but becomes yellow later during the day. This is most likely due to the accumulation of secretions during sleep with the consequent liberation of verdoperoxidase. This accumulated material is the first to be expectorated on arising and is then followed by the usual yellow sputum.

The character and consistency of the sputum may also yield useful information. In chronic bronchitis the sputum is usually mucoid, sticky, and grey or white in color. A pneumococcal infection is often characterized by scanty, extremely tenacious, blood-stained sputum. A foul odor is practically always indicative of a putrid lung abscess or gross bronchiectasis. Mucoid sputum which is stained a deep, pink color, the so-called "currant jelly" sputum, may occur with a pulmonary neoplasm; profuse, frothy, pink watery material is characteristic of pulmonary edema.

EXPECTORATION OF BLOOD

Blood may be mixed with sputum in varying amounts, or it may comprise the entire expectorate. Although the term hemoptysis has been used to describe both of these situations, it is important to distinguish between them. Some blood is frequently expectorated during acute pneumococcal pneumonia; this is usually mixed with very tenacious sputum which is rusty in color. Streaks and specks of blood in sputum occur commonly in acute respiratory infections, particularly during episodes of acute bronchitis. They probably result from rupture of vessels in the congested bronchial mucosa.

The expectoration of pure blood is a serious symptom. It may be the first manifestation of active pulmonary tuberculosis, and often there are no other associated symptoms. Aside from tuberculosis, the commonest causes of hemoptysis are a pulmonary infarction, bronchiectasis, mitral stenosis, bronchogenic carcinoma and pulmonary abscess. Frank hemorrhage only occasionally accompanies the bacterial pneumonias and is not a feature of viral or mycoplasmal pneumonias.

Bloody sputum loses much of its significance as far as the lungs are concerned if it is found to be associated with bleeding from a nonpulmonary source. If there is a history of bleeding from the nose or the gums or of the vomiting of blood, it is likely that some of the blood found in the sputum may have been aspirated into the larger bronchi and later expectorated. Abnormal bleeding in other parts of the body suggests that the hemoptysis may be a further indication of a generalized hematologic disorder.

BREATHLESSNESS

Breathlessness (dyspnea) or shortness of breath is an awareness of difficulty in breathing and is a cardinal symptom of cardiorespiratory disease.

A person is not usually aware of his breathing, unless his attention is directed to it, except under circumstances in which ventilation has increased considerably, such as in exercise, or in which a given level of ventilation requires increased effort. When assessing the significance of breathlessness, or dyspnea, it is essential to determine its mode of onset and severity. A sudden change in exercise tolerance has a different significance than a change that has taken place gradually over a number of years, in that it indicates that an acute process has developed.

The severity of breathlessness is assessed clinically by determining the minimum level of activity that is associated with breathlessness. A convenient classification is the following: (a) breathlessness on mild exertion, such as running a short distance or climbing a flight of stairs; (b) breathlessness while walking short distances on the level at an ordinary pace; (c) breathlessness while talking, shaving, washing, etc.; (d) breathlessness at rest; (e) breathlessness while lying down (orthopnea). The factors which are conducive to the subjective sensation of breathlessness are presented in Table 9.

Increased Awareness of Normal Breathing. Awareness of the act of breathing varies in degree from one person to another and even exists in a normal person if he "puts his mind to it." Patients often complain of "shortness of breath" even though there may be no organic reason for it. It must be presumed that the threshold of awareness of the breathing act has increased in these persons. It is not surprising that respiratory irregularities and sensations often arise

TABLE 9

FACTORS CONDUCIVE TO BREATHLESSNESS

A. INCREASED AWARENESS OF NORMAL BREATHING (PSYCHOGENIC)
B. INCREASED RESPIRATORY WORK
   1. Increased ventilation
      a. Exercise
      b. Hypercapnia
      c. Hypoxic hypoxia
      d. Metabolic acidosis
   2. Altered physical properties
      a. Increased lung elastic resistance, e.g., pneumonia, congestion, atelectasis, pneumothorax, pleural effusion
      b. Increased chest wall elastic resistance, e.g., kyphoscoliosis, obesity
      c. Increased bronchial nonelastic resistance, e.g., emphysema, chronic bronchitis, bronchial asthma
C. ABNORMALITY OF RESPIRATORY MUSCLES
   1. Muscular disease
      a. Muscular weakness, e.g., myasthenia gravis, thyrotoxicosis
      b. Muscular paralysis, e.g., poliomyelitis, Guillain-Barré syndrome
      c. Muscular wasting, e.g., muscular dystrophy
   2. Reduced mechanical advantage of muscles
      a. Marked inspiratory position, e.g., emphysema
      b. Marked expiratory position, e.g., obesity

from emotional states, since one of the chief subsidiary functions of the respiratory system is the expression of emotion. Weeping, sobbing, laughing, sighing and groaning are all produced by distortion of the respiratory rhythm. Minor respiratory effects of emotion are seen in the breathlessness of fear or wonder, the shout of elation, the sigh of satisfaction, the gasp of exasperation and the rapid breathing of anger. Variations of these psychophysical effects sometimes occur as symptoms in patients who are emotionally unstable and may be associated with respiratory distress or "shortness of breath." Usually this consists of a sensation of suffocation, choking or oppression in the chest and is often accompanied by other evidences of fear.

A very common complaint is the inability to take a full, satisfactory, deep breath. Introspective people worry about this and try to take deep breaths; the result is that they execute a series of imperfect sighs. The complaint is rarely related to organic disease, and it can almost always be readily cured by explaining that it is a habit due to too close attention to a function that should be unconscious and automatic. Nevertheless, some people are so obsessed by this difficulty that dizziness or faintness and numbness and tingling in the extremities may develop as a result of hyperventilation. In severe or prolonged cases tetany may develop because of the depletion of carbon dioxide with consequent alkalosis. This "hyperventilation syndrome" occurs most commonly in neurotic women and should be suspected if a respiratory alkalosis and a normal arterial oxygen tension are present and there are no signs pointing to organic diseases of the heart, lungs, blood or nervous system.

Increased Respiratory Work.   The rate and depth of respiration are relatively constant during rest, and one is accustomed to his own particular respiratory pattern. In any given person, awareness of the breathing act depends to a large extent on his past experiences. For instance, a person who exercises regularly becomes accustomed to the respiratory effort required for such activity, and he does not characterize such an experience as breathlessness; yet, a less active person may experience dyspnea when he is called upon to perform an equivalent amount of exercise. Awareness of breathing can also be induced in normal subjects by the addition of an artificial resistance so that the respiratory muscles must perform more work to achieve the same ventilation.

Breathlessness is a prevalent symptom in diseases which affect the tracheobronchial tree, the lung parenchyma, the pleural space or the chest wall. On the other hand, in chronic respiratory conditions in which the respiratory rate and depth have been altered for a long period of time, the subject may again become accustomed to the changed pattern of breathing so that the sensation of breathlessness is absent.

Abnormality of Respiratory Muscles.   Breathlessness may also be experienced if the respiratory muscles are abnormal. Under such circumstances, the ability to perform mechanical work may be diminished. This occurs when the muscles are weak, paralyzed or wasted; when breathing takes place in an inspiratory or an expiratory position; and perhaps when the muscles are required to function under hypoxic or ischemic conditions.

The key factor appears to be whether or not the level of ventilation or effort is recognized as being appropriate to the activity. The mechanism by which the inappropriateness is recognized has not been established. It has been suggested that a misalignment between the intrafusal and extrafusal fibers in the respiratory muscles are responsible for the reflex response and that breathlessness is recognized when there is an altered length-tension relationship in the respiratory muscles. When the muscles of breathing are required to perform an inappropriate amount of work, these receptors send impulses to the higher centers through pathways that have not yet been defined.

CHEST PAIN

Pain in the chest is a very common complaint. It very often induces great apprehension because the patient usually thinks this indicates a serious disease of either the lungs or the heart. In most cases no such disease exists, for although it is true that disease of the lungs may produce pain or discomfort in the chest, there are many other causes of chest pain. Consequently, it is important to determine the actual anatomical source of the chest pain. In order to do this, it is important to understand the distribution of the nerve dermatomes over the chest wall and to consider the many possible sources of chest pain.

The Dermatomes.   If nerve roots are irritated as a result of mechanical pressure or infection, pain is frequently felt over the corresponding areas of the skin of the thoracic and abdominal walls supplied by the dorsal roots of the spinal cord. These areas are known as dermatomes. There is a divergence of opinion regarding the exact distribution of dermatomes. Figure 62 illustrates one mode of distribution which has been described. There is no doubt that there is some overlapping of the individual dermatomes; they have been simplified in this illustration.

In determining the source of any chest pain, it is best to suspect and, as far as possible, to examine each component part of the chest from the skin inward. In the following discussion, trauma and other obvious surgical lesions which cause pain are not considered.

The Skin.   Pain is not uncommonly localized in the skin of the chest wall. The cause may be obvious if the pain is caused by a bruise, a boil or a carbuncle. If the pain is caused by inflammation of a posterior root ganglion (herpes zoster), it may develop long before the appearance of the characteristic vesicular rash. Pain due to irritation

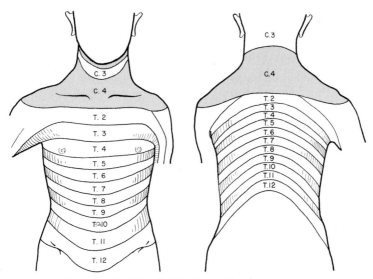

FIGURE 62.   The distribution of the dermatomes.

of the nerve roots is frequently accompanied by hyperalgesia over the corresponding area of skin.

The Ribs and Cartilages. Occasionally a rib may be fractured by a paroxysm of coughing, and this results in localized pain which is accentuated by breathing and coughing as well as tenderness over the affected area. A paroxysm of coughing may also cause a fracture or dislocation of a rib cartilage.

An acutely painful costal cartilage, usually at the costochondral junction, but occasionally in other areas, may develop following a strain on the chest wall, in association with respiratory infections, or even without apparent cause. Pain arising from this source is reproduced exactly when the involved costochondral junction or an area over a painful cartilage is compressed.

Tietze's syndrome is an uncommon cause of costal cartilage pain. This benign condition of unknown etiology may persist for years and consists of pain over one or more costochondral or sternoclavicular junctions and is associated with tender swelling in the affected area.

Osteomyelitis of the ribs of either tuberculous or pyogenic origin and malignant tumors in the ribs, which are usually secondary to cancer of the prostate or the lungs, are rare causes of chest pain. This source of the pain is diagnosed by the presence of tenderness, redness or swelling immediately over a rib.

The Nerves. Actual disease of the intercostal nerves as a cause of chest pain is hard to demonstrate because it is difficult to know whether the pain arises in the nerves, the muscle or the fibroid connective tissue.

Several diseases can involve the posterior nerve roots and lead to chest pain. Herpes zoster, a viral infection of the posterior root ganglions, is characterized by pain which is associated with exquisite hyperesthesia in the area of the distribution of the intercostal nerves or the nerve dermatomes. An eruption consisting of a cluster of small vesicles in the same area usually appears a few days after the onset of the pain. The pain, together with the hyperesthesia, may persist for a period of time after the rash has healed, but the condition may still be recognized by the brownish discoloration of the skin which is characteristic of a healed herpes infection.

Pressure on the posterior nerve root or on the nerve trunk by some disease process causes "root pain" which is usually referred to the peripheral distribution of its dermatome. The pressure on the nerve root is usually due to some manifest organic disease of the vertebrae, such as tuberculosis, degenerative arthritis or a neoplasm.

The Muscles. Pain originating in the thoracic muscles is often confused with pleurisy, since it is generally aggravated by deep breathing. Patients frequently became very anxious because they think that the pain is cardiac in origin, especially if the pain is over the lower left costochondral junctions, which is where many think the heart is located.

Fibrositis should be suspected as the cause of chest pain if there is localized tenderness on deep pressure at the site of the pain or if the pain is reproduced by putting the involved muscle groups into action against resistance.

The Pleura.   Only the parietal layer of the pleura is a source of pain. Irritation of pain fibers in the parietal pleura is referred to the chest wall and characteristically is sharply localized, superficial, knife-like or "catching" in character. It is aggravated by respiratory movements, particularly those of deep inspiration, coughing, sneezing and yawning.

Pain of pleural origin may be associated with any severe disease within the thorax, or it may be due to inflammation of the pleura itself. On the other hand, pleural pain can occur in conditions other than inflammation of the pleura, and inflammation of the pleura does not always necessarily produce pain.

The Diaphragm.   Pain arising from the diaphragmatic pleura is mediated through the phrenic and the intercostal nerves. The central portion of the diaphragm is innervated by the third, fourth and fifth cervical nerves so that irritation of this area results in a sharp pain which is referred to the shoulder on the same side. The pain fibers from the peripheral portion of the diaphragm and its posterior third travel via the fifth and sixth intercostal nerves; irritation of these areas results in pain along the costal margin, which projects into the epigastrium, the subchondral and the lumbar regions.

"Bornholm" disease (epidemic myalgia), an acute febrile illness caused by the Coxsackie B group of viruses, is characterized by fever, profuse sweating, a frontal headache and the sudden onset of an excruciating pain in the subcostal and upper abdominal regions, which has been so severe that it has been called "devil's grip." The pain is due to involvement of the intercostal muscles and the diaphragm, but pleural involvement has been reported in some epidemics.

The Lung Parenchyma.   The lungs are usually regarded as insensitive organs, and if pulmonary disease is accompanied by pain, it is likely that the parietal pleura is secondarily involved. Pain in association with a pneumothorax or a massive collapse of the lung is most likely due to traction on the parietal pleura by adhesions attached to the moving visceral pleura. There are, however, some situations in which pain apparently originates in the lung, pleural involvement not being readily apparent. For instance, a pulmonary neoplasm which does not appear to be involving the pleura sometimes give rise to a deep aching pain. Similarly, an acute atelectasis may be associated with a sudden violent pain, even though it is not associated with a pleural rub or an effusion.

The Tracheobronchial Tree. A raw burning sensation over the sternal area which is aggravated by breathing and coughing often occurs in persons suffering from acute tracheobronchitis.

The Aorta. A dissecting aortic aneurysm produces a severe retrosternal pain which radiates to the back, is sudden in onset and rapidly becomes agonizing.

The Heart. Pain due to cardiac disease need rarely be confused with pleural or pulmonary pain. Ischemia or hypoxia of the myocardium results in excess acid metabolites which result from anaerobic tissue metabolism and stimulate the nerve endings in the myocardium. The resulting impulses are sent through the cardiac plexus to the upper five or six thoracic sympathetic ganglia, through the white rami of the second to fifth thoracic nerve roots into the spinal cord, from which they reach the skeletal nerves via their respective posterior roots.

Cardiac pain is typically substernal and is brought on by exertion. "Angina of effort" is a pain resulting from ischemia of the myocardium due to an inadequate coronary blood flow; it is often described as a heavy, vise-like gripping sensation. It frequently radiates and is referred mainly to the base of the neck and the jaw, over the shoulders, the pectoral muscles and down the arms. For some reason, pain is referred more frequently down the left arm rather than the right. The pain of angina of effort forces the patient to rest which usually results in the subsidence of the pain, but it is also frequently relieved or prevented by nitroglycerine.

The pain resulting from an occlusion of one of the coronary arteries has the same distribution as that of angina of effort, but it is usually much more severe and "crushing." It may develop without preceding exertion and frequently develops while the patient is resting. In contrast to angina of effort, it does not disappear if the patient rests or takes nitroglycerine but may continue for minutes or hours, often requiring powerful analgesics for its relief.

The Pericardium. Inflammation of the pericardium may produce chest pain which is situated in either the substernal area or the left mammary region. The pain may vary from a dull burning discomfort to a feeling of severe pressure which simulates a myocardial infarction. It frequently becomes aggravated if the patient lies in a supine position or extends his neck. The explanation for this phenomenon is not apparent.

Neither the visceral pericardium nor the internal surface of the parietal pericardium contains any pain fibers, and only the lower part of the external surface of the parietal layer of the pericardium is sensitive. A lesion which affects the lower part of the pericardium frequently involves the adjacent diaphragmatic pleura so that, in addition to the characteristic substernal pain of the pericarditis, pain may also be felt in the neck and shoulder.

The Pulmonary Vessels. Patients with pulmonary hypertension may develop chest pain on exertion which simulates, in many respects, the pain of angina of effort. Similarly, a pulmonary embolus may cause pain which is similar to that of a myocardial infarction. It has been suggested that this pain is due to either dilatation of the pulmonary artery or ischemia of the myocardium of the right ventricle.

Psychogenic Pain. Despite the lack of obvious organic disease, a patient may complain of a nondescript chest pain or one which is much like that due to organic disease. Such patients are frequently apprehensive about the possibility of cardiac or pulmonary disease. Anxious patients often also may complain of lancinating pains in the chest which are sharp and fleeting and are often described by the patient as "stabbing." They are generally caused by muscle spasm and are usually inconsequential.

SIGNS

When certain properties of the lung and thorax are altered by disease processes, characteristic physical signs can be elicited by the clinician during the physical examination of the respiratory system. These abnormal physical signs, taken in conjunction with an analysis of the patient's symptoms, help the physician to arrive at an accurate diagnosis of the underlying disease process. The following discussion deals with the mechanisms involved in the production of the more important of these abnormal physical signs.

When a pathological process involves either the lung or the chest wall, the properties of the thorax are altered with respect to size, distensibility and sound transmission.

SIZE

Any alteration in the size of one lung is reflected by a shift of the mobile mediastinum from its normal midline position within the thorax. The mediastinum may be shifted from its normal midline position by a lesion of the lung parenchyma, a disease affecting the pleural space, distortion of the bony chest cage or an abnormality of the diaphragm.

When one lung becomes affected by either fibrosis or atelectasis, the mediastinum shifts toward the affected side because the end-expiratory intrapleural pressure is lower on this side (Fig. 63).

Conversely, if fluid or air collects in a pleural space, the mediastinum is displaced toward the opposite side (Fig. 64) because the end-expiratory intrapleural pressure on the affected side rises. The mediastinum shifts to the opposite side, which has a considerably lower intrapleural pressure.

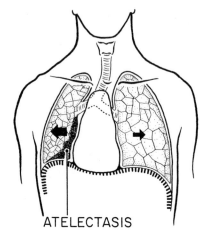

FIGURE 63.   The mechanism of the shift of the mediastinum in atelectasis.

FIGURE 64.   The mechanism of the shift of the mediastinum in a pleural effusion.

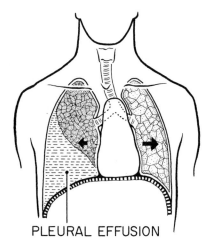

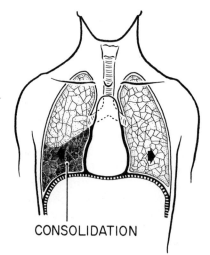

FIGURE 65.   The position of the mediastinum in consolidation.

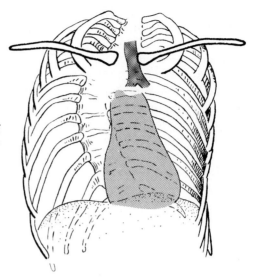

FIGURE 66. The position of the mediastinum in severe kyphoscoliosis.

In contrast, when consolidation of a portion of the lung develops, there is no change in the size of the affected lung, and as shown in Figure 65, the mediastinum remains in its normal midline position.

Distortion of the chest cage, as in severe kyphoscoliosis of the thoracic spine, generally causes displacement of the mediastinum toward the side of the lung which is compressed (Fig. 66).

If the abdominal contents herniate into the thoracic cavity through one of the foramina of the diaphragm, the mediastinum may be displaced to the opposite side because the intra-abdominal pressure, which is normally greater than the intrapleural pressure, is

FIGURE 67. The mechanism of the shift of the mediastinum in herniation of abdominal viscera.

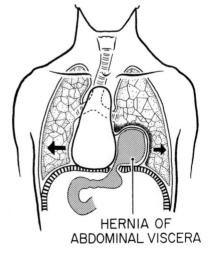

HERNIA OF
ABDOMINAL VISCERA

transmitted into the affected hemithorax so that the end-expiratory intrapleural pressure on the unaffected normal side is lower (Fig. 67).

If both lungs are diseased, the situation may be different. The position of the mediastinum will depend on the lung which has the most disease. Thus, if fibrosis or atelectasis is present in both lungs, the mediastinum will be shifted toward a more involved lung; and if there is a bilateral pleural effusion or pneumothorax, it will be shifted toward the side which is least involved. Understandably, if consolidation is present in both lungs, the mediastinum will still occupy a central position. Similarly, in emphysema, in which both lungs are usually equally hyperinflated, the mediastinum remains in its normal midline position. On the other hand, if there is hyperinflation of one lung, such as occurs with a check-valve obstruction of a major bronchus, the mediastinum is shifted to the opposite normal side.

MOVEMENT

All disease processes that affect the lung parenchyma, the pleural space or the chest cage alter the distensibility of the lungs and thoracic cage so that movement is affected. Consequently, the earliest manifestation of bronchopulmonary disease is diminished movement of that part of the chest wall which overlies the diseased area.

Chest movement is diminished when there are regional variations in the forces applied to the chest wall by the respiratory muscles, as in muscular dystrophy or poliomyelitis; when the chest wall itself offers an increased resistance to distention of the lung, as in obesity or kyphoscoliosis; when there is a regional increase in the resistance to distention of the lung, as in consolidation, fibrosis and atelectasis; or when the lung is compressed by fluid or air in the pleural space.

Chest movement is also reduced when the lungs are hyperinflated because of an increased resistance to expiratory airflow or a loss of elastic recoil, as in emphysema. In these conditions the chest cage enlarges to assume a more inspiratory position and exhibits restricted movement on both sides. In this position the intercostal muscles are less efficient and the accessory muscles of respiration assume a more positive role during inspiration. The diaphragm is depressed by the hyperinflated lungs so that when it contracts, the lower thorax may actually be drawn inward during inspiration.

SOUND TRANSMISSION

Sound consists of rapidly moving vibrations in the air. In order that sound may be heard, the frequency of vibrations must be within a certain range and above a certain minimal intensity.

Pitch.   The number of cycles of repetition that occur in one second is known as the "frequency" of a sound, and this accounts for the *pitch* of a musical note. Low frequencies produce a low note; high frequencies produce a high note. The pitch of a sound also depends on the length and diameter of the tube in which it is produced. The shorter and narrower the tube, the higher the pitch. Since each succeeding branch of the tracheobronchial tree is shorter and narrower than its predecessor, the pitch of the sound produced within succeeding branches becomes higher and higher, finally reaching a peak in the terminal bronchioles.

Intensity. The *intensity* of a sound, or its loudness, depends on both the energy with which it is transmitted and its frequency. Sound loses its intensity if it has to pass through one medium, such as air, into another medium, such as water, because the sound waves are reflected and absorbed by the fluid-air interfaces.

Timbre. The *timbre* of a sound is distinct from its pitch or intensity, in that this represents its character or quality. It depends on the relative proportion between the fundamental tone and the overtones. It is by means of the timbre that one is able to distinguish between sounds of the same pitch and intensity which are produced by different instruments. In the respiratory system sounds result from phonation or breathing, or they may also be imparted to the chest by means of percussion.

Vocal Sounds. Voice sounds are produced by the vibrations of the vocal cords in the larynx, which acts like a reed instrument. The sound is then carried upward into the oral cavity and the paranasal sinuses, thereby increasing its intensity and producing a particular tonal quality. The vocal sound is also carried downward through the tracheobronchial tree as far as the chest wall, causing the thorax to vibrate in unison with the laryngeal sounds. It is thought that the major portions of the vibrations are conducted within the lumen of the bronchi, and the remainder are conducted down along the bronchial walls. The sound produced within the trachea has been estimated to have vibrations of approximately 400 cycles per second, whereas that produced within the terminal bronchiole has vibrations of approximately 1700 cycles per second.

Breath Sounds. Most of the breath sounds which are produced within the tracheobronchial tree during inspiration and expiration are conducted within the lumen of the bronchi in a manner similar to vocal sounds. The passage of air into and out of the bronchial tree during respiration is illustrated in Figure 68. During inspiration, eddies and turbulence are produced when the air current strikes the sharp borders of the bronchial bifurcations. As the air moves outward during expiration, it mixes with air currents coming from other small airways and strikes against the wall of the parent bronchus, creating turbulence and small eddies, but presumably these are less than those which occur during inspiration because the outgoing air does not encounter any sharp bifurcations.

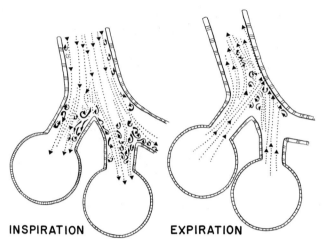

INSPIRATION   EXPIRATION

FIGURE 68.   The production of turbulence in the airways during inspiration and expiration.

It is believed that the alveoli act as a "selective transmitter" of sound in that they dampen the high frequency vibrations produced in the bronchial tree. In this way sounds with a frequency of 100 to 150 cycles per second are allowed to pass through the alveoli to the chest wall, while those with a higher frequency are not. If the lung becomes diseased, and the number of normally functioning alveoli diminishes, this "selective transmitter" property is believed to be affected, so that the higher frequency vibrations are transmitted to the chest wall. The transmission of sound is affected by changes in the density of the chest cage and its contents. In the physical examination of the chest, the transmission of sound is assessed by percussion, palpation and auscultation.

PERCUSSION

Percussion of the chest produces vibrations of the chest wall and the underlying lung parenchyma. As is shown in Figure 69 these vibrations penetrate medially into the thoracic cavity and also radiate laterally over the chest wall. The heavier the percussion stroke, the deeper the penetration and lateral radiation of these vibrations so that, ultimately, the whole thoracic cavity can be made to vibrate. The pitch of the sound produced by percussion enables the examiner to determine the ratio between air-containing tissue and solid tissue that exists in the area underlying the percussing finger. Percussion over normal air-containing tissue produces slow vibrations so that the resultant sound has a low pitch and is relatively long in duration. Percussion over an area in which the ratio of air-to-solid tissue is in-

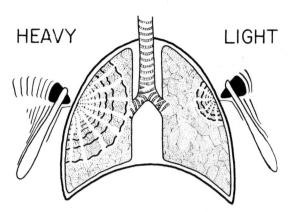

FIGURE 69.   The vibrations produced by light and heavy percussion of the chest wall.

creased produces a sound with a lower than normal pitch. This is the sound heard over a large collection of air in the pleural space or in emphysema, in which there is a generalized overdistention of air-containing alveoli. On the other hand, percussion over an area in which the air-to-solid tissue ratio is lower than normal, as in atelectasis or consolidation, produces a high-pitched or dull sound. Since the normal chest wall is approximately 1 inch thick, the vibrations produced by light percussion will only penetrate a short distance if there is obesity or if the thickness of the musculature of the chest wall is increased; therefore, percussion over a lesion which is deep within the lung will not result in abnormal sounds.

PALPATION

The vibrations produced over the chest wall by vocal sounds are called *vocal fremitus.* When the vibrations are felt by the palpating hand they are known as *tactile fremitus,* and when they are heard by means of a stethoscope they are known as *auditory fremitus.*

The intensity of vocal fremitus is the same over both lungs, except over the right upper lobe. Here, the intensity of the fremitus is increased because the large bronchi are situated close to the chest wall. Vocal fremitus is somewhat less intense in women and in children than it is in men, presumably because their voices are less resonant.

Vocal fremitus increases in intensity when the underlying lung parenchyma becomes more dense as a result of a disease process. When the alveoli are filled with inflammatory exudate, as in pulmonary consolidation, the vibrations produced by the spoken voice are clearly felt and heard over the overlying chest wall, provided the bronchus is patent. Presumably, loss of the "selective transmitter"

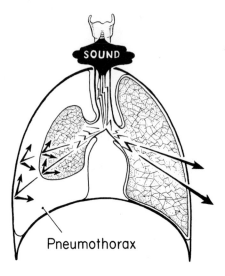

FIGURE 70. The reflection of sound waves at tissue-air interfaces in a pneumothorax.

property of the lung parenchyma permits the higher frequency vibrations to pass through to the chest wall.

Vocal fremitus decreases in intensity when either fluid or air is present in the pleural space because the sound vibrations passing through the underlying lung parenchyma are reflected and absorbed by the increased number of fluid-air interfaces (Fig. 70). Most of the sound vibrations which manage to pass through the visceral surface of the fluid or air are reflected by the parietal surface, and the vibrations are either diminished in intensity or completely dissipated before they finally reach the chest wall. Vocal fremitus will also be diminished if the chest wall is very muscular or obese because of the increased mass of tissue and distance through which the sound must travel.

AUSCULTATION

Breath Sounds. The breath sounds heard over the chest wall during auscultation differ considerably, both in quality and intensity, from those actually produced by the turbulence created by the movement of air within the tracheobronchial tree.

The sounds which are heard during auscultation over normal lung parenchyma are called *vesicular breath sounds*. The inspiratory sound is easily heard, but the expiratory sound is fainter and is approximately one-third the length of the inspiratory note. Vesicular breath sounds are heard normally everywhere, except for the apex of the right lung, where the bronchi are closer to the chest wall and are covered by a smaller amount of lung tissue. Here, the breath sound is bronchovesicular.

A *bronchovesicular breath sound* always implies that some of the alveoli in the underlying area of the lung are normal. Figure 71 demonstrates how the breath sounds change as the proportion of diseased to normal alveoli increases and the altered "selective transmitter" properties of the pulmonary alveoli allow high-frequency vibrations to pass through the chest wall to the stethoscope. First, the expiratory note increases in intensity and pitch and progressively lengthens until it is as long as inspiration. Then, the inspiratory sound increases in pitch and intensity until it equals that of the expiratory sound. As long as the end of the inspiratory sound blends with the beginning of the expiratory sound the breath sound is bronchovesicular. However, in a *bronchial breath sound* there is a gap be-

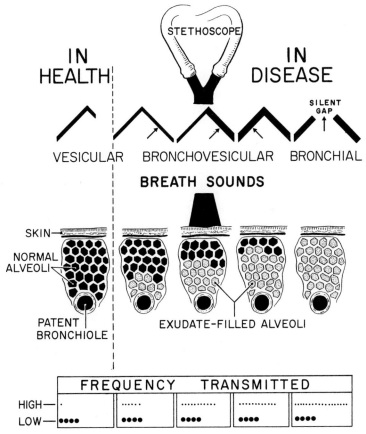

FIGURE 71. The changes which breath sounds undergo as an increasing number of alveoli become diseased. Note that the inspiratory sound increases in pitch and intensity until it equals that of the expiratory sound. As long as the end of the inspiratory sound blends with the expiratory sound it is bronchovesicular. In bronchial breathing there is a silent gap between end-inspiration and beginning of expiration.

tween the end of inspiration and the beginning of expiration. The sound is high-pitched and loud, inspiration and expiration being equally affected with respect to pitch, intensity and duration, and is identical to that normally heard during auscultation over the trachea. When a disease process in the lung involves all of the alveoli in the area, bronchial breathing becomes evident. As pointed out earlier this breath sound is heard over an area of consolidation as long as it is in close apposition to a patent bronchus.

Adventitious Sounds. Certain sounds produced by pathological processes within the lungs and the tracheobronchial tree are called adventitious sounds. These are never detected over healthy lung tissues; their presence indicates that a pathological process has developed in the underlying lung or pleura.

A *rhonchus,* derived from a Latin word meaning wheezing, is a musical sound produced within the lumen of the tracheobronchial tree. Whenever a portion of the tracheobronchial tree becomes narrowed, the resistance to airflow increases and turbulence and eddy formation may develop. Since the bronchi normally become shortened and narrowed during expiration, there will be more turbulence during this phase of respiration. Consequently, rhonchi are usually more pronounced during expiration.

A rhonchus that is only heard during the expiratory phase of breathing implies that the wall of the affected bronchus is still flexible, and capable of widening and lengthening during inspiration. A rhonchus that is heard during both expiration and inspiration suggests that the lumen of the affected bronchus is narrowed during both the inspiratory and expiratory phases of respiration. Occasionally, minor degrees of bronchial obstruction may not produce rhonchi during normal respiration. Under such circumstances, rhonchi may be elicited if the patient expires forcibly or coughs vigorously.

The pitch of a rhonchus provides a clue as to its site of origin, and it is generally felt that high-pitched rhonchi originate in small bronchi and bronchioles, and low-pitched rhonchi in large bronchi (Fig. 72). It has recently been demonstrated that the pitch of a rhonchus is not necessarily dependent on the diameter or the length of the affected bronchus but is related to the linear velocity of airflow through a constriction, which, in turn, is determined by the driving pressure and the degree of obstruction present. However, the mass of a bronchus probably also determines the pitch of a rhonchus, and a very low-pitched sound most likely arises in the large bronchi. High-pitched rhonchi are frequently heard during an attack of bronchial asthma; in this situation, the jets of air are forced through the constricted peripheral bronchioles by the high expiratory pressure within the chest.

A *rale* is a short, interrupted, nonmusical, explosive or bubbling

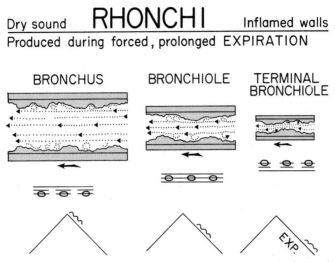

FIGURE 72. The origin of rhonchi and their pitch. Low-pitched rhonchi in early expiration originate in large bronchi; high-pitched rhonchi in late expiration originate in small bronchioles.

sound which is most readily heard during inspiration. Rale is the French word for rattle; it was originally believed that this sound was due to the bursting of bubbles of fluid within the bronchi. This may still explain rales which are heard when secretions are present in the trachea or the larger bronchi, but it has been suggested that rales originating in the peripheral airways result from the sudden rush of air through bronchioles which had closed during expiration and were opened abruptly during inspiration.

If there is only a minimal amount of parenchymal or bronchiolar disease, rales may not be detected during an ordinary deep inspiration, but they can often be elicited by having the patient inspire and expire deeply and follow with a cough. Often rales are produced just after the cough or at the beginning of the next inspiration. These "post-tussic" rales are presumably produced by the sudden rush of air through bronchioles where sticky walls had become adherent during the compressive phase of the cough.

The pitch of a rale depends on the type of lesion and on the diameter of the chamber producing the sound (Fig. 73). Rales may be classified clinically into three types, depending both on their pitch and on the phase of inspiration in which they predominate (Fig. 74). If the larger or medium-sized bronchi are diseased, as in a case of purulent bronchitis, low-pitched or coarse rales occur predominantly during the initial part of inspiration; if smaller bronchi are involved, as in bronchiectasis, medium-pitched rales occur predominantly in the middle phase of inspiration. If the peripheral bron-

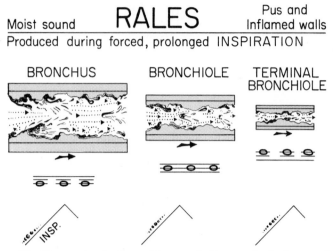

FIGURE 73.   The origin of rales and their pitch. Low-pitched rales in early inspiration originate in larger bronchi. High-pitched rales later in inspiration originate in smaller bronchioles.

chioles or the alveoli are involved, as in pulmonary congestion, or fibrosing alveolitis, high-pitched or fine rales occur predominantly during the last part of inspiration. It has therefore been suggested that the temporal position of the rales during inspiration may yield information regarding the anatomical location of the disease process. Unfortunately, it is difficult to obtain evidence to substantiate this obviously important hypothesis.

In diffuse fibrosis localized in the lung parenchyma, a creaky, interrupted dry sound may occasionally be heard. This characteristically extends uniformly throughout the whole of inspiration and expiration (Fig. 75). It has been suggested that this sound is caused by the stretching and relaxing of fibrous tissue during respiration.

A *pleural rub* is a loud, dry, creaking, coarse, leathery sound and is diagnostic of pleural irritation. It is produced by the rubbing of the inflamed surfaces of the two pleural surfaces against one another during respiration and is therefore present predominantly during the latter part of inspiration and the early part of expiration. Since the greatest movement of the lungs, and therefore the greatest excursion of the pleural surfaces, occurs over the lower lobes, friction rubs are most frequently detected over the lower areas of the chest wall and only occasionally over the upper areas of the chest wall.

Signs Associated with Air or Fluid in the Pleural Cavity.   Since there is no air in the pleural space, the sound heard over the posterior chest wall when two coins are clicked together over the anterior chest wall is muffled and faint. When there is a large collection of air, the sound is heard clearly and has a metallic quality. This *coin click* is

RALES

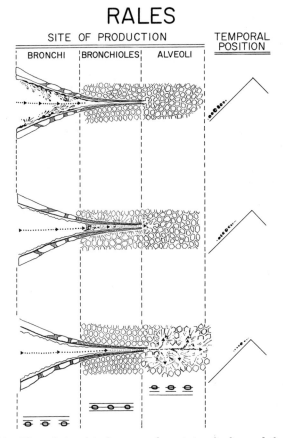

FIGURE 74. The relationship between the origin of rales and their inspiratory temporal position.

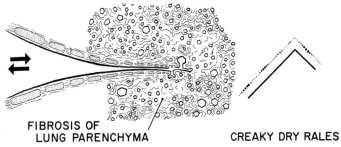

FIBGURE 75. The creaky, dry rales produced by pulmonary fibrosis.

presumably heard because the lung is almost completely collapsed by the air in the pleural space, and the number of interfaces at which the sound might be reflected is reduced.

When both air and fluid are present in the pleural cavity, a splashing sound may be produced when the chest is shaken abruptly. When detected by auscultation it is called a *succussion splash*.

When a bronchopleural fistula is present, a gurgling sound may be detected during inspiration. This is probably caused by air entering the pleural fluid through the fistula.

SECONDARY MANIFESTATIONS

In addition to the cardinal symptoms and signs associated with respiratory disease there are a number of secondary phenomena which may in turn further compromise respiratory function. The most important of these are the result of inadequate gas exchange, increased pulmonary vascular resistance, and constitutional or systemic derangements.

SIGNS OF INADEQUATE GAS EXCHANGE

When gas exchange becomes inadequate, hypoxia develops, either alone or in combination with hypercapnia. Both hypoxia and hypercapnia result in certain symptoms and signs and are attended by secondary effects which further compromise respiratory and cardiac function.

HYPOXIA

Although hypoxia does not produce a characteristic clinical picture, it occupies a central position in the pathogenesis of many of the manifestations of respiratory insufficiency. The severity of the signs and symptoms which develop depends on the degree of the oxygen deficiency and its duration. In some patients, mental confusion, hyperpnea, dyspnea and cyanosis may be dominant features; in others these findings may be minimal or absent.

Cyanosis. Cyanosis is a diffuse, bluish discoloration of the skin and mucous membranes and develops as a result of an increase in reduced or otherwise unoxygenated hemoglobin in the capillaries. It is best detected where the coverings over the capillaries of the skin or mucous membrane are thinnest and most transparent.

There are normally about 2.0 to 2.5 grams of reduced hemoglobin per 100 ml. of blood in the capillaries. It has been suggested that cyanosis does not become perceptible until the mean concentration of reduced hemoglobin in the capillaries doubles. For example, in a normal person whose hemoglobin content is 15 grams per cent and whose arteriovenous oxygen difference is 5 volumes per cent, the arterial and venous oxygen saturations are 97 and 74 per cent. This means that there is 0.45 gram of reduced hemoglobin in the arterial blood and 3.90 grams in the venous blood. The average amount of reduced hemoglobin in the capillaries is considered to be the mean of the sum of the arterial and venous values and is therefore $\frac{0.45 + 3.90}{2}$, or 2.18 grams per 100 ml. of blood.

If, in this same subject, pulmonary insufficiency were present so that the oxygen saturation was reduced to 80 and 50 per cent in the arterial and venous bloods respectively, there would be 3.0 grams of reduced hemoglobin in the arterial blood and 7.5 grams in the venous blood. The reduced hemoglobin content in the capillaries would then be $\frac{3.0 + 7.5}{2}$, or 5.25 grams per 100 ml. of blood.

These calculations indicate that cyanosis does not develop until the oxygen saturation of the arterial blood falls to approximately 80 per cent. This means that cyanosis cannot be perceived in patients suffering from respiratory disease until the arterial oxygen tension is approximately 50 mm. Hg. Thus, hypoxia may be severe before cyanosis can be detected.

The severity of the cyanosis increases with the amount of hemoglobin in the blood, for at a given oxygen saturation there will be a greater amount of reduced hemoglobin if the hemoglobin level is high. Thus, a patient who is suffering from polycythemia and whose hemoglobin concentration is greater than 20 grams per cent will develop cyanosis at a lesser degree of hypoxia than does a normal person. The converse situation is also important; in patients suffering from anemia, hypoxia may be extremely severe before cyanosis develops. Clearly then, the presence of cyanosis does not necessarily indicate the existence of severe hypoxia, particularly if polycythemia is present; even more important, hypoxic states do not necessarily produce cyanosis.

There are other conditions in which grave tissue hypoxia may be present without the warning signs of cyanosis. For instance, it is difficult to detect cyanosis in a patient with carbon monoxide poisoning when a non-oxygen-carrying hemoglobin is formed. Under these circumstances, severe tissue hypoxia may be present even though the skin remains pink and the blood is bright red. Similarly, in histotoxic hypoxia, as in cyanide poisoning, the arterial blood may be well oxygenated, but the tissues are unable to utilize the oxygen which is brought to them.

Conversely, cyanosis may develop in the absence of any associated underlying disease. This is true particularly in the extremities if the cutaneous arterioles become narrowed as a result of either a cold environment or nervous influences. Vasoconstriction slows the flow of blood through the capillaries so that more of its oxygen is extracted by the tissues and the amount of reduced hemoglobin in the capillaries is increased.

The problem becomes even more serious when it is realized that the clinical assessment of the degree of cyanosis is notoriously difficult, even for an observer with an artistic eye. The recognition of cyanosis depends on color perception, which is subject to wide variations from one observer to another. In addition, cyanosis becomes more difficult to detect if the skin overlying the capillaries is thickened and pigmented or if the number and size of the capillaries are reduced. Most examiners, although able to recognize well-developed cyanosis, are usually inconsistent in their judgment about the presence of cyanosis in different patients or even in the same patient on separate occasions. Despite all of these problems, many physicians regard cyanosis as the most characteristic sign of hypoxia and depend upon its presence or absence to decide whether hypoxia is present. Clearly these considerations point to the many pitfalls that exist if the judgment of arterial hypoxemia depends entirely on the presence of cyanosis. The presence of hypoxia can be established only by an analysis of the oxygen tension and oxygen saturation in the arterial blood. This is especially true in anemic patients who may have hypoxia severe enough to threaten life without the clinical development of cyanosis.

Since local cyanosis can be present even though the oxygen tension of the arterial blood is normal, clinicians have classified cyanosis according to the mechanism by which it is produced. They have suggested that cyanosis is either central, by which is meant that cyanosis is the result of a disturbance of pulmonary or cardiac function, or peripheral, in which case there is a local cause such as a slowing of the peripheral circulation by cold or increased vasomotor activity. Inspection of the undersurface of the tongue helps to differentiate these two types, for cyanosis which is peripheral in origin is unlikely to occur there. It must be stressed that this is an etiological classification and not an anatomical one, as is so often assumed, particularly by students. It is obvious that the peripheral portions of the body, such as the fingers and the tip of the nose, become cyanosed in both the central and the peripheral types of cyanosis. It is probably better to classify cyanosis on the basis of whether it is associated with a low arterial oxygen tension or a normal one.

Respiratory Manifestations.   Hypoxia is one of the major stimuli to ventilation. Just as some clinicians use cyanosis to judge the presence of hypoxemia, others use the presence or absence of breathlessness, or of hyperpnea, as criteria for the diagnosis of hypoxemia. The extent to which a hypoxic ventilatory drive contributes to the breathlessness of respiratory insufficiency is difficult to ascertain. Nevertheless, many patients claim some relief of dyspnea and demonstrate an increased effort tolerance when given oxygen. Since dyspnea is a purely subjective sensation and can be caused by a variety of factors, its presence or absence cannot be used as an indication of whether hypoxia is present or not. Similarly, the hyperpnea cannot be used as an indication of hypoxia, for the ventilatory response to hypoxia varies considerably in different persons. Under normal circumstances, the arterial Po_2 must fall below 60 mm. Hg before ventilation is stimulated noticeably. However, it has been demonstrated that the effect of a low arterial oxygen tension is enhanced by hypercapnia, and levels of hypoxia not ordinarily associated with an increased ventilatory drive may be effective stimuli in patients with carbon dioxide retention. In such persons, hypoxemia may become the major stimulus to respiration, and oxygen administration may result in hypoventilation and increasing hypercapnia, eventually leading to coma.

Cardiovascular Manifestations. Hypoxia plays an important role in the production of the cardiovascular component of respiratory insufficiency. An increase in pulse rate is also often used clinically as a guide to the diagnosis of hypoxia, and it is likely that this is a much more reliable index than are the changes in respiration. An acute reduction in the arterial oxygen tension may produce an increase in the pulse rate, even though it does not stimulate respiration. Unfortunately, from the diagnostic point of view, there are many other conditions besides hypoxia, such as fever, hypotension, pain, venous congestion and even drugs, which tend to increase the pulse rate. Furthermore, in some cases of prolonged hypoxia, the pulse rate may diminish rather than accelerate. It is, however, probably correct to suspect that hypoxia is present if the pulse rate decreases by ten or more beats per minute within a few minutes after starting the administration of 100 per cent oxygen.

Hypoxia causes an increase in cardiac output, dilates peripheral blood vessels, including the cerebral vessels, and constricts pulmonary blood vessels. Pulmonary vasoconstriction due to hypoxia is ordinarily readily reversible, but in some persons chronic hypoxia may lead to considerable structural change, with a further increase in pulmonary vascular resistance, which may ultimately result in the development of right-sided heart failure.

Aside from the effects of acute hypoxia on vasomotor tone, the most prominent effect on the peripheral vasculature seen in chronic hypoxia is an increase in the capillary density of skeletal muscle. The adaptive role of such proliferation in terms of oxygen transport is obvious, but its importance in patients with respiratory disease has not been ascertained.

Hematologic Manifestations. A prominent effect of hypoxia is the development of secondary polycythemia, which is mediated by an increased erythropoietin production. The extent of the increase in red blood cell mass is often masked by an increase in extracellular fluid and plasma volume so that the hematocrit value may be normal. In contrast to the primary form of polycythemia, splenomegaly, leukocytosis and thrombocytosis are absent. Information about the relative importance of polycythemia, either as a compensatory mechanism by which the capacity for oxygen transport is increased or as a deleterious factor which contributes to the pathogenesis of right-sided heart failure by increasing blood viscosity, is currently not available.

Metabolic Manifestations. The metabolic changes which are operative in the increased erythropoietin production or the pulmonary vasoconstriction seen with hypoxia are not known. There is currently no evidence to suggest that chronic hypoxia interferes with the metabolism of carbohydrate, fat or protein under resting conditions. It has been suggested that anaerobic metabolism, as judged by changes in blood lactate and pyruvate concentration, is increased during exercise in patients with chronic respiratory insufficiency but whether such changes are of greater magnitude than those observed in patients with similar degrees of debility due to other diseases has not been established.

Central Nervous System Manifestations. Acute hypoxia causes visual disturbances, incoordination, dysarthria and even coma. In normal persons, the inhalation of 10 per cent oxygen causes a reduction in the cerebral vascular resistance and an increase in the cerebral blood flow; as a result, the oxygen tension of the cerebral tissues does not fall as much as it might otherwise. Nevertheless, symptoms related to cerebral dysfunction are the commonest manifestations of acute or chronic hypoxia.

When a patient becomes acutely hypoxic, he usually becomes very restless, but he may exhibit somnolence and lassitude or a sense of comfort, well-being and self-satisfaction which is often associated with outbursts of hilarity or obstreperousness. The neuromuscular coordination frequently suffers, as is evidenced by clumsiness and a slowed reaction time, and judgement may become impaired to such an extent that the entire clinical picture resembles one of drunkenness.

Acclimatization to Hypoxia. Most of the information regarding acclimatization to chronic hypoxia has been gleaned from studies on subjects who have resided at high altitudes for long periods of time. In these subjects, hyperventilation is a characteristic finding. As a result, the alveolar and arterial carbon dioxide tensions are decreased, and there is a proportionate fall in the bicarbonate content so that the pH is maintained at an approximately normal level. The rate of formation of red blood cells increases as a consequence of the lowered arterial oxygen tension, and the consequent rise in hemoglobin content results in an increased oxygen capacity of the blood. The effects of acclimatization to altitude on the cardiovascular system are difficult to evaluate. A moderately brief exposure to high altitude causes a distinct increase in cardiac output, but it is normal in persons who have resided at a high altitude for a long period of time.

In patients who are chronically hypoxic at sea level, particularly those suffering from cyanotic heart disease, the ventilation tends to be increased, but there is a wide variation among different subjects. For a given degree of hypoxia, the ventilation increases less in a person who resides at sea level than it does in one who has become acclimatized to a high altitude. In hypoxic persons at sea level the bicarbonate content of the arterial blood tends to be reduced but to a lesser extent and for a different reason than in dwellers at high altitudes. In contrast to the hypocapnia which the latter exhibit, the arterial carbon dioxide tension is usually within normal limits in patients with congenital heart disease. On the other hand, patients with a congenital right-to-left cardiac shunt tend to be in a state of metabolic acidosis. This may be an advantage, since the acidosis shifts the oxyhemoglobin dissociation curve, thereby assisting in the unloading of oxygen to the tissues.

Just as in those who reside at a high altitude, there is an increased formation of erythrocytes in many patients who are hypoxic due to respiratory insufficiency. This secondary polycythemia results from stimulation of the kidney to produce erythropoietin, which in turn stimulates the bone marrow. The increased oxygen-carrying capacity of the blood, and therefore its oxygen content, at a particular partial pressure of oxygen allows the required amount of oxygen to be given off to the tissues without producing too great a fall in the partial pressure of the oxygen in the blood. In patients who are suffering from both chronic hypoxia and hypercapnia, the hematologic response is variable. A good correlation has, as yet, not been made between the hematologic response and the blood gas tensions. Nevertheless, it has been suggested that at a given level of hypoxia, the red blood cell mass does not increase as much in these patients as it would in an equally hypoxic healthy subject at a high altitude. The role which either infection or hypercapnia plays in altering the hematologic response to hypoxia has not been adequately elucidated.

HYPERCAPNIA

In patients with respiratory insufficiency hypercapnia is always associated with hypoxia unless the patient is inhaling a concentration of oxygen greater than that of room air. For this reason it is sometimes difficult to separate the effects of hypercapnia from those due to the associated hypoxia. When present, hypercapnia is the consequence of an inadequate alveolar ventilation. The alveolar, and therefore the arterial, carbon dioxide tension is intimately related to and dependent upon both the alveolar ventilation and the level of metabolism. For any given level of metabolism (and therefore of carbon dioxide production) a change in the alveolar ventilation results in an inverse alteration of the alveolar and the arterial carbon dioxide tensions. A decrease in the alveolar ventilation with no change in the metabolism leads to an elevated arterial carbon dioxide tension. Similarly, hypercapnia will develop whenever carbon dioxide production increases without a proportionate increase in alveolar ventilation.

Ventilatory Manifestations. An acute rise in arterial P_{CO_2} is the most outstanding of all the known chemical influences on ventilation. On the other hand, acclimatization to an elevated P_{CO_2} occurs in patients with chronic respiratory disease, and changes in arterial P_{O_2} may become the prime stimulus to ventilation. Thus, patients with chronic carbon dioxide retention exhibit a lower than normal ventilatory response to further increments of P_{CO_2}, and it would appear that the sensitivity of the medullary respiratory center to further changes in arterial P_{CO_2} is diminished in these patients. The decrease in ventilatory response to CO_2 may not necessarily reflect a diminished sensitivity of the respiratory center. Instead, this may be due to the increased buffering capacity of the blood and extracellular fluid resulting from retention of base bicarbonate so that a given change in carbon dioxide tension does not produce the usual increase in hydrogen ion concentration. Since the ventilatory response to changes in carbon dioxide tension and hydrogen ion concentration are not readily distinguished from each other, the result is an apparent diminished ventilatory response to carbon dioxide.

The disturbances in the mechanics of breathing (and elevated CO_2 production in relation to the alveolar ventilation) may also play an important role. If the work of breathing is elevated, any increase in ventilation may be inadequate to eliminate the carbon dioxide being produced.

Retention of carbon dioxide may occur in previously healthy persons if the alveolar ventilation falls because of respiratory center depression as a result of a head injury, a cerebrovascular accident or the ingestion of excessive amounts of barbiturates, tranquilizing agents or anesthetics. In patients suffering from chronic respiratory disease the manifestations of acute carbon dioxide retention are frequently precipitated by the development of an infection or heart failure or by the administration of oxygen or sedatives. Although such patients appear to be able to tolerate mild elevations of the carbon dioxide tension for long periods of time, severe retention of carbon dioxide leads to the development of a vicious circle which may have serious consequences. Chronic carbon dioxide retention may also reduce the sensitivity of the respiratory center so that ventilation falls and leads to further carbon dioxide retention, a further fall in ventilation with its consequent additional carbon dioxide retention, and eventually the development of coma and even death.

Central Nervous System Manifestations. An elevation of arterial P_{CO_2} results in cerebral vascular dilatation, an increased cerebral blood flow, a rise in cerebrospinal fluid pressure, narcosis and coma. The level of arterial P_{CO_2} at which these effects appear is highly variable among different persons. Headache on arising is a very common symptom and is probably related to the effects of progressive carbon dioxide retention and hypoxia during sleep. Occasionally mental aberrations such as hallucinations, hypomania, or catatonia prompt the admission of patients with hypoxia and hypercapnia to psychiatric institutions. Other unexplained neurologic manifestations include asterexis (flapping tremor), convulsions, papilledema and an apparent exophthalmos.

Cardiovascular Manifestations. As has been pointed out, hypercapnia results in cerebral vasodilatation and an increase in cerebral blood flow. On the other hand, hypercapnia (or the acidosis associated with it) causes constriction of the pulmonary vessels, thereby aggravating and increasing the level of pulmonary hypertension which may be present. The response of the peripheral vasculature to carbon dioxide depends upon the balance struck between its local and central effects. Although carbon dioxide normally produces local peripheral vasodilatation, this is usually masked by the vasoconstriction resulting from stimulation of the sympathetic nervous system. When carbon dioxide retention is severe, generalized vasodilatation predominates, hypotension is a common occurrence, and the patient may be in a shock-like state.

SIGNS OF INCREASED PULMONARY VASCULAR RESISTANCE

As a result of alterations in the pulmonary vasculature, the resistance within the vessels frequently increases so that the pressure in the pulmonary artery rises. Although factors such as obstruction or obliteration of the pulmonary vascular bed may be prominent in pulmonary disease, pulmonary vasoconstriction plays an important role and the level of pulmonary hypertension usually correlates well with the degree of oxygen unsaturation. The physical signs which indicate that the normal vascular hemodynamics have become altered are produced by the pulmonary hypertension. Examination of the lungs themselves provides no indication of the presence of pulmonary hypertension. Signs indicative of this abnormality are found during examination of the heart.

The intensity of the second sound in the pulmonic area is caused by the closure of the aortic and pulmonary valves and yields a great deal of information regarding the possibility of pulmonary hypertension. During inspiration, the second sound in the pulmonic area is often split into two parts because of a delayed closure of the pulmonary valve due to increased filling and prolonged systole of the right ventricle during inspiration. This pulmonic split second sound is normally readily detected in most children, but it may also be present in many older normal persons. When pulmonary hypertension is present, or when there is right ventricular failure due to pulmonary disease, the second sound may not split during inspiration. In addition, the second pulmonic sound is very much louder than normal, and if it is severe, this loud sound may be transmitted to the apex.

Other auscultatory signs of pulmonary hypertension are a high-pitched early systolic ejection click which is probably due to accentuated ejection vibrations in the pulmonic area and a presystolic gallop rhythm.

An increased pulmonary vascular resistance poses a very heavy burden on the right ventricle in that it must work harder to force blood through the pulmonary vascular bed. As a result, it frequently hypertrophies. A prominent pulsation along the left border of the sternum, associated with a conspicuous retraction over the left ventricle giving the anterior chest a rocking motion synchronous with the heart beat, is suggestive of right ventricular hypertrophy.

When right-sided heart failure develops the condition is called cor pulmonale. There is no exact correlation between the severity of the pulmonary hypertension and the development of cor pulmonale. In general, however, it has been said that a sustained mean pulmonary artery pressure above 40 mm. Hg is associated with both a significant alteration in the electrocardiographic tracing and the radiologic evidence of enlargement of the right ventricle.

EXTRAPULMONARY MANIFESTATIONS

Respiratory disease may also be manifested in symptoms and signs which originate in distant sites. The most important of these are constitutional symptoms, clubbing of the digits, pulmonary osteoarthropathy and some systemic manifestations which occur on rare occasions in patients suffering from a pulmonary malignancy.

CONSTITUTIONAL SYMPTOMS

Patients with respiratory disease may complain of various constitutional symptoms, such as fever, sweating, anorexia, weakness and loss of weight.

Fever.   Under most circumstances, the body temperature represents a balance between the heat produced by the body and that which is lost. Fever is associated with respiratory disease whenever there is infection, degeneration of tissue or extensive trauma and probably results from both an increased heat production and a reduced heat loss. The fever may be continuous, remittent, and oscillating or intermittent with a normal temperature for a varying length of time.

The patient may feel cold even though his body temperature is normal or even above normal. He may develop "shaking chills" during which his teeth chatter and he shivers so violently that he shakes the bed. The skin feels cold because of peripheral vasoconstriction and a diminished peripheral blood flow. Vasoconstriction reduces heat loss through radiation while heat production is increased because of the increased muscle tone and activity associated with shivering.

Sweating.   Under ordinary or basal conditions no sweat is secreted except possibly a small amount from special glands in the feet, hands and axillae. One stimulus to an increase in sweating is an elevated body temperature. In patients suffering from a respiratory disease, anxiety and worry about breathing difficulty may cause profuse sweating because of overactivity of the sympathetic nervous system. Occasionally there may be drenching "night or slumber sweats" in which the night clothes become thoroughly soaked. The explanation of this phenomenon is unknown, although an elevated body temperature might initiate corrective measures for heat loss. If the body temperature is not elevated, overactivity of the sympathetic nervous system for some unknown reason or a resetting of the hypothalamic thermostat at a lower level during the night leads to measures designed to increase the loss of heat.

Anorexia, Weakness, Fatigue and Weight Loss.   Anorexia, weakness, easy fatiguability and weight loss are frequent complaints during acute pulmonary infections as well as in patients suffering from some types of chronic respiratory disease.

Weakness and loss of weight may be encountered in acute or chronic respiratory disease if the caloric intake does not increase concomitantly with the expenditure of energy. In patients suffering from respiratory disease, an increased expenditure of energy is often the result of a high oxygen consumption by the respiratory muscles or the elevated metabolism which occurs during a fever. In addition, there may be an excessive loss of protein because of infection, tissue destruction, malignancy or trauma. Finally, an elevated body temperature by itself increases the caloric requirements of the body.

Anorexia associated with respiratory disease is difficult to explain. If the respiratory disease is severe, the mere act of eating may be so tiring and energy-consuming that the patient may lose all desire to eat. Consequently, a relative anorexia may exist simply because of the effort which is required for eating.

CLUBBING OF THE DIGITS

Clubbing of the fingers and the toes is an important manifestation of certain types of intrathoracic disease and is therefore of great diagnostic significance. It is most commonly associated with an intrathoracic malignancy such as a bronchogenic carcinoma or a pleural mesothelioma. Clubbing of the digits may also occur in association with suppurative disease of the lung, such as lung abscess, empyema and bronchiectasis; in certain congenital lesions of the heart or pulmonary vasculature associated with a right-to-left shunt; and in subacute bacterial endocarditis. Occasionally clubbing is seen in patients suffering from disease of the liver or the gastrointestinal tract, particularly those characterized by chronic diarrhea, such as ulcerative colitis and steatorrhea.

Clubbing consists of a painless, nontender enlargement of the terminal phalanges of the fingers and toes and is usually a bilateral condition (Fig. 76). Initially there is hypertrophy of the soft tissues covering the root of the nail so that the angle formed by the root of the nail and the nail bed (normally about 160 degrees) becomes 180 degrees or more (Fig. 77). As clubbing progresses, the skin becomes stretched and glistening. The nail gradually thickens, becomes curved and develops longitudinal ridges, and the pulp of the terminal phalanx enlarges and develops a bulbous appearance. In the advanced stages of clubbing, the nail is thickened, ridged and curved both longitudinally and laterally, and its distal end overrides

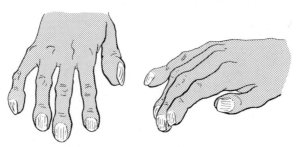

FIGURE 76. Clubbing of the fingers.

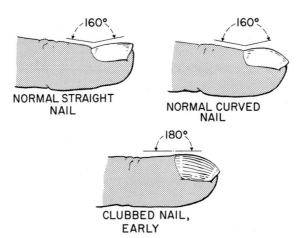

FIGURE 77. The "base angle" in a normal digit, a digit with a curved nail and a digit with early clubbing.

the end of the finger. An example of advanced clubbing of the fingers is illustrated in Figure 78.

Clubbing of the digits usually progresses slowly, often taking months or years to develop. Occasionally it may develop acutely in the course of a week or so if the underlying intrathoracic lesion is an acute septic process. Regression and even disappearance of digital clubbing may take place if the underlying lesion is eradicated by either medical or surgical treatment.

Pathogenesis of Clubbing. All types of digital clubbing show the same pathological changes, no matter what the underlying cause.

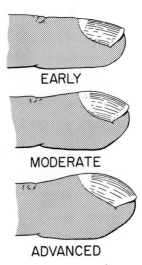

FIGURE 78. The progressive changes seen in finger clubbing. The nail thickens and becomes curved and overrides the end of the finger; the pulp of the terminal phalanx enlarges and has a bulbous appearance.

These consist of proliferation of the fibroelastic tissue, interstitial edema, and dilatation and engorgement of the arterioles and venules. There is evidence of an increased blood flow through dilated arteriovenous anastomoses which are very prevalent in the pulp of the terminal phalanges.

Although several theories have been advanced, the exact mechanism leading to clubbing in apparently unrelated diseases is as yet unexplained and still open to conjecture. Until recently, the most attractive explanation for the development of digital clubbing was that tissue hypoxia causes an increase in the number of arteriovenous anastomoses in the digits. This concept is supported by the fact that changes similar to clubbing may develop when a right-to-left shunt is experimentally produced in animals. Although tissue hypoxia may be the mechanism by which clubbing develops in pulmonary conditions or in cardiovascular or even hepatic conditions associated with a right-to-left vascular shunt, it is difficult to imagine how hypoxia could occur in patients with steatorrhea or ulcerative colitis. In addition, digital clubbing is rarely associated with severe chronic anemia, which should lead to considerable tissue hypoxia.

Some investigators believe that clubbing will occur whenever the left ventricle delivers more blood than is necessary to meet the needs of the tissues and that the digital blood pressure and blood flow is elevated so that the growth of the digital tissues is increased.

Chronic infection has also been proposed as one of the factors in the development of clubbing, since it is often present in suppurative pulmonary diseases. However, infection is usually associated with an elevation of both the sedimentation rate and the plasma globulins, which frequently results in rouleaux formation of the erythrocytes. Tissue hypoxia may be present under these circumstances because of peripheral vasodilatation and increased blood flow and because the erythrocytes in the rouleaux may not have time to release their oxygen to the tissues.

Reflex neurogenic factors have been implicated in digital clubbing because surgical removal of a pulmonary tumor often leads to a lessening in the degree of digital clubbing. It is obvious, however, that such an operative procedure may also result in a reduction of any venous admixture, and therefore of any hypoxia; improvement could easily be explained by such a mechanism.

HYPERTROPHIC PULMONARY OSTEOARTHROPATHY

Clubbing of the digits may progress to a condition called hypertrophic pulmonary osteoarthropathy, in which the gross, bulbous, enlarged terminal digital phalanges and thickened curved nails are associated with a painful, tender thickening of the wrists, the ankles and the long bones of the forearms and the legs.

The basic pathologic process is a proliferating subperiostitis with subperiosteal new bone formation which involves symmetrically the distal segments of the long bones of the arms and legs and a thickening of the connective tissue. In advanced situations the bones of the hands, feet, face and ribs may be involved and result in a clinical picture which may superficially resemble acromegaly. The joints of the knees, ankles and wrists often develop an effusion which is clear and viscous and may be associated with a synovitis.

Hypertrophic pulmonary osteoarthropathy is most frequently associated with carcinoma of the lung, particularly those in the periphery of the lung, or with central necrosis, the commonest cell type being squamous.

RARE SYSTEMIC MANIFESTATIONS

When a lung tumor metastasizes to distant sites such as the bones, liver, brain or adrenal glands, manifestations which are related to the tissue or organ involved may develop. However, bizarre systemic manifestations which bear no relationship to the site of metastases are occasionally seen in patients suffering from bronchogenic carcinoma although they are not unique for bronchogenic carcinoma and have been recorded with primary tumors in other parts of the body.

Many of these systemic manifestations appear to be mediated or influenced by hormone-like polypeptides that are secreted by bronchogenic tumors of the anaplastic or "oat cell type." A variety of endocrine disorders have been described, the most common being *Cushing's syndrome*, which is apparently produced by a substance similar to corticotropin. The syndrome of hyponatremia and a high osmolarity of the urine is apparently due to excessive production of a polypeptide resembling antidiuretic hormone. The *Carcinoid syndrome*, which consists of facial flushing, diarrhea and wheezing has been reported in association with oat cell carcinoma and is due to the production of a substance similar to 5-hydroxytryptamine. Hypercalcemia, polyuria, and weakness may be present and even coma may rarely occur as a result of secretion of a parathyroid-like hormone.

A number of people with hypertrophic pulmonary osteoarthropathy have an associated gynecomastia. An abnormal estrogen metabolism has been implicated as a causative factor for the breast changes.

Neuromuscular disorders may also develop in association with bronchogenic carcinoma. Cortical degeneration with a loss of Purkinje cells in the cerebellar cortex results in the rapid loss of function. In addition, peripheral neuropathy which may be purely sensory or mixed (with sensory and motor components) occasionally occurs.

Certain dermatologic disorders may also be associated with a bronchogenic carcinoma. Dermatomyositis, in which an erythematous rash predominantly affecting the face and upper thorax is associated with weakness of the muscles of the shoulders and hips, occasionally develops in patients suffering from a bronchogenic carcinoma and often appears several months before the lung cancer is discovered. Acanthosis nigricans, a rare skin disease consisting of darkly pigmented verrucal lesions predominantly in the skin folds of the body, usually signifies intra-abdominal cancer, but it also has been reported in association with lung cancer.

Section Three

THE ASSESSMENT OF RESPIRATORY DISEASE

THE CLINICAL ASSESSMENT

THE RADIOLOGIC ASSESSMENT

THE LABORATORY ASSESSMENT

Chapter 10

The Clinical Assessment

From the foregoing section, it is apparent that by eliciting the symptoms and signs which result from disturbances of the respiratory system the examiner is in a position to arrive at a tentative conclusion concerning the pattern and general nature of the patient's disease. A careful interview of the patient and a painstaking physical examination are the essential methods of arriving at the preliminary diagnosis; while confirmation and refinement of this diagnosis may involve radiologic and laboratory investigation.

INTERVIEWING THE PATIENT

To obtain an accurate description of a patient's problem, it is most important to establish proper rapport with him. The examiner should introduce himself to the patient and explain that he wishes to discuss the details of the patient's illness; in addition to exhibiting interest, the clinician should be unhurried, tactful and considerate during the interview. It is essential that he use words or phrases that the patient can understand. He also should avoid asking leading questions, for this often may result in an incorrect reply, although leading questions may occasionally be necessary to elicit certain pertinent points, particularly if the patient is garrulous.

A detailed account of the illness often makes it possible to arrive at a presumptive diagnosis. The entire historical aspect of the patient's illness should be recorded in an orderly, consecutive fashion under the following headings: the presenting complaints which led him to seek medical attention; his personal and family history; his previous illnesses and medical examinations; a review of his non-respiratory systems; the medications he has taken or is taking; and finally, the history of the present illness.

217

PRESENTING COMPLAINTS

The presenting complaints are in effect a capsule account of the patient's illness. These are the symptoms which prompted him to seek medical advice and should be recorded chronologically. It is best to begin by asking the patient when he last felt well and then noting each symptom in the order of its onset. With this information the examiner can determine whether he is dealing with a chronic, a subacute or an acute illness and whether it has remained stationary, progressed in severity or has been complicated by subacute or acute exacerbations.

PERSONAL HISTORY

The patient's background, living habits and environment may have some bearing on the development of his illness. The date of birth, birthplace and various countries in which he resided or visited should be listed in chronological order, together with the amount of time spent in each area. There is a higher incidence of chronic bronchitis and emphysema in highly industrialized areas with atmospheric pollution. Certain countries are notorious for endemic disease, especially those which are fungal in origin. Histoplasmosis is endemic in the valleys of the great rivers, such as the Mississippi, the Ohio and the St. Lawrence; coccidioidomycosis is found in the arid deserts of southern California, Arizona and northern Mexico; and the incidence of schistosomiasis is high in Puerto Rico, Central America and Egypt.

His socioeconomic status and that of his parents should be elicited. The patient may have spent his earlier years in extreme poverty; the associated malnutrition and poor hygienic standards are factors which may have predisposed to the development of childhood pulmonary tuberculosis. Certain ethnic groups, such as the Canadian Indian and the Eskimo, are especially susceptible to diseases such as tuberculosis.

A detailed and complete occupational history, together with the duration of each term of employment, may point to the pattern of disease which is present. For instance, underground work in a mine, even 20 or 30 years previously, may have been responsible for the development of silicosis. An occupation involving exposure to a high level of air pollution with smoke, dust, or fumes may lead to the development of chronic bronchitis and emphysema; those involved in the manufacturing of fluorescent light bulbs to berylliosis; and inhalation of asbestos fibers predisposes to asbestosis, fibrosis and also pulmonary malignancy. Farming may be associated with the development of a variety of respiratory diseases, including the nitrogen dioxide induced acute interstitial pneumonitis resulting from exposure to fumes in a silo; the hypersensitivity reaction induced by fungal spores in mouldy hay (farmer's lung); the histoplasmosis of chicken farmers; and the asthma associated with the inhalation of grain dust. The patient's habits may influence his ability to resist disease. Worries over financial difficulties or anxiety caused by pressure of work will influence personal habits significantly. Exhausting labor, especially in poorly ventilated surroundings, and insufficient rest may play a role in reducing resistance. Susceptibility to disease may be increased by an inadequate protein intake, as may occur in those who diet injudiciously to lose weight, or in chronic alcoholics who sacrifice food for alcohol. By contrast, gross overeating leading to obesity may lower the patient's resistance to infection and may also lead to respiratory insufficiency and cardiac failure.

Cigarette smoking has been linked to the development of bronchogenic carcinoma and is particularly important in the pathogenesis and perpetuation of chronic bronchitis. For reasons which are as yet not fully understood, the incidence of chronic bronchitis or bronchogenic carcinoma in pipe and cigar smokers is only slightly higher than in nonsmokers. A history of the patient's smoking habits is clearly essential and should include the age at which smoking began and the current daily consumption of cigarettes, cigars or pipe tobacco. If the patient has stopped smoking, the date should be recorded and the reasons noted, for it may have been because of cough, breathlessness or wheezing.

Close contact with pets or flowering plants may be important. Diseased pigeons or budgerigars may be the cause of the acute interstitial pneumonitis associated with psittacosis, or exposure to bird droppings may have led to a hypersensitivity reaction in bird fanciers. Attacks of bronchial asthma may be precipitated by exposure to the dander of dogs, cats or horses as well as the pollen of flowering plants.

FAMILY HISTORY

All serious illnesses which may have affected any member of the patient's immediate family should be recorded along with the cause of death of any deceased relative. This is important because it may direct attention to a possible hereditary predisposition to certain diseases, such as cystic fibrosis or asthma, or it may indicate contact with an infectious disease, such as tuberculosis, during some period of the patient's life.

PREVIOUS ILLNESSES AND MEDICAL EXAMINATIONS

The past illnesses of the patient, including the infectious diseases of childhood, should be recorded. If he is suffering from asthma, there may be a history of infantile eczema, atopic dermatitis or allergic rhinitis. Measles or pertussis in childhood, especially if prolonged or complicated by pneumonia, may have led to bronchiectasis, which should be suspected if there is a history of recurrent pneumonia affecting the same lung. On the other hand, a bronchogenic carcinoma should be suspected if a middle-aged or elderly person has recently had repeated pneumonias involving the same lung. A pulmonary abscess may follow a dental extraction, upper respiratory tract surgery or aspiration of a foreign body.

A previous injury or operation on the chest may be the cause of a fibrothorax or cardiorespiratory insufficiency in later life.

REVIEW OF NONRESPIRATORY SYSTEMS

An inquiry into the nonrespiratory systems is important because certain respiratory illnesses may be the consequence of disease processes which primarily affect other organs.

NERVOUS SYSTEM

A cerebral metastasis from a pulmonary neoplasm, a cerebral abscess secondary to bronchiectasis, or an attack of tuberculous meningitis may cause severe intractable throbbing headaches, vertigo, diplopia, drowsiness, confusion, disorientation, syncopal attacks or convulsions. On the other hand, many of these symptoms may also be caused by hypoxia and carbon dioxide retention. Occasionally a patient with severe chronic respiratory insufficiency is admitted to a neurological ward because an expanding intracerebral lesion is suspected. Paresthesia associated with muscle wasting and weakness of the limbs may be due to a peripheral neuropathy, which occasionally complicates a bronchogenic carcinoma.

The thought that the respiratory symptoms are due to some incurable organic disease may engender symptoms of anxiety and apprehension in the patient with respiratory disease, and as a result, he may develop insomnia and become irritable, depressed and highly emotional. Occasionally emotional disturbances lead to numbness and tingling in the extremities and faintness as a result of chronic hyperventilation.

CARDIOVASCULAR SYSTEM

Cough and dyspnea are also symptoms of cardiovascular disease. Orthopnea and an increase in the number of pillows used during recumbency suggest the onset of left ventricular failure. A recent attack of severe substernal pain followed by dyspnea suggests a myocardial infarction and possible pulmonary congestion. An increase in dyspnea, and bilateral ankle swelling may point to the development of right-sided heart failure secondary to a respiratory disease. An attack of pleuritic chest pain in a patient who has heart failure or a swollen, painful and tender limb suggests the possibility of a pulmonary embolus.

GASTROINTESTINAL SYSTEM

Difficulty in swallowing may be due to a stricture or a malignant process in the esophagus and may lead to aspiration of esophageal contents. Aspiration also may occur when there is a hiatus hernia or a dilated esophagus due to achalasia of the esophageal sphincter.

Anorexia and vague dyspeptic complaints may be associated with active pulmonary tuberculosis or a chronic bronchopulmonary disease, such as bronchiectasis. A postprandial epigastric pain which is relieved by the ingestion of food and alkali suggests peptic ulceration which is occasionally seen in association with emphysema. Chronic diarrhea may indicate the development of amyloidosis if the patient is suffering from a suppurative pulmonary disease, a carcinoid tumor of the bowel, tuberculous ulceration of the bowel or adrenal insufficiency caused by either tuberculosis or tumor metastases.

GENITOURINARY SYSTEM

Frequency, dysuria and hematuria may be due to renal tuberculosis. Hematuria may also be produced by a renal carcinoma. A painful or swollen testicle may indicate a tuberculous or malignant involvement. Amenorrhea often accompanies pulmonary tuberculosis as well as many other wasting diseases.

METABOLIC SYSTEM

Weakness, fatigue and weight loss are frequently present in chronic respiratory disease. Considerable weight loss may occur in active pulmonary tuberculosis or malignancy, and excessive weight may lead to alveolar hypoventilation and the symptoms of hypoxia and carbon dioxide retention.

LOCOMOTOR SYSTEM

If clubbing of the fingers has been noted by the patient, the time of its onset should be established. A recent onset suggests a malignancy. Pain and tenderness in the lower parts of his forearms and legs may be due to hypertrophic pulmonary osteoarthropathy. A fine tremor may indicate that hyperthyroidism may be the cause of dyspnea. On the other hand, a flapping tremor of the hands, similar to that which occurs in hepatic coma, is also seen in severe carbon dioxide retention and acidemia. Painful, tender, discolored areas of erythema nodosum commonly occur over the extensor surfaces of the legs and may be due to tuberculosis or sarcoidosis. The onset of weakness in specific groups of muscles may suggest poliomyelitis, infectious polyneuritis or a myopathy associated with pulmonary malignancy.

MEDICATIONS

It is important to know which medications the patient is taking or has taken in the past, since some of the patient's symptoms may have resulted from side effects caused by these drugs.

THE HISTORY OF PRESENT ILLNESS

With the background information obtained by judicious questioning as suggested in the foregoing sections, one is equipped to tackle the part of the history which deals with the respiratory illness itself.

A chronological history of the respiratory illness should be obtained beginning from the time the patient last felt "completely well." The evolution of the illness and the symptoms, with their mode of onset as well as their course, should be carefully noted. If the illness is acute, a day-by-day or even hour-by-hour account of the events should be elicited. If it is chronic, the month-to-month or year-to-year progression of events is important.

The following discussion deals with the type of questions that should be asked by the physician in order to describe each of the major symptoms of the respiratory disease. The mechanisms of development and significance of each symptom have already been discussed in Chapter 9.

COUGH

If cough is present, its approximate time of onset and its progress should be determined. If it is associated with acute exacerbations, the frequency and duration of attacks and whether they are becoming more frequent, more prolonged or more severe, as well as any known precipitating factors, should be determined. If fairly constant, one should note the effect of smoking, seasonal weather changes, dust or irritating fumes. A cough which is aggravated by a change in posture suggests bronchiectasis.

A harassing cough of recent onset suggests that an acute infection is present. Recurrent episodes of cough with free intervals between attacks is a feature of recurrent bronchitis. Chronic cough which persists for more than three months of every year and is not associated with localized bronchopulmonary disease is a feature of chronic bronchitis.

Paroxysms of coughing and wheezing which awaken the patient and are relieved by expectoration of sputum are common in obstructive lung disease. A severe paroxysm of prolonged coughing may result in dizziness, faintness or even syncope (see Chapter 9).

EXPECTORATION

Cough may be nonproductive initially and then be associated with the onset of the expectoration of sputum. Children and some adults usually habitually swallow their sputum and may not recognize or admit that they ever produce any sputum.

Although it may be difficult to be accurate, an approximate estimate of the amount of sputum expectorated during a 24-hour period should be obtained. The patient can generally give a rough estimate if the questioner asks him to relate the amount to a common measure such as a cup, a half cup, tablespoon or teaspoon.

Pinkish, frothy, watery sputum is characteristic of acute pulmonary edema. The mucoid sputum of chronic bronchitis is usually white or gray, and because it is quite viscous, it may be difficult to expectorate. In septic lesions of the lungs, such as bronchiectasis or a lung abscess, the sputum is usually thick and yellow, may have an unpleasant taste and occasionally has an offensive odor. This purulent sputum is generally less viscous than mucoid sputum and therefore is easier to cough up. The sudden expectoration of a very large quantity of pus suggests that a lung abscess may have eroded into a major bronchus.

The presence or absence of a postnasal discharge should be noted and its duration ascertained. The patient will recognize this as "phlegm" in the back of the throat, and if present, its color and consistency should be noted. Generally, the patient attempts to expectorate this material by hawking and clearing his throat rather than by coughing. Such a discharge may induce a chronic cough by irritating the posterior pharyngeal wall.

HEMOPTYSIS

The expectoration of blood is an alarming symptom and usually prompts the patient to seek medical advice. In discussing blood spitting with the patient, it is important to determine whether the material that was expectorated consisted entirely of blood or whether it was sputum that was only stained, streaked or spotted with blood.

The term "hemoptysis" should only be applied to the expectoration of frank blood. When this occurs it is generally bright red initially and gradually darkens and diminishes in amount over the next few days. The amount of blood expectorated should be ascertained, although this is often exaggerated by the patient.

Hemoptysis may occur in pulmonary tuberculosis, bronchiectasis, bronchogenic carcinoma, pulmonary infarction and mitral stenosis. A recent painful tender swelling of a lower extremity may indicate a thrombophlebitis which was followed by a pulmonary thromboembolism. This is commonly observed in elderly patients who have been confined to bed for long periods because of congestive heart failure, multiple fractures or extensive surgery. There is evidence suggesting that the incidence of thromboembolism is high in women taking oral contraceptive pills.

Sputum that is stained with blood is important, for it may be due to a bronchogenic carcinoma; but streaks or spots of blood in the sputum may also be of less consequence and may be due to the hyperemic bronchial mucosa which develops during acute infections of the tracheobronchial tree.

Blood spitting may also occur in patients suffering from certain blood dyscrasias, such as hemophilia and leukemia. Thus, one should inquire about episodes of bleeding from other orifices, the gums or into the skin. Similarly, it may occur as a result of hypoprothrombinemia in patients who are taking maintenance anticoagulant therapy following a myocardial infarction. The upper respiratory tract may also be the source of expectorated blood. The patient may have had epistaxis, and the blood may have been aspirated into the trachea and then expectorated.

Occasionally, a patient may be uncertain whether blood was coughed up from his lungs or was vomited. The distinguishing feature of hemoptysis is that the expectorated blood is generally bright red and frothy, because it is mixed with air, as opposed to hematemesis in which the blood is generally dark with no froth and often contains food particles. Blood originating in the stomach is also usually associated with the passage of black, tarry stools.

BREATHLESSNESS

If breathlessness on exertion is present, its time of onset in the illness and its progress should be noted. It may have remained fairly stationary over the course of the illness, gradually increased in severity, or increased episodically during acute exacerbations of the illness. The breathlessness may develop spontaneously even without exertion, as in asthma, and between attacks the patient may be completely free of breathlessness.

An accurate assessment of the severity of breathlessness is generally fairly difficult to obtain because this is affected by the amount of physical activity the patient undertakes and his fitness. The degree of dyspnea can be roughly approximated, however, if the type of exertion that induces breathlessness is described, especially if a similar exertion was previously carried out without difficulty. The degree of exertional dyspnea can generally be assessed by determining if breathlessness is noted while walking up a slight incline or a flight of stairs, while walking at a normal pace on level ground, while performing such ordinary activities as dressing and shaving, or even while sitting quietly at rest.

If the patient is breathless while lying down (orthopnea) and requires several pillows in order to be comfortable, the possibility of pulmonary congestion due to left-sided heart failure must be considered. However, a person who is suffering from chronic obstructive lung disease may also be more comfortable in an upright position. Breathlessness which awakens the patient may also be cardiac or bronchial in origin. If it is due to left ventricular failure, it may be relieved after he sits up, or he may be in such distress that he rushes to an open window in a frantic effort to obtain fresh air for his relief. If the nocturnal attack of breathlessness is due to the accumulation of secretions during sleep, the breathlessness usually subsides after he expectorates the secretions.

CHEST PAIN

The time and mode of onset of chest pain and its relationship to the other respiratory symptoms should be ascertained. Acute chest pain is associated with a fractured rib, a fibrinous pleurisy secondary to pneumonia or a pulmonary infarct. The pain usually develops gradually if it is caused by fibrositis of the intercostal muscles or herpes zoster.

The anatomic site, area of radiation and the characteristics of the pain are helpful. If the diaphragmatic pleura is involved, pain may be felt along the superior ridge of the trapezius muscle of the affected side as well as along the costal margin. The squeezing, anterior chest pain of myocardial ischemia is usually induced by exertion and relieved by rest and generally radiates into the neck and down one or both arms. The raw, burning discomfort of acute tracheitis is generally situated over the upper anterior portion of the chest. Pain due to pleuritic involvement is usually sharp and knife-like and is aggravated by deep breathing or coughing. On the other hand, the pain caused by fibrositis of the intercostal muscles is also aggravated by deep breathing and coughing. Pain due to nerve root irritation is generally burning in character.

UPPER RESPIRATORY SYMPTOMS

An abnormality in the upper respiratory tract may be an etiological or an aggravating factor in the patient's illness. The patient may complain of episodic attacks of profuse watery nasal discharge, nasal obstruction, paroxysmal sneezing spells, irritation of the eyes or marked tearing. These symptoms suggest that the rhinitis is allergic. Nasal obstruction which varies from one side to the other suggests mucosal swelling which may also have an allergic basis. Nasal obstruction which is constantly present on one side may be due to a deviated nasal septum. A purulent postnasal discharge indicates infection. Attacks of an acute sinusitis are often associated with pain and tenderness of that part of the face overlying the affected sinus.

If the patient complains of hoarseness, one must determine its duration, especially if it was preceded by an upper respiratory infection. If the hoarseness developed immediately after an operation on the thyroid gland, the possibility of an injury to one of the recurrent laryngeal nerves should be considered. Hoarseness due to laryngeal ulceration is an occasional complication of active cavitary pulmonary tuberculosis. A localized growth on one of the vocal cords, whether benign or malignant, is a fairly frequent cause of hoarseness.

CONSTITUTIONAL SYMPTOMS

Feverishness, chilly sensations, excessive sweating, anorexia, weakness, easy fatiguability and weight loss may be associated with any chronic pulmonary disease but are especially common in pulmonary tuberculosis, bronchiectasis, pulmonary abscess and bronchogenic carcinoma. "Slumber sweats" in which the patient wakes from his sleep in a drenching sweat requiring a complete change of night clothes may also occur in these diseases. Severe shaking chills, chattering of the teeth and involuntary shaking of the limbs may occur with bacterial infections, particularly a pneumococcal pneumonia.

EXAMINATION OF THE PATIENT

After obtaining the detailed history of the patient's illness, the physician is able to synthesize the pertinent aspects of the history into patterns suggesting several possible diagnoses. These diagnostic possibilities may now be strengthened and perhaps confirmed by examination of the patient. The following account presents the methods used to demonstrate the abnormal physical signs produced by respiratory disease. A mastery of these methods is essential in order to arrive at a correct diagnosis.

Proficiency in the clinical examination can only be attained by repeated examination of healthy persons so that even a minimal abnormality can be recognized in patients. Just as a functional inquiry into the nonrespiratory system is important in the history of the respiratory illness, a thorough and complete physical examination of the patient is of equal importance. The physical examination should be carried out in an orderly, systematic and consistent manner in every patient so that no abnormal physical sign will be missed. It is through errors of omission that failures in diagnosis occur. Although it is not within the scope of this discussion to cover the complete physical examination, it is obvious from the previous sections that respiratory disturbances may produce signs and symptoms which are referrable to other systems. In addition, abnormal physical findings in organs other than the lungs frequently yield valuable clues as to the nature of the respiratory illness.

In the following discussion, a detailed description of the examination of the respiratory system is presented. The mode of the examination of the remaining systems will not be included, and only those findings which may be helpful in assessing findings in the respiratory system will be referred to.

GENERAL OBSERVATION

Inspection of the patient, the initial phase of the physical examination, should be conducted conscientiously and meticulously before attempting to elicit signs of disease. Much that is learned from inspection is acquired automatically and unconsciously. For instance, most persons can make a fairly accurate guess at the age of a casual acquaintance but are quite unable to describe the physical evidence upon which the judgement is based. Even lay people habitually scrutinize an associate and decide from what they see that he "looks well" or "does not look well." In a similar way, experienced clinicians unconsciously gather valuable impressions, an occult faculty which largely accounts for what is termed "clinical intuition."

In the following discussion some of the more common abnormalities which may be seen are enumerated and briefly discussed. A single observation may be of little value, but in combination with other signs it may be of considerable value in arriving at a final assessment of the underlying respiratory disease.

THE HEAD

It is impossible to enumerate all the factors that may be detected from even a casual glance at a patient's face, but one can usually determine whether or not the patient is in distress and whether it is mental or physical in origin. From the facial expression, one often involuntarily estimates the mental capacity, general character, temperament and mood of the patient. More specific facts such as the presence of respiratory distress, pallor, plethora, cyanosis, pigmentation, a rash, jaundice, edema, venous dilatation, emaciation and obesity should also be noted.

The presence or absence of respiratory distress is particularly important, and one should ascertain whether there is inspiratory or expiratory difficulty, inspiratory collapse and expiratory distention of the external jugular veins, audible wheezing, obvious contraction of the sternomastoid muscles or other accessory muscles of respiration, or widening of the alae nasae during inspiration. In obstructive lung diseases such as asthma, chronic bronchitis and emphysema respirations may be rapid, gasping and shallow in character with the lips pursed during expiration. In an attempt to relieve the respiratory difficulty, the patient may assume a characteristic posture with the trunk bent forward and both hands pressed on the thighs if sitting or, if standing, against a chair or desk.

The breathing pattern should also be noted. Normal persons breathe at a rate of 12 to 18 respirations per minute, and an increased rate is called "tachypnea." A slow, deep, regular type of breathing, called Kussmaul breathing, is seen in patients suffering from metabolic acidosis. An irregular respiratory rhythm, such as Cheyne-Stokes respirations or Biot's respirations — which are occasionally seen in normal persons during sleep and in the very obese even while awake — is usually of grave significance in the presence of respiratory, cardiovascular or renal disease.

Localized neurological signs may be suggestive of a cerebral abscess secondary to a pulmonary abscess or bronchiectasis or perhaps a metastasis from a bronchogenic carcinoma. Delirium, confusion, irrational behavior and hallucinations may occur in severe acute respiratory infections or severe hypoxia and carbon dioxide retention. Meningismus may be indicative of tuberculous meningitis, which may be associated with miliary tuberculosis or, rarely, a pneumococcal meningitis.

THE EYES

Exophthalmos in a dyspneic patient may be due to hyperthyroidism or compression of the trachea by a substernal toxic thyroid gland. Fundoscopic examination may reveal engorged veins and swelling of the optic discs which occasionally develops during acute respiratory failure or small, yellowish, round miliary lesions in the choroid, which are diagnostic of miliary tuberculosis.

The pupils may be affected by respiratory disease. Irritation of the cervical sympathetic ganglia by a bronchogenic carcinoma in the apex of the lung, the so-called "thoracic inlet tumor," or by the pressure of enlarged metastatic lymph nodes may cause dilation of the pupil of that side. With progression of the disease the sympathetic ganglia are paralyzed, and the affected pupil becomes constricted; the palpebral fissure becomes narrower, and there is an absence of sweating on the affected side of the face, the so-called "Horner's syndrome." Argyll Robertson pupils, which are indicative of syphilis, may be associated with an aneurysm of the aorta compressing a bronchus.

THE NECK

Engorgement or visible pulsations of the veins of the neck in a patient who is propped up at an angle of 45 degrees (i.e., the veins are at a higher level than the right auricle) are abnormal and indicate that the venous pressure is elevated. Bilateral jugular venous distention is usually due to congestive heart failure, although it may also be produced by obstruction of the superior vena cava when it is associated with visible collateral veins over the neck and anterior chest wall. As mentioned earlier, distention of the jugular veins, particularly during expiration, is not unusual in patients suffering from severe obstructive lung disease.

A painful stiff neck due to cervical disc degeneration may be associated with irritation of the cervical nerve roots and upper chest pain. An enlarged, hard, fixed thyroid gland may be carcinomatous and may be the source of a pulmonary metastasis. Cervical lymphadenopathy may be due to tuberculosis, malignancy, sarcoidosis, infectious mononucleosis or one of the lymphomas. Scars on the neck may be the result of draining sinuses or operative removal of a tuberculous adenitis.

Palpation is used to determine the position, resiliency, consistency, size and anatomic relations of the various masses which may, or may not, have been obvious on inspection. This serves to differentiate between lymph nodes, the thyroid gland or some soft tissue which may be of no significance. Palpation of the neck for enlarged nodes should be carried out with the finger tips, using gentle pressure and a rotary movement, in the posterior and the anterior triangles of the neck and the submental region. In addition, one should palpate the supraclavicular areas, where the finding of an enlarged node aids in the diagnosis of bronchogenic carcinoma, and the area directly behind the clavicular insertion of the sternomastoid muscle for the scalene node.

THE EXTREMITIES

Clubbing of the fingers and toes is an important manifestation of respiratory disease. In the lateral aspect or profile of the terminal phalanx of a finger the angle between the proximal end of the nail and the soft tissues covering its root is approximately 160 degrees. The earliest sign of digital clubbing is hypertrophy of the soft tissue so that this "base angle" is obliterated and becomes 180 degrees or greater. The normal "base angle" and that seen in digital clubbing are shown in Figure 77.

Obliteration of the base angle is a constant feature throughout the progress of the condition, and its further progression is shown in Figure 78. As the clubbing becomes more severe, the skin overlying the nail bed becomes stretched and glistening and loses its normal wrinkles so that it looks as if it had been polished by a nail buffer. The nail itself then gradually thickens, becoming curved and developing longitudinal ridges. At the same time, the pulp of the terminal phalanx enlarges and eventually becomes blunted and bulbous. In the advanced stage, the nail is thickened, ridged and curved longitudinally and transversely, and the distal end of the nail overrides the end of the finger so that it resembles a parrot's beak. The nail is easily depressed and gives the impression of lying on a bed of fluid.

Clubbing of the digits should not be confused with the curved nails occasionally found in perfectly healthy people. As is seen in Figure 77, the curved nail superficially resembles moderately advanced clubbing and is frequently mistaken for it. However, it can be distinguished from clubbed digits because the "base angle" is normal, always remaining at about 160 degrees.

The thumb and index finger are usually first affected, and the other fingers become involved as the condition progresses. The condition is usually bilateral, although unilateral clubbing and even unidigital clubbing has also been described. Since the terminal phalanges of the toes are normally misshapen, clubbing of these digits is not as obvious as in the fingers. The appearance of the terminal phalanx of the big toe more closely approximates that of the fingers, however, and it is this digit which should be examined for clubbing. The appearance of the normal and the clubbed big toe is shown in Figure 79.

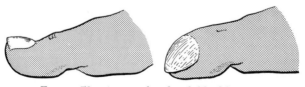

FIGURE 79.   A normal and a clubbed big toe.

Hypertrophic pulmonary osteoarthropathy is the final stage in the progression of digital clubbing. In this situation painful, tender thickening of both the ankles and the wrists is present in conjunction with gross digital clubbing. There is inflammation of the subcutaneous tissues, the capsule and the synovial membrane of the wrists and ankle joints and a periostitis of the lower ends of the long bones in the arms and legs. The presence of hypertrophic pulmonary osteoarthropathy is highly suggestive of pulmonary malignancy.

THE UPPER RESPIRATORY TRACT

As described earlier, diseases which affect the upper respiratory tract may be a factor in diseases of the lower respiratory tract. A searching examination of the mucous membranes of the nose, mouth, tongue, pharynx and larynx should therefore precede the examination of the lungs.

The Nose. The patency of each nasal passage should be tested by having the patient sniff through one while the other is obstructed. In addition the nasal speculum with a head mirror which reflects light into the nasal passages or an electric otoscope should be used to examine the interior of the nose. A deviated nasal septum may lead to nasal obstruction and may be a factor in the production of a chronic infection. Nasal polyps, which have a glistening grape-like appearance and are usually associated with an allergic diathesis, may cause unilateral obstruction. Healthy nasal mucosa is smooth, pink and glistening in appearance, but an inflamed mucous membrane is dull and very red. Allergic nasal mucosa appears swollen and pale. A thin, watery and clear nasal discharge is present in allergic rhinitis. With inflammations the discharge is thick and yellow or green. A yellow or green exudate or postnasal discharge points to a purulent infection. Fresh blood in one of the nasal passages may indicate the source of a recent episode of hemoptysis.

The presence (or absence) of a postnasal discharge and whether it is mucoid or purulent should be noted.

The Mouth. The buccal mucosa should be carefully examined for eruptions, petechiae, pigmentation, cyanosis or the reddish purple color associated with polycythemia. An odorous breath may result from improper oral hygiene and pyorrhea or from chronic infection of the tonsils, adenoids or nasal mucosa. In addition, septic diseases of the lungs, such as bronchiectasis and lung abscess, pyloric obstruction secondary to a duodenal ulcer, or gastric carcinoma may make the breath malodorous. The condition of the gums and teeth should be checked, for poor dental care and pyorrhea may be the factors in the development of bronchopulmonary diseases.

The Larynx. The larynx should be examined indirectly, particularly if the patient complains of hoarseness or a croupy cough or if stridor is evident. This causes very little discomfort to the patient and enables the examiner to obtain a functional assessment of the vocal cords. In this procedure, the patient's tongue is held out with some gauze, and a warmed laryngeal mirror is placed against the soft palate in front of the uvula. With reflected light from a head mirror, the epiglottis, the arytenoid regions and the vocal cords can be viewed. Direct examination of the larynx is carried out by inserting a laryngoscope into the patient's throat while he is lying in a supine position. This procedure is more uncomfortable but is necessary if a biopsy of one of the vocal cords is indicated.

Stridor which is suggestive of laryngeal obstruction is a high-pitched, harsh, inspiratory sound. Aphonia associated with a type of cough which seems to have lost its explosive character suggests paralysis of one of the vocal cords. Unilateral vocal cord paralysis develops as a result of pressure or injury to one of the recurrent laryngeal nerves, such as by a bronchogenic carcinoma. During quiet respiration, the affected vocal cord will occupy a position midway between adduction and abduction and will fail to move toward the midline during phonation.

THE CHEST

There are wide variations in the general contours of normal thoracic cages, but the bony structure of the chest cage is normally symmetrical. Its symmetry is largely related to a straight thoracic spine so that deformities of the thoracic spine such as scoliosis, kyphosis and kyphoscoliosis can produce corresponding alterations in the chest cage. These may be easily overlooked unless the thoracic spine is routinely examined, by both inspection and palpation of the spinous processes. The extent of disfiguration which the chest undergoes varies with the degree of deformity of the thoracic spine.

Other deformities of the thorax such as the funnel-chest and pigeon-breast are usually of no serious significance, although severe grades of funnel-chest may so distort and compress the mediastinum that cardiac and respiratory embarrassment may develop in later years.

An additional important observation is the presence of inspiratory "indrawing" of the intercostal spaces which is frequently seen over the lower lateral part of the chest cage. This will be evident on both sides of the chest in cases of chronic obstructive lung disease, or it may only be visible on one side if there is fibrosis of the underlying lung. The sudden onset of unilateral intercostal indrawing suggests atelectasis secondary to bronchial obstruction.

Movement. Since there is no absolute standard of normal chest movement, only a definite departure from the average can be re-garded as significant. Unequal movement of the two sides of the chest suggests that there is a disease process underlying the chest wall which moves less. In chronic obstructive lung disease the chest is barrel-shaped, tending to move up and down "as a whole." The move-ment of the chest cage laterally is restricted, but both sides move equally. Although the costal margin normally moves outward during inspiration, it may occasionally move paradoxically, i.e., inward during inspiration and outward during expiration, in conditions in which the diaphragm has been depressed.

Cardiac Impulse. The apical impulse of the heart can be seen frequently in the fifth left intercostal space, approximately 8 cm. from the midline of the sternum. It may not be visible if hyperin-flation of the lungs is present. Its exact position is extremely import-ant in the differential diagnosis of the underlying respiratory disease.

Collateral Veins. Engorged superficial veins over the chest wall, the neck and the upper extremities, often associated with an edematous, plethoric face, are indicative of an elevated venous pres-sure resulting from superior vena caval obstruction. This is frequently caused by a pulmonary neoplasm with metastatic involvement of the mediastinal nodes or by the pressure of an expanding tumor such as a thymoma in the anterior mediastinum. If there is partial obstruction of the superior vena cava, the engorged veins may be considerably fewer in number and only slightly dilated, but they enlarge strikingly when the patient performs the Valsalva maneuver.

EXAMINATION OF THE CHEST

The physical examination of the chest should answer the follow-ing questions:

1. Is there an abnormality in the thorax?
2. If an abnormality is found, is the pattern one of partial airway obstruction, consolidation, fibrosis, atelectasis, a pleural effusion or pneumothorax?
3. Does the disease process affect one lung or both lungs?
4. If disease is present in both lungs, is it predominant in one lung or are both lungs equally affected?
5. Is the volume of the affected lung or lungs decreased, in-creased or unchanged?
6. Is pulmonary hypertension present?
7. Is there an impairment in pulmonary function?

In order to answer these questions a knowledge of the boundaries of thoracic contents is essential, for this provides the examiner with a mental picture of the lobe or segment involved in a disease process. With this in mind, the surface anatomy of the chest will now be re-viewed.

LANDMARKS

The spinous processes of the thoracic vertebrae and the sternal angle enable the examiner to orient himself with regard to the position of the underlying thoracic contents. In the erect subject with head bent slightly forward, the first thoracic spine is the lower of two prominent projections at the junction of the neck and the thorax, the upper projection being the spinous process of the seventh cervical vertebra. The kidney angle, which is at the junction of the posterior end of the costal margin and the sacrospinalis muscle, is situated at the level of the twelfth thoracic spine.

The sternal angle, or angle of Louis, is at the same level as the bifurcation of the trachea and indicates the approximate upper level at which the lungs meet anteriorly and the upper limit of the atria of the heart. In order to demonstrate an increased venous pressure in the arms, therefore, they must be elevated above the level of the sternal angle. If the pressure is normal, the veins collapse when the arms are elevated to this level. The sternal angle also serves as a landmark for the identification of the costal cartilages and the ribs. The second costal cartilage articulates with the sternum at the sternal angle, and palpation from this level identifies ribs, cartilages or intercostal spaces.

TOPOGRAPHICAL LINES

Certain conventional topographical lines are also used to demarcate various areas of the chest wall. The "midclavicular line," as the name implies, runs vertically downward over the anterior chest wall from the middle of the clavicle to the lower costal margin. The "anterior axillary line" runs vertically downward from the origin of the anterior axillary fold, and the "posterior axillary line" runs downward from the termination of the posterior fold. The "midaxillary line" runs vertically downward over the lateral aspect of the chest wall from the middle of the apex of the axilla to the lower costal margin, midway between the anterior and posterior axillary lines. The "midscapular line" runs vertically downward from the middle of the inferior angle of the scapula to the kidney angle.

SURFACE MARKINGS

The apices of both lungs are closely covered by pleura and lie in the root of the neck in an area which starts at the lower end of the sternoclavicular junction, curves upward to about one inch above the clavicle and then descends to the lower end of the clavicle at the junction of its lateral and middle thirds.

The anterior border of the right pleural space can be indicated by a line drawn from the sternoclavicular joint to the center of the angle of Louis and then down the sternum as far as the xiphisternal joint. The surface markings of the anterior border of the right lung correspond almost exactly to that of the right pleura, for the lung lies just a little inside it. The anterior border of the left pleural space is indicated by a line drawn from the left sternoclavicular joint to the center of the angle of Louis and then down to the level of the fourth costal cartilage, where it turns laterally to the left border of the sternum and then runs downward to the seventh costal cartilage. The anterior border of the left lung occupies a position slightly inside the pleura until the fourth left costal cartilage is reached; then it turns laterally along the fourth costal cartilage to a point about 3 cm. from the left sternal border. From here it again turns downward and ends at the sixth costal cartilage, about 2.5 cm. from the border of the sternum.

The inferior borders of both pleural spaces correspond to a line starting at the lower ends of both anterior margins and then running backward, crossing the sixth ribs at the midclavicular line, the eighth ribs in the midaxillary line and the twelfth ribs in the midscapular line, finally ending about 2.5 cm. lateral to the twelfth thoracic spine. The posterior part of these lines is fairly horizontal and passes through the kidney angle, ending at the medial ends of the twelfth ribs. The inferior borders of both lungs correspond to those of the pleura in its anterior part, crossing the midclavicular and midaxillary lines at the sixth and eighth ribs, respectively. Thereafter, they cross the mid- scapular line at the tenth rib posteriorly and end at the level of the tenth thoracic spine. The posterior borders of the pleurae and lungs run parallel to one another, that of the lung being just lateral to the pleural border.

Fissures. The situation of the various lobes of both lungs is illustrated in Figures 80 to 82. The major or *oblique fissures* in both lungs separate the upper and lower lobes. The course of the oblique fissures can be mapped out on the surface of the chest wall by a line starting at the second thoracic spine posteriorly and running obliquely downward, curving around the chest wall over its posterior, lateral and anterior aspects. It crosses the midaxillary line at the fifth rib and ends anteriorly at the inferior border of the sixth costal cartilage, midway between the midsternal and midclavicular lines. If the pa- tient stands erect and places his hands behind his neck, the position of the scapulae is such that their vertebral borders correspond to the posterior parts of the oblique fissures.

The minor or *transverse fissure,* which is present only in the right lung, separates the middle lobe from the upper lobe. The lingular

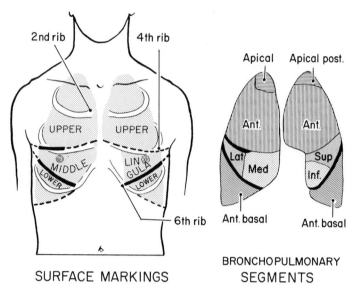

FIGURE 80. Surface markings of the lungs (anterior aspect). The underlying bronchopulmonary segments are also shown.

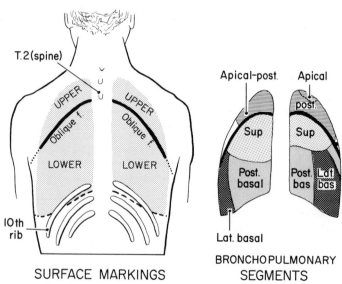

FIGURE 81. Surface markings of the lungs (posterior aspect). The underlying bronchopulmonary segments are also shown.

segment of the left upper lobe corresponds morphologically to the right middle lobe and it possesses its own bronchus, although a true fissure is generally absent. The transverse fissure can be outlined on the chest wall by a line starting at the anterior border of the lung at the level of the third or fourth intercostal space. It then passes laterally, in a slightly upward direction, ending at the point where the oblique fissure crosses the midaxillary line.

Bronchopulmonary Segments. The *bronchopulmonary segments* lie within the confines of the boundaries of the lobes. The anterior segment of both upper lobes underlies an area in the upper anterior chest between the levels of the clavicle and the transverse fissure. The apical segment of the right lung occupies the area of the lung above the clavicle anteriorly, and a small area posteriorly in the apex of the lung. The remainder of the posterior aspect of the right upper lobe is occupied by its posterior segment. The apical posterior segment of the left upper lobe underlies an area similar to that of the apical and posterior segments of the right upper lobe.

The medial segment of the right middle lobe is situated in the part of the middle lobe which occupies the anterior surface of the chest, and the lateral segment occupies the remaining portion of the middle lobe area in the anterior portion of the axilla. The lingular segment of the left upper lobe which has two segments, a superior and an inferior, occupies a position on the left anterior chest wall which is identical to that of the middle lobe of the right lung. The superior segment occupies approximately the upper half of the lingular area.

The surface anatomy of the bronchopulmonary segments of the two lower lobes is very similar. The superior or apical segment occupies the upper part of the posterior aspect of the lower lobe, its upper boundary being the oblique fissure and its lower boundary corresponding approximately to the spinous process of the seventh thoracic vertebra. The remainder of the posterior aspect of the lower lobe area is occupied by the posterior basal segment. The axillary aspect of the lower lobe area is occupied by the lateral basal segment, and that part of the lower lobe area on the anterior chest wall is occupied by the anterior basal segment. The medial basal segment of the right lower lobe lies next to the mediastinum and has no comparable area over the surface of the chest wall.

The apex beat of the heart, which corresponds to the apex of the left ventricle, is normally situated in the fifth left intercostal space, approximately 8 cm. from the midline of the sternum. The left border of the heart, formed by the left atrial appendage and the left ventricle, starts one inch from the left border of the sternum at the level of the second costal cartilage and runs laterally to the apex of the heart. The right border of the heart, formed entirely by the right atrium,

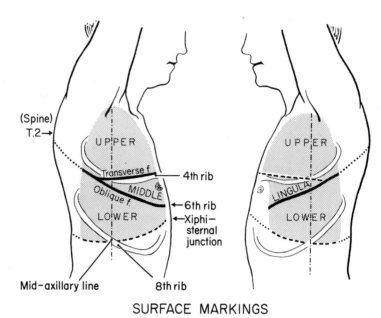

SURFACE MARKINGS

FIGURE 82.   Surface markings of the lungs (lateral aspect).

corresponds to a line which is slightly convex to the right, running between the third and sixth costal cartilages, about one-half inch from the right border of the sternum. The superior border of the heart, formed by the right and left atria, corresponds to a line drawn between the upper ends of the left and right borders. The inferior border of the heart, formed chiefly by the right ventricle and partly by the left ventricle, is located by a line joining the lower ends of the left and right borders and passing over the xiphisternal joint. Normally, the borders of the pericardial sac correspond to those of the heart.

PALPATION

Position of the Mediastinum. An alteration in the relative volume of the two lungs is reflected by a shift of the mediastinum from its normal midline position, and this can be determined by palpation of the position of the trachea and the cardiac impulse.

The trachea is normally in the midline position, except for elderly persons in whom it may normally be shifted to the right because of pressure on it by an unfolded, atheromatous ascending aorta. A shift of the trachea from its midline position is indicative of intrathoracic disease.

The tracheal position should be determined while the patient

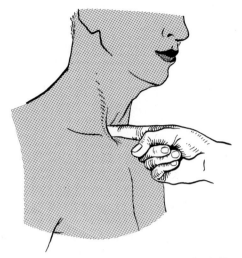

FIGURE 83. Palpation for the position of the trachea. The tip of the fully extended finger is inserted just medial to the sternoclavicular joint; the part of the trachea just before entrance to the thoracic inlet is the most mobile and reflects shifts of the mediastinum.

is either in a sitting position or recumbent in bed, his neck slightly flexed so that the sternomastoid muscles are relaxed, and his chin in the midline position. The examiner is only interested in the lowest part of the trachea, just before it enters the thoracic inlet, which is the most mobile part of the trachea. Small shifts of the mediastinum may be less obvious if the trachea is palpated at a higher level in the neck. As is shown in Figure 83, the tip of the examiner's fully extended index finger is inserted into the suprasternal notch just medial to the sternoclavicular joint and is gently pressed back toward the cervical spine, first on one side and then the other. If the trachea is in its normal midline position, the examining finger will strike only soft tissue on both sides of the trachea. If the trachea is deviated from its normal position, the examining finger will encounter the firm cartilaginous ring of the trachea on the side to which the mediastinum has shifted and soft tissue on the other side.

To determine the position of the apical impulse, the lower left anterior chest is palpated with the palm of the hand, which is moved from the midaxillary line toward the sternum until the impulse is felt. Using the tips of one or two fingers, the most lateral definite systolic impact should be defined. The apical impulse may be difficult to palpate, especially in sthenic or obese subjects and also in patients suffering from chronic obstructive lung disease, although the action of the heart may be seen and felt in the epigastrium.

The intensity of the cardiac impulse should also be noted while the palm is over the left inframammary region. Normally, a localized systolic thrust is felt, but a heave is imparted to the ribs if left ventricular hypertrophy is present. In right ventricular hypertrophy there may be a thrust just to the left of the sternum and simultaneous retraction over the left ventricle so that a rocking motion is produced.

If the apical impulse is more than 8 cm. from the midsternal line in the fifth left interspace, the heart is either hypertrophied or displaced. The finding of a centrally placed trachea in the presence of a shift of the apical impulse to the left is, in all probability, due to left ventricular hypertrophy. The trachea and apex beat may be displaced by an abnormality of the bony thoracic cage, a lesion of the lung parenchyma, a disease of the pleural space or an abnormality of the diaphragm. In chest cage deformity they are displaced to the side of the compressed lung. In a pulmonary condition, such as atelectasis or a local fibrosis, they are displaced to the side of the lesion, but in a pleural effusion or pneumothorax they are shifted to the opposite side. When there is herniation of abdominal contents into the thorax, the mediastinum is also shifted to the opposite side.

The Site of Chest Pain. Determination of the source of chest pain requires a careful and systematic search for tender areas. Starting well away from the painful area the tip of the thumb should be pressed firmly, following along the course of both the ribs and the intercostal spaces. A grating sensation at the site of the fracture will be associated with a localized area of exquisite tenderness if there is a rib fracture. Acute, localized tenderness when pressure is applied to the junction of the affected cartilage and the rib with the hands on either side of the dislocated cartilage is indicative of subluxation of a costal cartilage.

Fibrositis of one of the intercostal muscles is also associated with a localized area of tenderness within the affected intercostal space. A small peripheral pulmonary embolus may cause acute pleuritic pain which is associated with exquisite tenderness in the adjoining intercostal space.

If the chest pain suggests nerve root irritation, hyperalgesia should be sought. By drawing the point of a needle or a pin across the skin both from above and below the painful area at intervals along the side of the chest, the level at which the skin irritation becomes more acute is noted. In this way, one can often outline and identify the affected dermatome.

Movement of the Chest Cage. Reduced distensibility of a portion of the lung is reflected by diminished movement of the overlying area of the chest cage. Diminished movement of a part of the chest is the earliest evidence of pulmonary disease, often developing before any other clinical abnormality can be detected.

Assessment of chest movement is accomplished by stretching the skin of the chest wall toward the middle of the chest with the examiner's hands while the patient is breathing quietly and, then, allowing the hands to follow the chest movement while the patient inspires deeply. The examiner's elbows and shoulders should be maintained in a relaxed state and only the wrists used to apply pres-

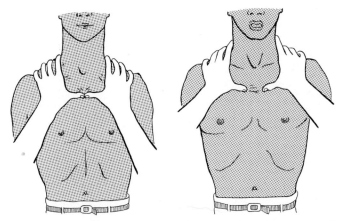

FIGURE 84. Examination of the movement of the upper lobes. Both hands move an equal distance with inspiration.

sure to the chest wall, as this allows the shoulders to act as a fulcrum which helps to exaggerate the movement of the hands. Provided both areas are healthy, both hands will move an equal distance away from each other. The extent of movement varies in healthy persons, and it is the comparison of the two sides that is important. If one of the sides is diseased, then its movement will be decreased. On the other hand, if the disease process is minimal, movement may lag at the beginning of inspiration, but total movement may be equal bilaterally.

Movement of the upper lobes is assessed while the patient faces the examiner. The patient should turn his head away from the examiner's face to avoid the possibility of infection. Movement is checked over the anterior chest wall because the upper lobes are largely situated anteriorly under the first four ribs. The method of examining movement of the upper lobes is illustrated in Figure 84. The examiner places the palms of both hands firmly over the patient's upper anterior chest wall with fingers extended and overlying the trapezius muscles. The skin is then stretched by dragging the palms of the hands downward until the palms lie firmly over the infraclavicular areas while the extended fingers remain over the supraclavicular regions. Keeping the thumbs fully extended, the skin is pulled medially toward the sternum by the hands until the tips of both thumbs meet at the midsternal line. With the pressure on the stretched skin applied only by the wrists, and the elbows and the shoulders relaxed, the hands are allowed to follow the movement of the skin as the patient inspires deeply.

The middle lobe of the right lung and the lingular segment of the left upper lobe underlie the corresponding fifth and sixth ribs. Inspiratory expansion of this portion of the chest wall takes place in

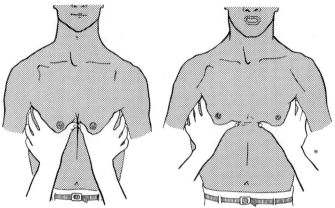

FIGURE 85.   Examination of the movement of the middle lobe and lingula. Both hands move an equal distance with inspiration.

both an anteroposterior and a lateral direction, but it is primarily the lateral expansion of these ribs which is tested (Fig. 85). Movement of the middle lobe and lingula is assessed while the patient faces the examiner. The widely outstretched fingers of both hands are placed over the posterior axillary folds high up in the axilla, with the palms lying flat against the chest wall. The underlying skin is then pulled medially until the outstretched thumbs meet at the mid-sternal line, the pressure once again being applied only by the wrists, and the hands are allowed to follow the chest movement.

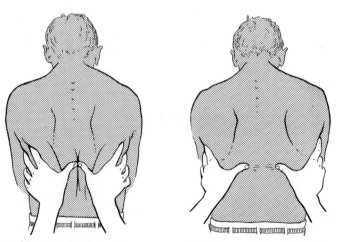

FIGURE 86.   Examination of the movement of the lower lobes. Both hands move an equal distance with inspiration.

Movement of the lower lobes is assessed while the patient sits with his back to the examiner. Since these lobes underlie the corresponding seventh to tenth ribs, inspiratory expansion of this part of the chest cage takes place entirely in a lateral direction. As is shown in Figure 86, the examiner places both his hands high up in the axilla with the outstretched fingers overlying the anterior axillary folds. Both hands are then drawn medially, pulling the underlying skin with them until the outstretched thumbs meet in the midline over the vertebral spinous processes, and then they are allowed to follow the movement of the chest.

The lower lobes differ from the other lobes in that they also expand vertically because of the downward excursion of the diaphragm. Vertical movement of the lower lobes is assessed by percussing the descent of the diaphragm, a procedure which will be discussed later.

Because it is dome-shaped, the diaphragm also causes inspiratory elevation of the lower ribs during inspiration. In examining for this action of the diaphragm, the examiner stands beside the supine patient and places both his hands lightly over the lower anterior chest wall while both thumbs overlie the respective costal margins, their tips almost meeting in the midline over the xiphoid process. As is shown in Figure 87, the examiner's thumbs move away from each other for an equal distance when the patient inspires deeply if the dome shape of the diaphragm has not been altered. If, instead of being dome-shaped, the diaphragm were simply a flat sheet of muscle, contraction would cause the costal margins to move inward. This is what happens when the diaphragm becomes depressed by disease, such as hyperinflation of the lungs, or by fluid or air in the pleural space.

Fremitus.   Vibrations which are produced over the thoracic wall as a result of the conduction of vocal sounds through the tracheo-bronchial tree and lung parenchyma are known as "vocal fremitus."

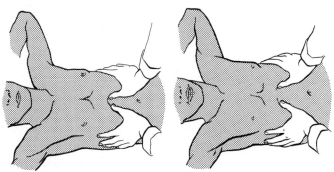

FIGURE 87.   Examination of the action of the diaphragm on the costal margins. Both hands move an equal distance with inspiration.

Although an alteration in the degree of fremitus can be detected by means of the stethoscope, the method which is traditionally used is palpation or "tactile fremitus." Using the side of the hand, the examiner can detect vibrations while the patient slowly repeats a combination of words such as "one, two, three" or "ninety-nine." Often there is a striking change from normal fremitus to an increase or decrease in intensity when the side of the hand reaches the diseased area.

All areas of both sides of the chest must be compared with one another. The intensity of the fremitus is normally uniform over healthy lungs, except for the apex of the right lung, where the intensity is frequently increased because the bronchi are closer to the chest wall. Tactile fremitus is less intense in women and children than it is in men, probably because their voices are less resonant. It also is less intense if there is a considerable amount of muscle or fat interposed between lung tissue and the palpating hand, but the decrease in intensity of the fremitus is uniform over the entire chest wall in such cases. Tactile fremitus increases in intensity whenever the density of the underlying lung parenchyma is increased, as in consolidation or extensive pulmonary fibrosis, as long as the underlying bronchi are patent. Tactile fremitus is diminished or absent when there is fluid or air in the pleural space or when obstruction of a bronchus has led to atelectasis.

PERCUSSION

Percussion is performed in order to determine whether there is an alteration in the density of the underlying area of lung or pleural space. There are two methods of percussion: direct and indirect. Indirect percussion, which is also known as mediate percussion, is used most commonly and is effected by placing the third finger of the left hand (the pleximeter) on the surface of the chest and tapping it with the third finger of the right hand (the plexor). Direct percussion, which is also known as immediate percussion, is effected without the interposition of a pleximeter, the chest wall being struck directly with the pads of one or two fingers. Direct percussion of the central part of the clavicles with the tips of one or two fingers is occasionally used to detect an abnormality in an upper lobe, but it provides little information compared to indirect percussion, especially if the underlying lesion is small.

The position of the fingers during the act of indirect percussion of the chest wall is shown in Figure 88. If the examiner is right-handed, the left middle finger is used as the pleximeter. The terminal phalanx of the finger is applied to the patient's chest wall with very little pressure, and the rest of the finger and the remaining four

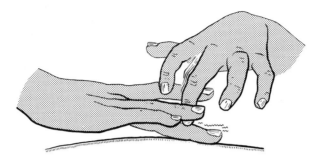

FIGURE 88.   Percussion of the chest.

fingers are raised slightly so that the percussion note is not dampened. Using the wrist as a fulcrum, with the elbow fixed in a semi-
flexed position, the plexor finger is brought down sharply at a right
angle to tap the terminal phalanx of the pleximeter finger in a rapid
staccato manner. The blows should be short, sharp and light, with
instantaneous recoil of the finger, because if the recoil is slow, the
sound may be dampened. If the percussion is too forceful, large areas
of the chest will be made to vibrate, so that the underlying pulmonary lesion may be missed. Conversely, if the lesion is small and
more than two inches beneath the chest wall, it may not be detected
by percussion.

The pitch of the sound produced during percussion is determined by the ratio of air-containing tissue to solid tissue in the area
directly beneath the percussing finger. Well-aerated lung parenchyma
produces a low-pitched resonant sound which is similar to that of a
muffled drum. A sound that is higher in pitch, with a dull to flat note,
implies that the amount of solid tissue beneath the percussing finger
is increased because of atelectasis, fibrosis, consolidation or fluid in
the pleural space.

In most cases, diminished movement will already have alerted
the examiner as to the side or particular area that is affected. It is a
good plan to percuss over the supposedly healthy lung first. The
pleximeter finger is moved slowly and continuously from the apex
down to the base, anteriorly in the axilla, and posteriorly with the
plexor continuously tapping rapidly and lightly. A practically continuous sound, having the same pitch throughout, will result if the
underlying lung is normal, and a change in pitch will be obvious.
The same procedure is then carried out on the side of the chest which
is suspected to be abnormal. If a disease process is suspected in the
lower part of the chest, percussion should be started at the apex,
proceeding downward toward the abnormal area. If an abnormality
in the upper part of the chest is suspected, percussion should be
started over the base of the lung. The borders of an abnormal area

should be outlined by percussing from above and below as well as from each side. To be certain that the pitch is truly altered, it should be compared to the corresponding area of the opposite side.

When a pleural effusion is present, the pitch of the percussion note is high, and it sounds very flat. Characteristically, at the upper level of the dullness there is a gradual blending into a resonant note indicative of the normal lung parenchyma above it.

A small collection of fluid in the pleural space may be difficult to differentiate from an elevated diaphragm. As long as the elevated diaphragm is not immobile and fixed by adhesions, the two may be distinguished from one another by having the patient inspire deeply. The upper limit of dullness may move downward if the impaired note is due to an elevated diaphragm but not if it is due to pleural fluid.

The percussion note over a pneumothorax is hyperresonant, the degree of resonance depending on the amount of air that is present in the pleural space. It must be remembered that air tends to rise so that a small collection of air will be evident only in the upper part of the chest cage.

If there is a hydropneumothorax, i.e., both air and fluid within the pleural space, the air is always situated above the fluid. In this case the upper limit of the flat note caused by the fluid ends abruptly and has a horizontal upper border, or conversely, the lower limit of the hyperresonant note has a horizontal lower border.

Percussion of Shoulder Straps. Percussion of the "shoulder straps" may detect an abnormality in the apices of the lungs, such as may occur with pulmonary tuberculosis or an early bronchogenic carcinoma. Percussion should be carried out from dullness to resonance. Beginning at the lateral end of the shoulder the pleximeter finger is moved continuously along the trapezius toward the neck until a zone of resonance is reached, and this border is then marked with a pencil. Percussion is then carried out moving laterally from the neck until a zone of resonance is reached, and this border is also marked with the pencil. The width of the resonant zones on both sides are then compared. The shoulder straps are normally equal and approximately 4 to 6 cm. in width. If the apex of one lung is diseased, the shoulder strap on that side will be considerably narrower or even obliterated.

Percussion of Diaphragmatic Movement. The inspiratory descent of the diaphragm may be assessed by means of percussion. This is carried out over the lower posterior surface of the chest wall while the patient is sitting. The pleximeter finger should be placed in a horizontal position so that it lies parallel with the plane of diaphragmatic dullness. It is easier to detect the change in note if percussion is carried out from the area of resonance to dullness—i.e., down from the lower lobe of the lung—until the abrupt, flat note produced by the solid intra-abdominal contents is reached, indicating the position of the diaphragm. The procedure is repeated while the patient holds his breath at full inspiration and at full expiration. If diaphragmatic movement is normal, the level of dullness will be lower during inspiration than during expiration, the extent being equal on both sides. If the diaphragm is paralyzed on one side, it will move paradoxically, rising above its resting level when a deep inspiration is made. The movement of the diaphragm can also be assessed anteriorly by percussing the upper level of liver dullness (normally at the level of the fourth right intercostal space) and noting its change in position from full inspiration to full expiration.

AUSCULTATION

Auscultation, the detection of breath sounds and abnormal sounds by means of the stethoscope, should be carried out over the entire chest.

Breath Sounds.   The student can best appreciate the soft rustling quality of the vesicular breath sound by listening through his stethoscope over the axillary region of his own chest wall. The inspiratory phase is easily heard, but the expiratory phase is considerably fainter, and its length is only about one-third of the inspiratory phase. As has already been pointed out, the "vesicular" breath sound is the type of breath sound heard normally over the entire chest wall, except for the right supraclavicular area which overlies the apex of the right lung. Here the breath sounds have a bronchovesicular quality because the bronchi are closer to the chest wall.

The student can best appreciate the bronchovesicular breath sound by listening through his stethoscope over the right supraclavicular area of his own chest. If bronchovesicular breath sounds are heard anywhere but over the right apex, it implies that the underlying lung parenchyma has become affected by a disease process which has altered its "selective transmitter" properties so that more of the high frequency vibrations in the bronchi pass through to the chest wall. As a result, the expiratory phase of the breath sound is longer, louder and higher in pitch than that of the vesicular sound. In chronic obstructive lung disease, such as asthma or emphysema, the breath sounds are often very faint and distant, and the expiratory phase is prolonged. The breath sound is often mistakenly thought to be bronchovesicular.

The student can gain an appreciation of bronchial breath sounds by listening over his own trachea at the upper part of the sternum where there is no lung tissue between the airway and the stethoscope. In this sound, the inspiratory and expiratory notes are equal in pitch,

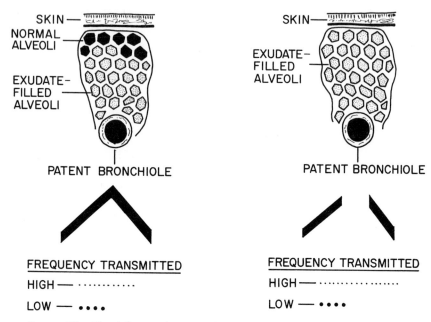

FIGURE 89.   The difference between the bronchovesicular breath sound (left) and the bronchial breath sound (right). The sound produced depends upon the proportion of diseased alveoli. Note that the bronchial breath sound has a silent gap between end-inspiration and beginning expiration.

intensity and duration and are separated by a silent interval or gap. This breath sound is called "bronchial." It means that a disease process has become extensive so that there is considerable loss of air-containing alveoli and that patent bronchi are surrounded by solid lung tissue. The intensity of the bronchial breath sounds will depend upon the diameter of the patent bronchus underlying the solid portion of lung. If for some reason the bronchus has become completely obstructed so that there is no movement of air within it, the breath sounds may be faint or even absent. The distinguishing feature between the bronchovesicular breath sound and the bronchial breath sound is that in the former the inspiratory phase runs directly into the expiratory phase, and in the latter there is a silent interval or "gap" between end-inspiration and beginning-expiration (Fig. 89).

Whispering Pectoriloquy. If one listens with a stethoscope while the patient whispers a combination of words such as "one, two, three," one may bring out small areas of consolidation or confirm the suspicion of consolidation. This characteristic high-pitched sound can be appreciated by the student if he listens with the stethoscope over his own trachea while whispering "one, two, three." By whispering, vibrations with a very high frequency are deliberately created in the bronchial tree. As long as the underlying lung parenchyma is healthy, none of these vibrations are transmitted to the chest wall because of the dampening effect of the "selective transmitter" property of the alveoli. However, if the underlying lung tissue is consolidated, it apparently loses its "selective transmitter" quality, and the whispered sound is transmitted to the chest wall with great clarity. "Whispering pectoriloquy" is a very helpful physical sign, particularly if the consolidated lesions are small and patchy, as in lobular pneumonia.

Egophany. A similar alteration in the quality of the sound heard on the chest wall takes place if the words "one, two, three" are spoken instead of whispered when there is consolidation of the underlying lung parenchyma. The words come through loudly and with great clarity but have a nasal bleating quality. This characteristic sign of consolidation is known as "egophany" or "bronchophany."

Adventitious Sounds. Abnormal vibrations produced by a pathological process in the tracheobronchial tree or the lung parenchyma are called "adventitious sounds." Their presence always indicates that some type of pathological process has developed in the affected area.

Rhonchi are prolonged musical or whistling notes which are produced within the lumen of the tracheobronchial tree. They are indicative of increased turbulence, presumably due to narrowing of the lumina of the tubes. Rhonchi therefore become more pronounced during the expiratory phase of respiration and especially during forced expirations or the expulsive phase of coughing.

The pitch of the rhonchus depends on the diameter of the bronchus in which the sound is produced. A rhonchus which has a low-pitched quality is produced in one of the larger bronchi; one that has a medium-pitched note is more likely produced within medium-sized bronchi; and a rhonchus which has a very high-pitched note is produced in a small bronchiole. If the bronchial obstruction is very slight, however, rhonchi may not be evident during quiet respiration and will only be elicited by having the patient expire forcibly through a wide-open mouth for as long as possible.

By listening over the chest wall while the patient carries out forceful expirations, the site of origin of the rhonchi may occasionally be detected. A persistent rhonchus which is localized to one portion of the chest wall is a very important finding, for it signifies a localized partial obstruction, which may be due to a new growth, bronchostenosis, an aspirated foreign body or secretions. On the other hand, rhonchi which are equally distributed over both sides of the chest are indicative of diffuse bronchial obstruction.

In contrast to the musical sound of rhonchi, which are best heard during expiration, *rales* are moist, short, disconnected bubbling

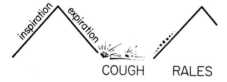

COUGH   RALES

FIGURE 90.   "Post-tussic" rales.

sounds which are heard most readily during inspiration. The pitch of a rale depends on the size of the chamber involved as well as on the type of lesion producing it. They may be classified according to their pitch and position during inspiration which, in turn, may yield information about their site of production. Low-pitched rales heard in the initial third of the inspiratory phase suggest that secretions are present in the large and medium-sized bronchi. Medium-pitched rales heard during the middle third of the inspiratory phase suggest that the smaller bronchi are involved, and high-pitched or fine rales heard during the terminal third of inspiration suggest that the lung parenchyma may be involved.

If the disease in the alveoli is very slight, rales may not be elicited by an ordinary deep inspiration. They can often be brought out, however, by having the patient inspire and expire deeply and then cough. As seen in Figure 90, a shower of very fine rales may then be heard during the initial phase of the ensuing inspiration. These *"post-tussic"* rales are probably produced by the separation of sticky bronchiolar walls which have become adherent during the compressive phase of the cough. Conversely, rales which are heard during ordinary breathing may disappear following a cough, indicating that the secretions producing the rales had been moved up higher in the bronchial tree by the act of coughing.

A *pleural rub* is a creaking, leathery sound which seems to be close to the examining ear and is heard at the end of inspiration and at the beginning of expiration (Fig. 91). The friction rub is diagnostic of pleural irritation and is most likely produced by the rubbing of the inflamed surfaces of the two pleural layers against one another during respiration. Since the excursion of the pleural surfaces is greatest

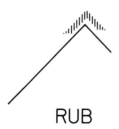

RUB

FIGURE 91.   The "pleural rub."

over the lower lobes, friction rubs are most frequently detected in the lower parts of the chest; they are only very occasionally heard over the upper areas.

Other Abnormal Sounds. A creaky, interrupted, dry sound which characteristically extends uniformly throughout the whole of inspiration and expiration may be heard when there is gross fibrosis affecting the lung parenchyma or the peribronchial tissues.

When air and free fluid are both present in the pleural cavity a splashing sound, which is easily detected by the stethoscope, may be produced. This *"succussion splash"* is demonstrated by shaking the patient abruptly while the examiner listens to the chest. If a bronchopleural fistula is present, one can often hear a gurgling sound which is caused by air escaping from the fistula into the fluid.

SIGNS OF PULMONARY HEART DISEASE

Respiratory disease may lead to an increase in the pulmonary vascular resistance and the consequent development of pulmonary hypertension and right ventricular hypertrophy. There are no abnormal signs in the lungs which are indicative of an increased pulmonary vascular resistance; this can only be elicited by the examination of the heart. In the following discussion only the methods of examination of the heart which are pertinent to the signs of increased pulmonary vascular resistance are presented.

Cardiac Impulse. The position and character of the cardiac impulse, if visible, should be noted during the inspection of the chest. The character of the cardiac impulse is as important as its location, for a heave over the hypertrophied right ventricle just to the left of the lower half of the sternum is frequently felt in cases of right ventricular hypertrophy and pulmonary hypertension. There is often an associated zone of conspicuous retraction over the left ventricle lateral to the heave which gives the precordium a characteristic rocking motion. In addition, systolic expansion of a dilated pulmonary artery may produce a visible pulsation in the left upper parasternal area.

The Heart Sounds. The second heart sound is caused by closure of the aortic and the pulmonic valves. The aortic component is best heard in the aortic area as well as the apex of the heart, and the pulmonic component is best heard in the pulmonic area. Palpation, particularly over the pulmonic area, may reveal vibrations associated with an accentuated pulmonic sound, indicating that pulmonary hypertension is present. On auscultation, the intensity of the second pulmonic heart sound should be noted because it is increased when pulmonary hypertension is present. The pulmonic second sound is normally split, and this is accentuated during inspiration because of a prolongation of right ventricular systole as a result of its increased filling during inspiration. If the split does not widen during inspiration, this further suggests the presence of pulmonary hypertension. On the other hand, a prolonged split of the second pulmonic sound during inspiration is probably caused by a delay in closure of the pulmonic valve, which is usually the result of either a bundle branch block or a mild pulmonary stenosis.

A high-pitched systolic ejection click in the pulmonic area is also indicative of pulmonary hypertension. This occurs during systole just after the opening of the pulmonic valve at the end of the period of isometric contraction. It is probably due to accentuated ejection vibrations, and it is almost invariably found in patients with large left-to-right shunts, mild pulmonary stenosis or dilatation of the pulmonary artery.

The presence of heart murmurs may yield evidence indicating the source of the respiratory symptoms. The typical apical diastolic murmur of mitral stenosis may indicate the possible origin of a recent hemoptysis, or atrial fibrillation may explain the cause of a pulmonary infarction.

ASSESSMENT OF PULMONARY FUNCTION

Just as the blood pressure is an essential component of the evaluation of cardiovascular function, assessment of the amount of disability present is an essential component of the clinical assessment of the respiratory system. A rough evaluation of the extent of disturbance of ventilatory function can be made while examining the patient.

The amount of disturbance in ventilatory function can be assessed in the office or at the bedside by analysis of the forced expiratory volume with a simple spirometer, the time taken to expire forcibly, or the flow rates achieved. In restrictive disease such as pulmonary fibrosis, the vital capacity is low. In obstructive lung disease, the forced expiratory volume is slowed, and the amount expired in the first second ($FEV_{1.0}$) is reduced.

The forced expiratory time can be measured by auscultation. After a maximum inspiratory effort, the patient expires forcibly for as long as possible through his widely opened mouth. One can time the length of the expiratory sound heard with the stethoscope from the beginning of the expiratory sound to its very end. In a normal subject the forced expiratory time is never more than four seconds. In moderate and severe obstructive disease it is always increased.

The peak expiratory flow rate can be assessed by determining whether the patient can blow out a burning match, which is held approximately 3 inches from his open mouth, with a forceful expiration. The test is incorrectly performed if the patient's lips are allowed to purse during the procedure. Inability to blow out a match is indicative of a marked degree of obstruction to airflow and has been shown to occur when the maximum breathing capacity is less than 40 liters per minute. However, the occasional patient suffering from a purely restrictive type of disease may also fail to blow out a match.

The extent of the disability should also be assessed when the patient is examined. This is done by having the patient undergo a form of activity to which he is accustomed, such as climbing a flight of stairs or walking, and noting when breathlessness and tachycardia develop.

These tests serve to establish a rough index of the disturbances in function produced by the respiratory disease. More specific studies of pulmonary function should always be carried out, for they are an essential component of the evaluation of any patient with respiratory complaints and also serve as a guide to therapy. The tests which can be performed and their interpretation have been described in Chapter 7.

ASSESSMENT OF THE INFANT AND CHILD

Although much of what has been discussed previously is applicable to the assessment of respiratory disease in infants and children, there are diseases which are peculiar to this age group and which require historical information of a different nature. The history must be obtained in large part from the parents, and since considerable probing may be necessary, the questioning requires much tact and consideration of personal feelings. In addition, although the approach to the physical examination is essentially the same as in the adult, examination of the child requires a greater degree of gentleness and patience in order to obtain optimal information.

HISTORY

When approaching the problem of a newborn infant with respiratory distress, detailed information regarding previous pregnancies and their outcome, as well as the present pregnancy and delivery, is essential. It is important to determine the gestational age of the infant, since the preterm infant (born before 37 completed weeks of gestation) has a 10 per cent chance of developing hyaline membrane disease. Both the quality and quantity of amniotic fluid must be ascertained. Foul-smelling, murky amniotic fluid suggests infection, and meconium staining of the amniotic fluid is suggestive of meconium aspiration. Excessive amniotic fluid (hydramnios) is often associated with a tracheo-esophageal fistula. Rupture of the amniotic sac with leakage of amniotic fluid for longer than 24 hours is associated with an increased chance of infection and is a likely cause of pneumonia in the newborn infant. There is an unusually high incidence of aspiration pneumonia and spontaneous pneumothorax in post-term infants (born after 42 completed weeks of gestation). This is presumably due to *in utero* aspiration of amniotic fluid, which, at this time, contains a large number of squamous epithelial cells.

The type of presentation and delivery is important, since a traumatic delivery or a breech presentation may be associated with CNS hemorrhage and subsequent respiratory distress. Conditions such as placenta previa, a prolapsed or entangled umbilical cord, or evidence of fetal bradycardia are often associated with asphyxia prior to birth and a flaccid, apneic and cyanotic infant. Similarly, excessive administration of medications such as morphine or Demerol to the mother immediately prior to delivery of the infant may cause respiratory depression in the infant. The Apgar score (Table 10), given one minute following delivery, is useful in assessing the condition of the infant immediately postpartum. Each of the five signs indicated in the table is rated from 0 to 2, and the total score calculated is known as the Apgar score.

Assessment of older children involves careful evaluation of growth development and a knowledge of both the previous and the current state of immunizations. Children are now routinely immunized within the first year or two of life against diphtheria, whoop-

TABLE 10

THE APGAR METHOD OF SCORING NEWBORN INFANTS*

SIGN	SCORE		
	0	1	2
Heart rate	Absent	Slow (below 100)	Over 100
Respiratory rate	Absent	Slow, irregular	Good, crying
Muscle tone	Limp	Some flexion of extremities	Active motion
Reflex irritability (response to catheter in nostril)	No response	Grimace	Cough or sneeze
Color	Blue, pale	Body pink, extremities blue	Completely pink

*The score is taken first 60 seconds after the complete delivery of the infant and may be repeated at 1- to 5-minute intervals until the total score reaches at least 8.

    Score: >7 Normal
               4–7 Suspicious
               <4 Marked abnormality

ing cough, tetanus, polio, measles, smallpox and mumps. The birth weight and the pattern of growth (in both height and weight) should be noted and compared to other children of the same age and sex on a special chart available for this purpose. Developmental milestones such as when the child first smiled, sat, walked, spoke words and spoke phrases should be noted. The first sign of any illness in childhood is often anorexia, so careful attention should be paid to recording the food and water intake of the patient. Since vitamin supplements are necessary in the first year of life, it is important to assess the adequacy of vitamin intake.

PHYSICAL EXAMINATION

It has been pointed out that examination of the child requires both patience and gentleness, particularly in the uncooperative age group from one to three years. Unlike the examination of the adult, it is the child who dictates the order in which the physical examination is conducted. Often most of the examination is best conducted while the child is being held by the mother, either sitting on her lap or held over her shoulder. Even so, the use of instruments should usually be left to the end of the examination, since such utensils as the stethoscope, otoscope and tongue blades often frighten the child.

Inspection is the most important part of the physical examination in the newborn. The frequency of breathing normally may vary from 30 to 60 breaths per minute in the first few days of life, and a rate above this range is definitely abnormal. Preterm infants often have Cheyne-Stokes respiration with periods of apnea lasting from 10 to 15 seconds. Apnea lasting longer than 15 seconds is abnormal and is usually associated with bradycardia.

The anteroposterior and transverse diameters of the thorax are nearly equal in the newborn. With time there is a greater increase in the transverse diameter, and the chest contour has adult proportions at the time of puberty. Because the infant's chest wall is very compliant, it is often easier to judge the degree of respiratory difficulty. Retraction in suprasternal, intercostal, and subcostal areas and even in the entire sternum may occur in association with respiratory difficulty. Flaring of the alae nasae is also a common sign. A typical sign of severe respiratory distress is the expiratory grunt which may or may not be heard without the aid of a stethoscope. The expiratory airway obstruction produced by the grunt prolongs the time for gas exchange within the lung and, in addition, may prevent collapse of alveoli and airways during expiration.

Frothy blood in the mouth suggests pulmonary hemorrhage. The presence of a laryngeal web or a congenital vascular ring which is compressing the trachea should be suspected if a baby tends to keep his head extended or has stridor. Newborn infants commonly demonstrate peripheral cyanosis, but central cyanosis is as difficult to judge as in the adult. Cyanosis and tachypnea in the absence of pulmonary disease suggests the presence of a cyanotic congenital heart disease. The presence of a scaphoid abdomen will suggest the possibility of a diaphragmatic hernia.

Inability to breathe without an oral airway is suggestive of atresia of the posterior nares (choanal atresia). A routine part of the physical examination on admission to the nursery should be passage of a #8 French catheter through each naris. It should be noted that the newborn infant is an obligate nose breather, and it may take several weeks before he learns to breathe through his mouth.

A shift of the apical impulse, with or without a similar shift of the trachea, in the newborn infant is highly suggestive of a pneumothorax. In children the high-pitched voice penetrates the chest wall poorly, and therefore vocal fremitus is not a reliable part of the examination. However, fremitus can be picked up through the chest wall during crying, but this makes auscultation difficult.

Percussion is also very difficult to interpret in the small infant, since the percussion note is easily transmitted by the small thorax. Infants tend to have a hyperresonant percussion note compared to adults, and it is only after the first few months of life that percussion becomes a reliable clinical sign.

Since auscultation is extremely difficult or impossible in a crying infant, this part of the physical examination should always be carried out first if the child is quiet, but the sight of the stethoscope may induce a crying episode, so the approach to each child must be individualized. The mother may have to gently restrain the hands of the curious infant who reaches for the stethoscope tubing, or alternatively, he may be induced to play with another object such as a reflex hammer or a tongue blade.

The child's head must be in a central position, since the mere turning of the head often results in a marked decrease in breath sounds on one side of the chest, even in the absence of chest disease. Breath sounds in small children and infants are more harsh, louder and sound closer to the ear (i.e., bronchovesicular in nature) than are breath sounds in adults. This is because of the thin chest wall and the proximity of the airways to the chest wall. Because the breath sounds radiate widely in the small chest, they may not be decreased when there is a loss of lung volume or even a pneumothorax. In premature infants with hyaline membrane disease breath sounds are often completely absent. An audible expiratory grunt may be picked up by holding the stethoscope in front of the infant's nares. Fine inspiratory rales are common immediately after birth and presumably represent the opening of unexpanded alveoli.

OTHER IMPORTANT ASPECTS OF THE GENERAL EXAMINATION

THE ABDOMEN

The abdomen should be palpated to determine whether there are any abnormal masses or enlargement of the liver or spleen. An enlarged liver may be caused by congestive heart failure, metastatic infiltration from a bronchogenic carcinoma, one of the lymphomas or an amebic abscess. A palpable spleen is found in association with one of the lymphomas or sarcoidosis as well as with septicemia or subacute bacterial endocarditis. A malignant condition involving the stomach, bowel, kidney or one of the ovaries may produce a palpable mass. A benign tumor of the ovary may be the cause of Meig's syndrome, a condition in which ascites and a unilateral hydrothorax develop. A hard, fixed, nodular prostate indicates a malignant process which may be the source of pulmonary metastases. A carcinoma of the rectum is easily acessible to the examining finger. A fistula-in-ano should make one suspect a tuberculous etiology if a pulmonary lesion is present.

EXTERNAL GENITALIA

The scar of an old primary chancre due to syphilis suggests the possibility of an aortic aneurysm, as does the finding of an enlarged nontender syphilitic orchitis. A tuberculous epididymitis makes one suspect the possibility of active pulmonary tuberculosis.

THE SKIN

Anemia is almost always suggested by the presence of pallor in the palms and finger pulps. For many reasons, this is a much safer guide to the hemoglobin content of the blood than the color of the face, for the face may be weather-beaten or disguised by cosmetics. The presence of cyanosis should be particularly noted. In addition, pigmentation in the skin creases suggestive of Addison's disease should be looked for.

In an allergic state, atopic dermatitis or urticaria may be present. Erythema nodosum may occur in association with a streptococcal sore throat, tuberculosis, sarcoidosis or coccidioidomycosis. Metastases from a bronchogenic carcinoma may develop in the subcutaneous tissues and may be felt as firm, nontender nodules. Chronic infiltrations in the skin may occur with sarcoidosis, fungus infection and histiocytosis "X." Icterus is occasionally associated with a pulmonary infarct.

THE EXTREMITIES

In addition to digital clubbing, a search for other signs in the extremities should be carried out. A painful, tender, thrombosed vein due to thrombophlebitis may account for the source of a pulmonary infarction. Congestive heart failure causes bilateral pretibial edema. A peripheral neuropathy develops on rare occasions as a complication of a bronchogenic carcinoma. Enlarged tender shafts of the long bones due to hypertrophic pulmonary osteoarthropathy in association with digital clubbing suggest the presence of either a bronchogenic carcinoma, one of the suppurative lung diseases or congenital heart disease. A diffuse pulmonary fibrosis is occasionally associated with the typical deformed joints of rheumatoid arthritis. The presence of degenerative arthritis of the large joints, together with Heberden node formation on the distal phalanges of the fingers, suggests the possibility of similar degenerative changes in the thoracic spine and may be the cause of chest pain.

SUMMARY

It must be emphasized that the abnormal findings which are elicited during the clinical examination of the chest indicate only that certain categories of disease are present as well as their approximate location. These findings do not yield any information about the exact etiology or nature of the disease. This may be inferred when the abnormal physical findings are taken in conjunction with the history of the illness. It is only by making a thorough inquiry into the chronological development of the symptoms, the duration of the illness and the nature of its progress, together with a careful, complete general physical examination, that it is possible to arrive at a presumptive clinical diagnosis of the disease. This, in turn, should be supplemented by an assessment of the effect of the disease on pulmonary function.

The morphological changes that are produced by certain disease processes usually result in fairly characteristic, abnormal physical signs. These are summarized in Table 11.

CONSOLIDATION

In this condition the alveolar air is replaced by fluid or tissue as a result of a bacterial or a viral pneumonia or invasion of the lung parenchyma by a malignancy, but the volume of the affected parenchyma remains unchanged. Characteristically, the trachea occupies a central position, and there is diminished movement, an impaired

TABLE 11

PHYSICAL SIGNS IN VARIOUS PATTERNS OF DISEASES*

	CONSOLIDATION†	ATELECTASIS†	LOCALIZED† FIBROSIS	PNEUMOTHORAX†	PLEURAL† EFFUSION	OBSTRUCTIVE LUNG DISEASE**
Size						
Trachea position	↔	→ (R)	→ (R)	→ (L)	→ (L)	↔
Apex position	↔	→ (R)	→ (R)	→ (L)	→ (L)	↓
Distensibility						
Movement	↓ (R)	↓ (R)	↓ (R)	↓ (R)	↓ (R)	↓ Bilateral
Sound transmission						
Percussion	↓ (R)	↓ (R)	↓ (R)	↑ (R)	↓ (R)	↑ Bilateral
Tactile fremitus	↑ (R)	↓ (R)	↑ (R)	↓ (R)	↓ (R)	↓ Bilateral
Breath sounds	Bronchial (R)	Diminished or absent (R)	Broncho-vesicular (R)	Absent (R)	Absent (R)	Prolonged expiration
Adventitious sounds	Whispering pectoriloquy and rales (R)		Rales (R)		? Rub (R)	Rhonchi

*Note that there is usually one sign that is significant in establishing the correct diagnosis.

**The signs are bilateral.

†The signs are those found when a right-sided lesion is present. If the lesion is left-sided, L should be substituted for R and R for L.

percussion note, an increase in tactile fremitus, bronchial breath sounds, whispering pectoriloquy and egophany, as well as fine inspiratory rales which are predominant in the terminal third of inspiration over the affected area.

ATELECTASIS

Collapsed, airless lung parenchyma occurs as a result of complete obstruction of its draining bronchus, because of a bronchogenic carcinoma, thick secretions or an aspirated foreign body. In this condition, therefore, the volume of the affected area is reduced. Consequently, the trachea is deviated to the affected side, and there is diminished movement, an impaired percussion note, diminished or absent tactile fremitus, and diminished or absent breath sounds over the affected area.

LOCALIZED PULMONARY FIBROSIS

Fibrosis confined to a segment or a lobe of the lung is usually the result of bronchiectasis or arrested pulmonary tuberculosis. In this condition, the trachea is deviated to the affected side, and there is diminished movement, an impaired percussion note, increased tactile fremitus, and bronchovesicular breath sounds of diminished intensity over the affected area. If there are retained secretions, medium-pitched rales will be heard predominantly during the middle third of inspiration. Unilateral diminution or loss of the "shoulder-strap" area of resonance is a valuable sign of fibrosis affecting the apex of the lung. Fibrosis due to arrested pulmonary tuberculosis is generally situated in the upper lobes, and that due to bronchiectasis commonly affects the lower lobes. In both conditions, both lungs may be affected, but one side is invariably affected more than the other.

DIFFUSE INTERSTITIAL FIBROSIS

This condition, which is also known as fibrosing alveolitis, is a diffuse fibrosis affecting both lungs and involving the interstitial tissues as well as the terminal bronchioles and alveoli. It is the end result of lesions resulting from the inhalation of a variety of irritating substances or fumes, such as silica, asbestos, nitrous dioxide, sulfur dioxide, fungal spores and possibly viral infections.

In this condition, the trachea is deviated to the side which is most affected, and this side of the chest will also show a greater degree of restricted movement. Generally, the lower lobes are chiefly affected, and in these areas there is an impaired note to percussion, increase in tactile fremitus, bronchovesicular breath sounds, and there are coarse inspiratory rales throughout inspiration but more predominant in the terminal third.

PNEUMOTHORAX

Air in the pleural cavity may develop spontaneously, or it may be traumatic in origin. The size of the affected side increases so that the trachea is deviated to the opposite side and there is diminished movement, hyperresonance on percussion, absent tactile fremitus and absent breath sounds over the affected area.

PLEURAL EFFUSION

The physical signs of a pleural effusion are the same whether it is serous, hemorrhagic or purulent in character. In this condition, the trachea is deviated away from the diseased side, and there is diminished movement, a flat note on percussion, absent tactile fremitus and absent breath sounds over the area involved. Bronchovesicular breath sounds are often heard at the upper limit of the fluid because of the compressed underlying lung. A pleural rub may also be present at this level. If there is only a thin layer of fluid present in the pleural cavity, signs produced by the underlying compressed lung parenchyma may become evident and may mimic consolidation so that the unwary examiner may assume the presence of a pneumonia. Occasionally, a pleural effusion, usually an empyema, is localized by pleural adhesions, and the signs of pleural effusion are sharply outlined.

CHRONIC OBSTRUCTIVE LUNG DISEASE

The findings in chronic bronchitis and emphysema are similar to those found during an acute attack of bronchial asthma, except that in this case the signs are present constantly. Expiration through pursed lips is a common feature, and the use of accessory muscles with marked inspiratory retraction of the supraclavicular areas and indrawing of the lower intercostal spaces may be evident.

A "barrel chest deformity" (i.e., the chest is in an inspiratory position with the ribs horizontal, kyphosis of the thoracic spine, a prominent sternal angle and wide subcostal angle) is frequently present, the anterior aspect of the chest moving up and down as a single unit during respiration (thoracic heave). The diaphragm may be so depressed that both costal margins are drawn inward during inspiration. The trachea lies deep in the neck but is in the midline position unless the patient is elderly, in which case it may be shifted to the right. The chest movement is restricted but equal bilaterally, there is hyperresonance throughout, and tactile fremitus is diminished over both sides of the chest. The breath sounds are vesicular and generally diminished in intensity or almost inaudible. Expiration is markedly prolonged and high-pitched sibilant rhonchi may be evident during quiet respiration or when the patient expires forcibly through a widely opened mouth.

COR PULMONALE

If pulmonary hypertension and right ventricular hypertrophy are present, there may be a left middle and lower parasternal systolic heave with a simultaneous lateral retraction of the precordium. The pulmonic sound is markedly elevated, and its split is narrowed or absent. If the lungs are markedly hyperinflated, the cardiac impulse will not be seen or felt; heart sounds are faint, but a marked pulsation may be seen and felt in the upper part of the epigastrium. When right-sided heart failure has developed, the jugular veins are distended, the liver is enlarged and tender and peripheral edema is evident.

Chapter 11

The Radiologic Assessment

After the examiner has obtained a complete history from the patient and has performed a thorough physical examination, he is usually able to arrive at a conclusion regarding the anatomical location of a pulmonary lesion and a tentative diagnosis. Further valuable information leading to a more definitive diagnosis can now be obtained by a radiologic assessment of the patient's chest. Although there are many bronchopulmonary diseases in which the x-ray examination is entirely noncontributory, most pulmonary lesions can be demonstrated radiologically long before their presence is detected by the usual clinical methods of examination. It therefore follows that a radiologic examination is an integral part of the assessment of a patient suffering from a respiratory disease. Apart from the place of radiography in the initial detection of disease, x-ray films and fluoroscopic examination also serve as a standard for following the course of disease and its response to therapy.

The radiologic examination may be considered as a twofold assessment. The static assessment consists of x-ray films of the thorax taken in the posteroanterior and lateral positions and, in addition, includes more detailed and specialized techniques when they are indicated. By these means the anatomical position of a lesion, and frequently the pathological diagnosis, may be established. This information may be supplemented by fluoroscopy of the heart and lungs during normal respiration and various breathing maneuvers, and this yields valuable information regarding the dynamic function of the lungs as well as the heart size.

THE ROENTGENOLOGIC APPEARANCE OF THE NORMAL CHEST

The thorax is an ideal region for a radiologic examination. The aerated lung parenchyma offers very little resistance to the passage of roentgen rays, and it therefore produces very radiant shadows. On the other hand, the soft tissues of the thoracic wall, the mediastinum, the heart and great vessels, and the diaphragm do not permit the rays to pass through to as great an extent and therefore appear as denser opacities on the x-ray film. The bony structures of the thorax — the ribs, vertebrae and sternum — are even less readily penetrated, and their shadows are consequently even more dense.

The appearance of the heart and the lungs on the x-ray film of the chest must be clearly understood before any attempt can be made to determine the existence of abnormalities or disease processes, particularly since normal x-ray findings vary considerably with age, sex and habitus and under different conditions of respiration in the same subject. The examiner must learn all the various appearances which may be considered normal by studying large numbers of x-ray films, just as he can learn to recognize normal breath sounds only by repeated stethoscopic examination.

THE HEART

In the posteroanterior view, the heart shadow comprises a series of arcs or curves which represent the margins of the various chambers and the great vessels (Fig. 92). The right heart border is formed entirely by the right atrium. Often the inferior vena cava can be seen entering the right atrium. The ascending arch of the aorta and the superior vena cava often overlaps it from the border superior to the right atrium. On the left side, beginning at the level of the diaphragm, the border of the left ventricle can be seen. Ascending superiorly, a gentle indentation, which is the site of the left atrial appendage, is encountered; immediately above this is a gentle curvature, convex to the left, caused by the undivided segment of the pulmonary artery. The most superior aspect of the left border of the cardiovascular sys-

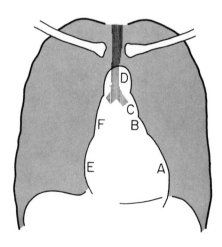

FIGURE 92. The roentgenologic appearance of the heart. *A*, Left ventricle; *B*, left atrial appendage; *C*, pulmonary artery; *D*, aortic knob and margin of descending aorta; *E*, right atrium; and *F*, superior vena cava.

tem is formed by the aortic knob, which is produced primarily by the transverse arch of the aorta.

On a lateral x-ray film of the chest, the posterior mediastinum is visualized as an area of radiolucency between the posterior border of the heart and the anterior aspect of the spine. The descending aorta is outlined in this space.

In the right anterior oblique position, the posterior border of the heart shadow is made up of the left and right auricles, with the superior vena cava above. The anterior border of the heart shadow is formed by the right ventricle.

The left anterior oblique position is particularly valuable for the visualization of the right ventricle, which lies along the diaphragmatic and the inferoanterior portion of the cardiac outline. The left auricle and the left ventricle form the posterior portion of the silhouette.

THE LUNGS

In the posteroanterior view of the chest, the trachea is a vertical translucent shadow situated in the midline, overlying the cervical vertebrae. The hila, or lung roots, are poorly defined areas of increased density in the medial part of the central portion of the lung fields. These are made up of the pulmonary blood vessels, the bronchi and a group of lymph nodes. The left hilum is partially obscured by the overlying shadow of the heart and great vessels, and it lies at a slightly higher level than the right hilum. In the middle third of the lung fields there is a series of linear reticular shadows which are wider and denser in the region of the hila, progressively decreasing as they move out toward the periphery. These linear markings are principally formed by arteries, but veins and lymphatics also contribute to them. A bronchus seen end-on forms a ring-like area of increased density with a central translucency, but a blood vessel seen end-on appears as a round solid shadow. In the peripheral portions of the lung these linear markings are much less obvious. They are usually similar in both lungs, but those on the left side are obscured by the heart.

Just as it was important to understand the surface anatomy of the chest in the physical examination, so it is necessary to have clearly in one's mind the anatomic location of each of the lobes and the delineation of the various bronchopulmonary segments.

BRONCHOPULMONARY ANATOMY

The trachea extends anteriorly from the lower edge of the cricoid cartilage to the level of the second costal cartilage, which corresponds posteriorly to the lower border of the body of the fourth thoracic vertebra. Here the trachea divides into the right and left major bronchi, which serve each lung.

The right major bronchus divides into three main branches, each serving an individual lobe of the right lung. From above downward these consist of a bronchus to the upper lobe, one to the middle lobe and one to the lower lobe. The left major bronchus divides into only two branches: one to the upper lobe and one to the lower lobe.

The lobar bronchi divide into smaller branches, which are known as *segmental bronchi*, each supplying a portion of a lobe called a *bronchopulmonary segment.* These are illustrated in Figures 93 and

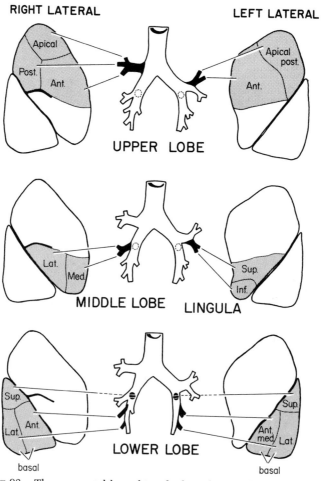

FIGURE 93.   The segmental bronchi and a lateral view of the bronchopulmonary segments.

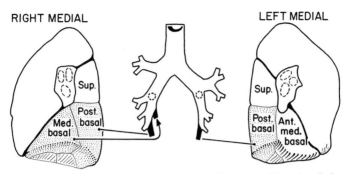

FIGURE 94.   The bronchopulmonary segments of the lower lobes (medial aspect).

94. A given segment has not only its own bronchus but, in addition, its own artery, vein and lymphatics. That is why a segmental resection can be carried out with impunity, for removal of a lung segment does not compromise the blood supply of other parts of the lung.

The Right Lung.   The bronchus supplying the upper lobe of the right lung arises from the lateral aspect of the right major bronchus about 2.5 cm. beyond the bifurcation of the trachea and almost immediately divides into three branches. The anterior branch supplies the anterior segment of the right upper lobe, which is situated anteriorly between the levels of the clavicle and the fourth rib. The apical bronchus supplies the apical segment of the upper lobe, which lies in the area above the level of the clavicle. The third branch, the posterior bronchus, supplies the posterior segment of the upper lobe, which lies posteriorly to the other segments of the upper lobe.

The middle lobe bronchus of the right lung arises from the anterior aspect of the right major bronchus about 2 cm. below the opening of the upper lobe bronchus. It runs in a downward and forward direction, finally dividing into two branches which supply the medial and the lateral segments of the middle lobe.

After giving off its branch to the middle lobe, the right main bronchus gives off the superior or apical branch posteriorly, then continues its downward course, and finally divides into four branches, each supplying a particular segment of the lower lobe. These are the anterior basal, the medial basal, the lateral basal and the posterior basal segments.

The Left Lung.   The bronchus to the upper lobe of the left lung arises from the anterolateral aspect of the left major bronchus about 5 cm. from the bifurcation of the trachea. Unlike the right major bronchus, it then splits into an upper and a lower division.

The upper division of the left upper lobe bronchus divides into two branches: one supplies the anterior segment, and the other supplies the apical posterior segment of the upper lobe. The anterior

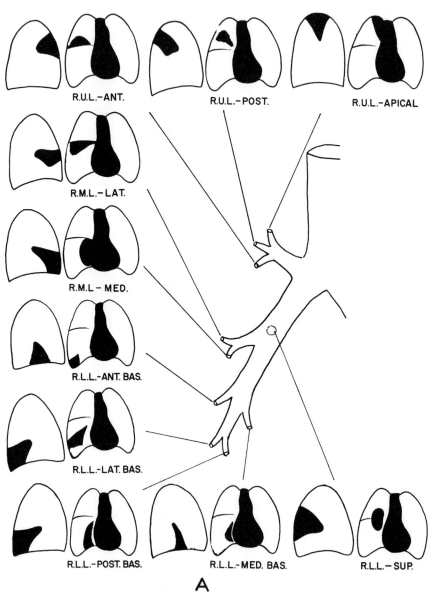

R.U.L.-ANT.   R.U.L.-POST.   R.U.L.-APICAL

R.M.L.-LAT.

R.M.L - MED.

R.L.L.-ANT. BAS.

R.L.L.-LAT. BAS.

R.L.L.-POST. BAS.   R.L.L.-MED. BAS.   R.L.L.- SUP.

A

FIGURE 95.   The roentgenographic appearance of infiltrations in the various bronchopulmonary segments on the   posteroanterior and lateral chest roentgenograms. A, Right lung.

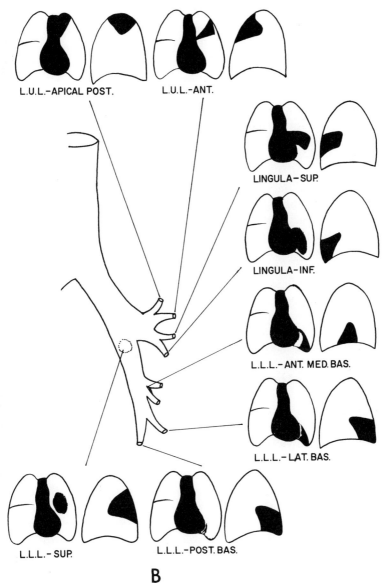

L.U.L.-APICAL POST.

L.U.L.-ANT.

LINGULA-SUP.

LINGULA-INF.

L.L.L.-ANT. MED. BAS.

L.L.L.-LAT. BAS.

L.L.L.-SUP.

L.L.L.-POST. BAS.

B

FIGURE 95. *Continued. B,* Left lung.

segment corresponds to that of the right upper lobe, whereas the apical posterior segment corresponds to both the apical and posterior segments of the right upper lobe.

The lower division supplies the lingula which, although actually a part of the left upper lobe, corresponds morphologically to the middle lobe of the right lung. The bronchus to the lingula divides into two branches, supplying the superior and the inferior segments of the lingula, which are situated one above the other.

The lower division of the left major bronchus continues its downward course in a manner similar to that of the right major bronchus to form the left lower lobe bronchus. This divides into four branches which supply the superior or apical segment, the anterior medial basal segment (which corresponds to both the anterior basal and the medial basal segments of the right lung), the lateral basal segment and the posterior basal segment.

The roentgenologic appearance of infiltrations in the various bronchopulmonary segments on the posteroanterior and lateral projections is illustrated in Figure 95, *A* and *B*.

The lobes of the lungs cannot normally be distinguished. It is of utmost importance, however, to have clearly in one's mind the anatomical location of each of the lobes and the delineation of the various bronchopulmonary segments. The major or oblique fissures of both lungs are usually seen only in the lateral view as a very thin dense line. The minor or transverse fissure on the right side is normally seen on the posteroanterior film as a fine hair-like line running transversely in either the third or the fourth intercostal space, and on the lateral view it runs horizontally from the hilum to the anterior margin of the chest cage. The position of these fissures is frequently of diagnostic value. For instance, if the right upper lobe is contracted or atelectatic, the fissure is drawn up; if the middle lobe is atelectatic, it is drawn downward. Similarly, when the lower lobe is collapsed, the major fissure is drawn downward and posteriorly.

The upper lobes mainly lie anteriorly. The lower lobes occupy the posteroinferior aspects of the chest. The right middle lobe lies in the inferior portion of the anteromedial aspect of the chest. The lobes overlap each other considerably, however, so that a clear localization of each lobe is not possible in the posteroanterior view of the chest. For this reason, a lateral view and occasionally oblique views are essential in order to delineate accurately the lobes of the lungs and their various bronchopulmonary segments.

THE DIAPHRAGM

The two hemidiaphragms are rounded, smooth, sharply defined shadows, the right one being normally situated one interspace higher than the left. The right leaf of the diaphragm merges with the shadow of the liver. The costophrenic angles are moderately deep, and they are approximately equal in size on the two sides.

BONY STRUCTURES

The ribs, the clavicles, the scapulae and portions of the humeri are reasonably clearly outlined on most x-ray films of the chest. Abnormalities in these structures should be carefully sought, for they are important aids in diagnosis. For instance, notching of the ribs is an important manifestation of coarctation of the aorta.

EXAMINATION OF THE CHEST ROENTGENOGRAM

It is important that the x-ray film should not be either overexposed or underexposed. The patient should be well centered before the exposure is made so that the sternal notch overlies the vertebrae. The outline of the vertebral column should be visible through the heart shadow. The ribs should show good bony detail, and the vascular markings should be visible from hilum to periphery. The cardiac outline—and if possible the transverse fissure, the left subclavian artery and the inferior vena cava—should be sharply defined.

It is essential that the examiner study an x-ray film of the chest in a systematic fashion. The actual sequence followed is probably not important. as long as it is systematic and thorough. The examiner should determine the size of the cardiac shadow and of the mediastinum as well as their contours. The position of the trachea and its branches and, if possible, their contours should be assessed. Note should be made of the position and the shape of the two hemidiaphragms, the depth, clarity and position of the two costophrenic angles and the appearance of the lateral borders of the lungs.

The size, shape and position of both hilar shadows should be noted. It is difficult to differentiate definitely between a normal and a pathologically enlarged hilum unless there are gross abnormalities. Enlargement of both hila suggests either that there is diffuse pulmonary disease which has led to an increase in the pulmonary artery pressure or that the lymph nodes in both hilar regions have become enlarged. A malignant disease should be considered if only one hilum is enlarged, particularly in association with a pulmonary lesion in an elderly patient. When the hila are enlarged and butterfly-shaped and there are associated increased pulmonary markings, the most likely cause is pulmonary congestion.

The size and extent of the pulmonary markings and the appearance of the lung fields bilaterally should then be examined with special reference to any abnormal shadows. If a lesion is seen, it is important to localize it to the particular bronchopulmonary segment which is involved. A lesion of the right middle lobe and the medial basal segment of the right lower lobe usually obliterates the cardiac border, whereas lesions of the posterior basal segment of the right lower lobe do not. The bony structure should then be studied for the appearance of the ribs bilaterally, the vertebrae, both clavicles, scapulae and humeri.

An assessment of the x-ray film in this manner usually confirms the diagnosis which has been established previously by the history and physical examination. It may, in addition, reveal the presence of pulmonary disease which has not been suspected. On the other hand, further special radiographic techniques may be required in order to establish the diagnosis.

ADDITIONAL ANCILLARY RADIOGRAPHIC TECHNIQUES

FLUOROSCOPY

When pulmonary disability is present, fluoroscopy may be a useful adjunct to the diagnostic roentgenogram, for it may provide information about the function of the respiratory system. Since fluoroscopy has serious potentialities as far as radiation is concerned, the physician who is performing this procedure should exercise the utmost precautions and use adequate protective devices.

Although it is clear that this examination yields considerable information about the heart, this will not be discussed except as it is related to respiratory disease.

The position of the trachea and the butterfly-shaped hilar markings should be noted. The lowest portion of the trachea may be normally displaced to the right by an elongated aorta in an elderly person.

Aeration and deflation of the lungs should be assessed during quiet breathing, during deep breathing and during a cough. If the lungs do not become less translucent during expiration, there may be either a loss of elasticity or a generalized partial bronchiolar obstruction of the check-valve type. If this finding is localized in one area of the lung, there may be obstruction of a bronchus by a malignant process or a foreign body. In diffuse obstructive emphysema, the retrosternal space is characteristically abnormally increased and translucent.

The resting level of the diaphragm at the end of a quiet expiration and the movement on both sides should be assessed during quiet breathing as well as during a deep inspiration. Diminished movement of the diaphragm may be associated with either localized or diffuse pulmonary disease. The diaphragms are depressed and show restricted movement in emphysema and occasionally may paradoxically move upward during inspiration.

If a hemidiaphragm does not move at all, it is important to determine whether it is paralyzed. Paralysis of the diaphragm is usually determined by the "sniff test." The diaphragm is apparently essential for the production of a sniff, and when it is bilaterally paralyzed, as it may be in poliomyelitis, the patient is unable to sniff. If the phrenic nerves are intact, a sniff results in a sharp downward movement of the diaphragm. If one of the leaves of the diaphragm is paralyzed, a sniff or even a normal inspiration may result in a paradoxical movement of the diaphragm. In such a situation, the normal hemidiaphragm descends while the paralyzed one rises during inspiration, being pushed upward by the increased intra-abdominal pressure.

A shift of the mediastinum toward one side during respiration means that the intrathoracic pressure on the affected side is less than it is on the other. Because this is most commonly seen when a bronchial obstruction is present on one side, it is often associated with failure of the lung fields on the affected side to darken during expiration.

INSPIRATION-EXPIRATION FILMS

Posteroanterior x-rays taken at maximum inspiration and maximum expiration, like fluoroscopy, are particularly useful in determining the presence or absence of mediastinal shift or localized air trapping such as occurs with a check-valve obstruction due to a foreign body or bronchogenic carcinoma. The expiration film may also be useful in demonstrating the presence or absence of a small pneumothorax because there is less radiolucency in the lungs at full expiration and the pneumothorax is then more readily evident. Clearly, this type of study also yields an indication of the extent of movement of the hemidiaphragms.

TOMOGRAPHY

This involves radiographing a single plane, whose thickness can be varied, at various depths within the lung. A series of films of the lung can be obtained at various planes as little as one centimeter in depth. Tomography is particularly useful in delineating the characteristics of a radiological shadow, particularly when it is deep-seated or underlies the clavicle or a rib.

Full chest tomography in which the x-ray beam is focused on the midsagittal plane of the whole chest has been used to study the status of the pulmonary vasculature. In normal subjects, the pulmonary vessels can be followed easily out to the periphery, but in patients with emphysema, particularly of the panlobular type, the peripheral segmental vascular markings may be very sparse or may taper rapidly as they proceed distally.

OBLIQUE VIEWS

Oblique views of the chest are most useful in the assessment of cardiac chamber size; they are occasionally also useful in localizing an abnormality. The lobes of the lungs overlap each other considerably so that a clear localization of each lobe is not possible in the posteroanterior projection of the chest. Occasionally oblique views are essential in order to delineate accurately the lobes of the lungs and their various bronchopulmonary segments. The appearance of the chest x-ray in the two oblique positions is shown in Figure 96. The right anterior oblique roentgenogram allows visualization of the lingula of the left lung and the right lower lobe, and the left anterior oblique view allows improved visualization of the right middle lobe and left lower lobe. The oblique views are taken with the correspond-

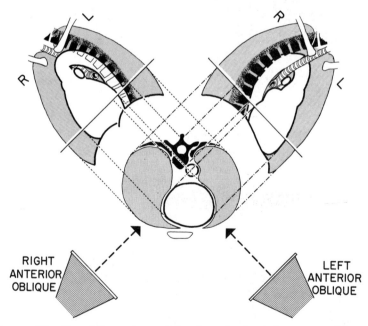

FIGURE 96. The oblique views of the chest. In the right anterior oblique, the lingula of the left lung and right lower lobe are visualized; in the left anterior oblique, the right middle lobe and the left lower lobe are visualized.

ing shoulder against the x-ray cassette. In a right anterior oblique view, the right lower lobe is situated posteriorly, and the lingula of the left lung is delineated anteriorly. In the left oblique view, the left lower lobe is situated posteriorly, and the right middle lobe is located anteriorly.

APICAL LORDOTIC VIEWS

A pulmonary lesion may be obscured on the conventional posteroanterior chest film because of the overlapping of the ribs. An abnormal shadow may be made more distinct if the film is taken in the lordotic position, which throws the clavicles above the lung fields.

STEREOSCOPIC FILMS

Stereoscopic films may also be used to localize pulmonary lesions. In this technique, two x-ray films of the chest are taken at the same time, and by making them overlap, a three-dimensional impression of the chest is obtained when they are viewed stereoscopically.

LATERAL DECUBITUS FILMS

If the presence of fluid in the pleural space is suspected but is not grossly evident in the ordinary film, it may become apparent on a film taken in the lateral decubitus position with the patient lying on the suspected side. If a pleural effusion is present, the fluid shifts to the most dependent position.

BRONCHOGRAPHY

An x-ray film of the chest made after either iodized oils or water-soluble iodized solutions are instilled into the tracheobronchial tree is called a bronchogram. The radiopaque iodized substances reveal in great detail the size and the appearance of the tracheobronchial tree. From knowledge of the segmental anatomy of the lung, the exact location of the bronchial disease can be established. In addition, bronchograms demonstate the form of the bronchi and test their patency, as evidenced by their ability to conduct the oil to the periphery of the lungs.

In a normal bronchogram, the bronchi beyond the early segmental branches divide at intervals of about 1 cm. The final branches lie about 1 to 2 mm. apart and are 1 to 3 mm. long. The filling terminates at about 3 mm. from the edges of the ribs in the posteroanterior view and at the same distance from the interlobar septa in the lateral view.

The walls of the peripheral branches are parallel, and the lumen decreases in caliber after branching.

In bronchiectasis, on the other hand, the bronchi are dilated, have an irregular outline and may be unable to conduct the oil to the periphery of the lungs because of obstruction by secretions, organic narrowing or obliteration. Only the larger bronchi or more proximal branches become filled, and a local dilatation of the proximal bronchus of the first to the fifth generation following the lobar division is usually found. The dilatation may be fusiform, tubular or cystic and may be slight in extent or quite gross.

In chronic bronchitis, the bronchial filling usually reaches further toward the periphery, and the changes are generally found in smaller bronchi and bronchioles. Dilatation of a peripheral bronchiole shows up as a circular shadow 1 to 3 mm. in diameter at the end of a small branch. There may be only a few or many such shadows.

ESOPHAGOGRAM

The esophagogram is an x-ray film of the chest taken while the patient drinks a mixture of barium. This is a very useful procedure, particularly when involvement of the mediastinum by a pulmonary malignant process is suspected. In such a situation, displacement of the esophagus may indicate the presence of enlarged mediastinal lymph nodes or metastatic involvement of the esophagus.

ANGIOGRAPHY

This is a technique whereby a radiopaque substance is injected into the blood stream, and x-ray films are taken during its passage through the right side of the heart, the pulmonary circulation, the left side of the heart and then the aorta. It is a very valuable procedure in the diagnosis of pulmonary thromboembolism, in which this examination usually demonstrates dilated major pulmonary artery branches as well as obstruction of a segmental or lobar branch of the pulmonary artery in acute episodes or irregular filling defects along the walls of arteries in more long-standing cases. If this procedure is repeated at intervals, these findings may disappear completely, which further confirms the diagnosis of an acute pulmonary vascular occlusion. Angiographic examination is also of value in cardiopulmonary disorders, particularly when there is a right-to-left shunt of blood.

This technique may also be utilized to demonstrate an obstruction of a major vein in the thorax, i.e., the superior vena cava, such as may occur with a bronchogenic carcinoma.

RADIOACTIVE ISOTOPE SCANS

Perfusion abnormalities can be assessed by scanning the lungs in the anterior, posterior and both lateral positions after the intravenous injection of I^{131} tagged macroaggregates of human serum albumin. The finding of diminished perfusion to an area of lung, particularly if the chest roentgenogram is clear or there is increased radiolucency in this area, is very suggestive of a pulmonary thromboembolism. This technique, which should be considered as an adjunct to angiography, is simple to perform and can be repeated at frequent intervals so that it may be used to assess progress of the disturbance. Under all circumstances, the interpretation of radioisotope scans of the thorax must be tempered with knowledge of the size (volume) of the lung or area of lung being scanned and that local hypoxia can influence the perfusion considerably. The relationship between ventilation and perfusion over various regions of the lung can be estimated by comparing count rates over the lungs obtained following the inhalation of xenon^{133} with that obtained following the intravenous injection of the same isotope (see Chapters 1 and 2).

SUMMARY

It is apparent that assessment of the deviation of the chest roentgenogram or other ancillary radiologic techniques from the normal enables the examiner to recognize an abnormal pattern in the respiratory system. From knowledge of the anatomy of the lungs, he is able to establish its exact location. Radiography is not only an important part of the initial assessment of the patient with respiratory complaints, but it is also of considerable value in following the course of a disease and its response to therapy.

Chapter 12

The Laboratory Assessment

From analysis of the patient's complaints, the abnormal findings detected on the physical examination, and any abnormalities that may be present in the chest roentgenogram it is usually possible to arrive at a presumptive diagnosis. This clinical diagnosis should be confirmed and the responsible agent identified, when necessary, by physiological, microbiological, histological and biochemical techniques. The physiological methods for testing respiratory function have been described in detail in Chapter 7. In this chapter we shall be concerned with the other laboratory techniques which are useful in establishing the etiology of respiratory disease and are based principally on bacteriologic and cytologic examinations of abnormal secretions and the histologic examination of diseased tissues.

ABNORMAL SECRETIONS

The secretions which are most commonly examined in patients suffering from respiratory disease are sputum, pleural fluid and discharge from a draining sinus.

SPUTUM

Abnormal bronchial secretions result from inflammation in either the lung parenchyma or the tracheobronchial tree or both. These secretions are usually expectorated as sputum or they may be swallowed and found in the gastric contents or aspirated from the bronchial tree by suctioning through a catheter or bronchoscope.

COLLECTION

The ideal time for the collection of sputum is shortly after awakening, for abnormal bronchial secretions tend to accumulate during a night's sleep. Care must be taken to reduce contamination with organisms which normally inhabit the oropharynx. Postnasal secretions can generally be "hawked up" and discarded before a specimen is collected. In addition, the patient should brush his teeth, wash his mouth and gargle with an antiseptic mouthwash. Following this, he should cough vigorously and expectorate the sputum into a sterile container.

The sputum should be sent to the laboratory with a minimum of delay. If the container is not sterile, and the specimen is allowed to remain at room temperature, there may be an overgrowth of saprophytic organisms. Thus, the culture may be contaminated and the antibiotic sensitivity tests invalidated.

Occasionally a patient may be unable to expectorate sputum because he is too ill, too old or too young to be cooperative. In such cases, a satisfactory specimen may be obtained by deliberately inducing the cough reflex by the application of a sterile cotton applicator or laryngeal mirror to the base of the tongue or by inserting a sterile suction catheter into the trachea. Secretions may also be aspirated directly from the affected bronchus through a bronchoscope. This procedure obviously has a therapeutic as well as diagnostic value. Bronchoscopic aspiration is particularly valuable for demonstrating malignant cells, tubercle bacilli and fungi.

Gastric Aspiration. Considerable quantities of sputum are unknowingly swallowed by patients. In addition, some patients with active pulmonary tuberculosis and only minimal infiltrations in the chest roentgenogram may have no cough or sputum. In such patients, the aspiration of gastric contents in the fasting state shortly after awakening is a valuable procedure, particularly for the detection of tubercle bacilli.

The presence of acid-fast organisms on smear of gastric contents is of no significance because saprophytic acid-fast mycobacteria are frequently seen in gastric contents. Only a positive culture is diagnostic of tuberculosis.

Induced Sputum. Recently an aerosol of a heated, hypertonic saline solution containing propylene glycol has been administered to induce bronchial secretions in patients who have radiological evidence of pulmonary infiltrates but no cough or sputum. Bacteriologic examination of the secretions may establish the diagnosis of active tuberculosis, and cytologic examination may point to a carcinoma of the lung.

Whether examination of induced sputum is superior to a culture of gastric contents for detecting tuberculosis is controversial. Studies have shown that a culture of induced sputum is more likely to be positive if the secretions are induced immediately after a gastric aspiration and that both techniques are more likely to be positive if the sputum is induced first, probably because some of the induced secretions are swallowed. This suggests that the induction of sputum, followed by aspiration of gastric contents, would be most fruitful in detecting tubercle bacilli.

MACROSCOPIC EXAMINATION OF THE SPUTUM

Volume.   The amount of sputum expectorated during a 24-hour period often provides useful information about the nature of the disease as well as its course and prognosis. A daily volume of over 100 ml. may be expectorated in such diseases as bronchiectasis, lung abscess and occasionally chronic bronchitis. The daily volume should gradually decrease if recovery is taking place. If it remains unchanged or increases in amount, it may indicate the disease is progressing unfavorably. A sudden decrease in volume may be due to obstruction of the draining bronchus, an event usually associated with a deterioration in the patient's condition. A sudden increase in volume may indicate rupture of a pulmonary abscess or an empyema into the bronchial tree.

Color and Consistency.   Mucoid sputum is translucent and glairy, has a viscid, tenacious consistency and is often gray among city dwellers and cigarette smokers. In acute pulmonary edema the sputum is pinkish, watery and frothy. Purulent sputum is generally yellow or green, and the color and consistency of mucopurulent sputum, which consists of a mixture of mucus and pus depends on the proportions of these ingredients. If a large collection of purulent sputum is allowed to stand in a conical glass, it often tends to separate into three layers. The top layer is usually frothy and discolored, the middle layer tends to be cloudy and watery, and the lower layer generally consists of a thick sediment of pus.

Blood in the sputum is easily recognized and may be in the form of streaks or small clots mixed in the sputum. In hemoptysis, the expectoration consists entirely of blood. The color of the blood depends on the interval between the actual bleeding and the expectoration of the sputum. Fresh blood is bright red, but it becomes dark if it is not immediately expectorated.

Odor.   The odor of the sputum should always be noted. Most specimens are odorless. Purulent sputum may occasionally have a sweet odor. A rotten, decomposed stench is indicative of an anaerobic putrefactive process, and infections caused by certain coliform organisms occasionally also produce a foul odor.

Abnormal Substances.   Occasionally foreign material which is related directly to the underlying disease may be expectorated, either alone or mixed with the sputum. Such substances can sometimes be recognized by their macroscopic appearance but it is usually necessary to identify them microscopically or chemically.

The sputum of city dwellers is polluted with carbon particles, and the sputum of coal miners is commonly stained by particles of coal dust or may be practically black if the miner is suffering from severe anthracosis.

Particles of calcium known as broncholiths may be found in the sputum. These usually originate from calcified tuberculous hilar lymph nodes which have eroded through the wall of a bronchus into its lumen or from calcium deposits in the lung parenchyma, as in silicosis and histoplasmosis. These calcium particles, usually minute and sand-like in size, are generally irregular, stony-hard and grayish white.

Dittrich's plugs may occasionally be found in the purulent sputum of chronic suppurative diseases, such as bronchiectasis and lung abscess. These yellow-white masses are inspissated, disintegrated, purulent material consisting of fatty acids and fat globules. They possess an extremely putrid odor and vary in size from that of a pinhead to a pea.

MICROSCOPIC EXAMINATION

Microscopic examination of sputum is essential in order to identify the organisms and their source, as well as the cells or minute abnormal substances that may be present. When an infection is present, microscopic examination of a gram-stained smear of secretions will indicate whether the organisms are predominantly gram-positive or gram-negative; this is of prime importance in order to institute proper antibiotic therapy promptly. A Ziehl-Neelsen stain may reveal the presence of acid-fast bacilli, indicating active tuberculosis, and occasionally fungi, such as *Actinomycosis israelii* or *Blastomyces dermatitidis*, can be demonstrated on smear. Proper identification of the pathogenic organisms, however, is achieved by culture of the specimen; this process will be discussed later.

Cytological Examination. This examination helps to determine whether the specimen is derived from the oropharynx or from the lower respiratory tract. Secretions from the upper respiratory passages contain flat, polygonal epithelial cells. Large round or oval histiocytes, often filled with carbon particles, are frequently seen in secretions from the bronchial tree. Ciliated, columnar cells which have been shed from the bronchial mucosa are often seen as well.

The sputum of a tuberculous infection contains numerous lymphocytes, whereas that of a nontuberculous bacterial infection contains predominantly polymorphonuclear neutrophils. Many eosinophils are frequently present in the sputum of patients suffering from bronchial asthma. Large numbers of erythrocytes in the sputum are indicative of either a recent hemorrhage or exudation of blood, as in the rusty sputum of pneumococcal pneumonia.

In bronchogenic carcinoma, examination of the sputum by a technician who has been specially trained in cytological examination often discloses malignant cells which have been exfoliated into the bronchial tree by the neoplastic process.

Abnormal Substances.   Purulent material should be routinely examined for elastic fibers, which indicate active destruction of pulmonary tissue such as may occur in pulmonary tuberculosis, bronchiectasis, lung abscess and pulmonary malignancy. To demonstrate these fibers, a fleck of purulent sputum is mixed with sodium hydroxide, which dissolves all the cellular material, thus allowing any elastic fibers to become visible under the low-power objective. They are slender, wavy, highly refractile threads of uniform diameter and of varying lengths, with split or curled ends. They are usually seen either singly or grouped together in small bundles.

The detection of oil droplets in bronchial secretions suggests lipid pneumonia or fat embolism. The oil droplets may be in the cytoplasm of macrophages or may be extracellular. They are easily recognized microscopically because they readily absorb a scarlet red dye such as Sudan III. Osmic acid stains vegetable and animal oils black and liquid petrolatum yellow.

Asbestos bodies are frequently found in the sputum of patients with asbestosis. These slender, elongated structures with bulbous ends range from 10 to 180 microns in size and stain a brilliant blue with potassium ferrocyanide. They are formed by the deposit of an iron-containing protein on an asbestos fiber.

PLEURAL FLUID

When fluid is present in the pleural cavity, it must be aspirated in order to determine its nature, and a pleural biopsy is obtained at the same time for histological examination.

COLLECTION

Aspiration of pleural fluid, or *thoracentesis,* should be carried out while the patient is in the sitting position if this is at all feasible. The site of aspiration and biopsy must be chosen with care. Both the upper limit of the fluid and the level of the opposite normal diaphragm should be determined by percussion. Aspiration should be carried out at a point midway between these two levels on the posterior wall of the affected side. If the fluid is encapsulated, its borders must be carefully outlined by percussion, and the needle is inserted into the center of the dull area.

The needle should be inserted through the intercostal space over the superior border of the rib, thus avoiding any accidental injury to the intercostal vessels and nerves. As much fluid as possible should be removed slowly; too rapid a withdrawal may result in acute edema of the underlying lung. Although it is preferable to keep the pleural cavity free of air, it may be necessary to allow air to enter through the needle if the patient should complain of chest tightness during the aspiration. A roentgenogram of the chest taken as soon as possible after the aspiration is of extreme value in determining whether there is an underlying pulmonary lesion.

MACROSCOPIC EXAMINATION

Volume. If the amount of aspirated fluid represents the total quantity in the pleural space, it yields valuable information concerning the extent of the underlying pathological process.

Appearance. A transudate is usually watery, pale yellow and either clear or slightly hazy. An exudate is generally deep yellow and turbid and feels thicker and stickier because of its higher protein content. The turbidity of pleural fluid depends upon the number of formed particles it contains, and it may vary from cloudiness to thick, creamy pus. When red blood cells are present, the color of the fluid varies from a reddish tinge to dark red. Fresh blood in the pleural fluid is generally the result of trauma, a pulmonary infarction or neoplastic process. An empyema fluid may vary from brown to yellow or green. Chylous fluid has a milky turbidity.

Coagulability. The degree of spontaneous coagulation of the pleural fluid after its aspiration depends on the amount of fibrin present. A transudate rarely coagulates, but exudates and neoplastic effusions can coagulate fairly rapidly.

Odor. Transudates and exudates are usually odorless, but the fluid may have a putrid stench if the pleural effusion is secondary to putrefactive changes in the lung.

CHEMICAL EXAMINATION

Specific Gravity. The specific gravity of the aspirated fluid helps distinguish between a transudate and an exudate. The specific gravity of a transudate is usually between 1.006 and 1.018, but that of an exudate, because of its greater protein content, is generally considerably higher than 1.018.

Protein Content. The protein content of pleural fluid may vary from 0.1 to 8.0 grams/per 100 ml. The protein content of a transudate is usually well under 2.5 per cent, but that of an exudate is always higher than 2.5 per cent.

Glucose Content.   In pleural effusions due to malignancy, pneumonia, fungal diseases and other infections, the pleural fluid glucose content is the same as that in the blood. In approximately 60 per cent of tuberculous effusions, the glucose content is less than 60 mg. per cent. In rheumatoid disease, the glucose content is always markedly reduced to 5 to 17 mg. per cent.

Other Chemical Examinations.   An additional feature of pleural effusions secondary to rheumatoid disease or other collagen diseases is the presence of the rheumatoid factor or lupus erythematosus cells in the fluid.

MICROSCOPIC EXAMINATION

Although not diagnostic in itself, the cellular content of pleural fluid is of considerable importance, and the predominant cell type may suggest the probable causative disease. Numerous polymorphonuclear neutrophils suggest a pyogenic infection, such as a bacterial pneumonia. A predominance of lymphocytes is suggestive of tuberculosis, although they can also be found in any chronic pleural effusion. Numerous eosinophils may be found in a pleural effusion due to a collagen disease or a parasitic infection, such as hydatid disease. Numerous erythrocytes may be found in pleural fluids caused by trauma, tuberculosis, pulmonary infarction or malignancy.

Malignant cells are present in about 50 per cent of effusions due to a neoplastic process involving the pleural surfaces. These cells are generally difficult to recognize, however, unless mitosis is present or the cells are arranged in a tissue pattern.

The centrifuged sediment of all pleural fluids should be smeared, stained and examined for bacteria. Bacteriologic examination is essential in order to identify the offending organism, and this can only be established by cultural methods. This is discussed in the following section.

BACTERIOLOGIC DIAGNOSIS

The bacteriologic examination of sputum, pleural fluid or material from draining sinuses by microscopic examination of a smear, culture and, under certain circumstances, animal inoculation is extremely important in arriving at a definitive diagnosis of a bronchopulmonary infection. Once the responsible organism has been determined, the correct antimicrobial therapy can be instituted.

Examination of a smear of the sputum which has been stained using the gram and the Ziehl-Neelsen methods should be carried out in all cases of pneumonia. Determination of whether the organisms in the sputum are predominantly gram-positive or gram-negative enables provisional administration of the appropriate antibiotic while awaiting the results of the sputum culture and sensitivity tests. Even then, the bacteriologic report should always be assessed critically and in the light of the clinical picture. One should remember that the bacteria grown may only be secondary invaders and not actually responsible for the disease and that organisms which grow profusely when cultured may be present in only small numbers in the bronchial secretions.

BACTERIAL INFECTIONS

The presence of gram-positive cocci in pairs or chains in a smear of the sputum is indicative of the presence of either pneumococci or a species of streptococci. Although no longer typed routinely, it is important to point out that type III and type VIII pneumococci are responsible for approximately 25 per cent of the deaths in pneumococcal pneumonia, despite adequate antibiotic therapy. The hemolytic streptococcus is the second commonest cause of bacterial infections. Although it may produce a primary type of pneumonia, it generally acts as a secondary invader following in the course of some other infection, such as influenza or measles.

Staphylococci are gram-positive cocci which occur in "grape-like" clusters. Because the *Staphylococcus aureus* is frequently present in the upper respiratory tracts of healthy, noninfected persons, large numbers of these organisms mixed with pus cells in the sputum has more diagnostic significance than the growth of staphylococci in a sputum culture. The *Staphylococcus aureus* acts most commonly as a secondary invader during the course of influenza or some debilitating disease, although it does so much less frequently than the hemolytic streptococcus. It may also develop as a result of the invasion of the blood from a primary focus in some other part of the body such as perinephric abscess, the pneumonia then being a part of a widespread infection.

Friedländer's bacillus is a very rare cause of pneumonia. It is occasionally found in the healthy oropharynx where it behaves as a saprophyte, but it can become pathogenic if the body resistance is lowered. *Hemophilus influenzae* generally produces a primary pneumonia in infants and children, and it is frequently demonstrated in the sputum of patients with chronic bronchitis.

MYCOBACTERIAL INFECTION

The sputum present in all bronchopulmonary diseases must be examined for acid-fast bacilli, since the radiologic opacities produced by nontuberculous diseases can be mimicked by pulmonary tuberculosis.

Mycobacterium Tuberculosis. Tubercle bacilli are usually readily demonstrated in active disease, but the organisms may be found only after repeated and persistent searching if the disease is chronic and indolent.

The detection of acid-fast mycobacteria, which morphologically resemble tubercle bacilli, by the direct microscopic examination of a smear of the sputum stained by the Ziehl-Neelsen method is generally accepted as positive proof of the diagnosis of pulmonary tuberculosis. However, it has been estimated that at least 100,000 bacilli must be present in 1 ml. of sputum before a single organism can be detected by the direct examination. If no tubercle bacilli are demonstrated in the sputum smear, it may be possible to demonstrate bacilli in a concentrated specimen of sputum. A large collection of sputum to which sodium hydroxide has been added is centrifuged, and the sediment is stained by the Ziehl-Neelsen method and examined for acid-fast bacilli.

When sputum containing tubercle bacilli is planted on a solid medium containing a mixture of egg and potato flour or starches and incubated at 37° C. for four to six weeks, a dry, wrinkled, grayish-yellow warty growth results. A Ziehl-Neelsen stain of a smear from this culture will show thousands of typical acid-fast mycobacteria.

Atypical Mycobacteria. The "atypical" or "anonymous" mycobacteria resemble the *Mycobacterium tuberculosis* morphologically but have different cultural characteristics and are found in soil, contaminated water and occasionally in human gastric contents. In the past they were considered to be saprophytes and not pathogenic to man. In recent years, however, it has been shown that some of them are capable of producing pulmonary disease which can mimic pulmonary tuberculosis.

Several classifications of these anonymous or atypical mycobacteria have been suggested, but the one used most commonly is based on distinctive cultural characteristics and divides them into four main groups (see Chapter 14).

Group I (*photochromogens*), when cultured, resemble *Mycobacterium tuberculosis* if kept in the dark but develop a vivid yellow color when exposed to light during the period of active growth; group II atypical mycobacteria (*scotochromogens*) are orange both in the dark and when exposed to light; group III atypical mycobacteria (*nonphotochromogens*) have little pigment, are ivory or buff in color, and are not affected by exposure to light; group IV atypical mycobacteria (*rapid growers*) also possess very little pigment and are not affected by exposure to light, but they are distinguished from the other groups by their very rapid rate of growth. In contrast to the first three groups, which require two or three weeks at room temperature, group IV mycobacteria become mature in a matter of two or three days.

Before deciding that the pulmonary disease is caused by one of the atypical mycobacteria, they should be demonstrated in very large numbers in the smear, and the identical strain should be grown repeatedly.

VIRAL INFECTION

Of the known filterable viruses that are capable of causing pneumonia in man, the most important ones are the myxoviruses and influenza A and B. Others are the respiratory syncytial virus, which has a predilection for children; adenoviruses 4 and 7; and parainfluenza 3. Despite improvement in the isolation techniques of viruses, however, they have only been identified in approximately 50 per cent of the nonbacterial pneumonias.

Viruses can be grown by inoculating the patient's throat washings, which are obtained during the early phase of the illness, into an embryonated egg as well as into ferrets or mice. A viral infection can be diagnosed by the virus neutralization test, which demonstrates the presence of antibodies capable of neutralizing the virus in the serum. Specimens are obtained as early as possible after the beginning of the illness, again about fourteen days later, and again about four weeks after the onset of the disease. The diagnosis of viral pneumonia is established on the basis of a serum viral-antibody titer which rises from the acute phase to the convalescent phase. In actual fact, this method provides a specific diagnosis in less than 25 per cent of the paired serum specimens which are submitted to the laboratory, and even then the diagnosis is established long after the pneumonia has run its natural course.

A viral etiology can also be established by the hemagglutination inhibition test, which is based on the ability of the virus to agglutinate erythrocytes, a reaction which can be inhibited by a specific antiserum.

MYCOPLASMA INFECTION

Mycoplasma pneumoniae is the most frequent cause of nonbacterial pneumonia in the civilian population. This organism shares the characteristics of both a virus and a bacterium in that its particle size is similar to that of viruses, but it also possesses enzyme systems which are similar to those of bacteria. The diagnosis of mycoplasma pneumonia is established by isolating the mycoplasma pneumoniae in the sputum. The demonstration of an increased specific antibody in the serum is also of value, but this procedure takes two to three weeks. In about 40 per cent of proven cases of mycoplasma pneumonia, a substance capable of agglutinating human group O erythrocytes appears in the serum at low temperatures but not at body or room temperature. These cold hemagglutinins frequently only appear during convalescence and may reach a titer of 1:32 in the average case.

The demonstration of cold hemagglutinins is not specific for mycoplasma pneumonia, since they may be elevated in approximately 20 per cent of the pneumonias caused by the adenoviruses and also occasionally in other pulmonary diseases such as pneumococcal pneumonia, tuberculosis and bronchogenic carcinoma.

Agglutinins to the streptococcus MG antigen may also be present in patients suffering from mycoplasma pneumonia, but these are even less specific than the cold agglutinins.

FUNGAL INFECTIONS

Although mycotic infections of the respiratory tract are very rare in relation to other pulmonary infections, they do occur with sufficient frequency to warrant consideration in the differential diagnosis of an obscure pulmonary lesion, particularly if the patient is known to have resided in a geographical area where a particular fungus infection is endemic. An accurate diagnosis of the mycotic infection can be established only by the isolation and identification of a fungus in bronchial secretions or from the histological examination of diseased tissues.

The presence of fungi in the sputum does not necessarily imply that these organisms are the primary or sole cause of the disease. They may be saprophytic, having accidentally contaminated the specimen, or they may have invaded some other pre-existing disease secondarily. This particularly applies to yeasts, which are frequently found in the sputum of patients with such chronic diseases as tuberculosis, bronchiectasis or bronchogenic carcinoma. *Candida albicans* and other members of the Candida family are normally inhabitants of the mouth. For this reason, the diagnosis of candidiasis is often difficult, especially since the advent of the widespread use of antibiotics and corticosteroids, which has increased their incidence in sputum cultures. On the other hand, certain other fungi, when isolated from the bronchial secretions, can definitely be considered to be primarily responsible for disease, particularly *Actinomyces israelii*, *Coccidioides immitis*, and *Blastomyces dermatitidis*.

Actinomyces israelii is present in the form of "sulphur granules," which consist of a dense tangle of gram-positive mycelia, in bronchial secretions or the discharge from sinuses. These whitish yellow amorphous masses are often visible to the naked eye if the pus is shaken in normal saline and examined against a dark background. The organism can be grown only under anaerobic conditions, a feature which distinguishes it from *Nocardia asteroides*, which can be grown only under aerobic conditions.

Blastomyces dermatitidis, the fungus responsible for North American blastomycosis, is a large, yeast-like cell. *Coccidioides immitis*, the cause of coccidioidomycosis, exists in nature in a mycelial form, but it becomes a large spherule once it invades the tissues. *Histoplasma capsulatum*, which is responsible for histoplasmosis, differs from all the other pathogenic fungi in that it is an intracellular organism and is confined to the cells of the reticuloendothelial system so that it is rarely found in the sputum.

Most pathogenic fungi can be identified only by cultural methods. They are isolated by culturing the sputum on either Sabouraud's agar at room temperature or on blood agar at 37° C.

RICKETTSIAL INFECTION

Coxiella burnetii, which is responsible for the pneumonia in Q fever, can occasionally be isolated by the injection of the patient's blood or urine into a guinea pig or into the yolk sac of a chick embryo. The diagnosis is usually made serologically by the complement-fixation and agglutination tests using *C. burnetii* yolk sac antigen. Complement-fixing antibodies usually appear during the first week of the illness, and agglutination antibodies usually appear during the second or third week.

The Weil-Felix reaction, an agglutination test using Proteus X=19, X=2 and X=K is frequently positive in most rickettsial diseases except Q fever.

HISTOLOGIC DIAGNOSIS

Under certain circumstances, an accurate diagnosis of the respiratory disease under study can be established only by histologic examination of the diseased tissue. Methods which may be used include biopsy of an endobronchial tumor through a bronchoscope; transbronchoscopic biopsy of the lung tissue in cases of bilateral pulmonary infiltrations; percutaneous needle aspiration of a solitary pulmonary lesion; surgical excision of enlarged mediastinal lymph nodes by mediastinoscopy; or biopsy of the diseased pulmonary tissue by means of an open thoracotomy.

BIOPSY OF ENDOBRONCHIAL LESIONS

Endobronchial biopsies are performed through a bronchoscope, a speculum which enables the examiner to inspect the interior of the trachea and the major bronchi as well as the orifices of their larger subdivisions. The smaller bronchi and their peripheral radicles cannot be visualized, but one may obtain valuable information by brushing or aspirating secretions from these areas for bacteriologic and cytologic studies.

Bronchoscopy is indicated whenever there are any symptoms or signs of a localized bronchial obstruction. It is imperative that this procedure be carried out if there is the least suspicion of a bronchogenic carcinoma, for over 50 per cent of these tumors can be visualized with the bronchoscope, and many more are diagnosed from examination of aspirated bronchial secretions.

LUNG BIOPSY

A lung biopsy is often necessary in order to arrive at an etiological diagnosis when there is roentgenologic evidence of diffuse pulmonary infiltrations or certain types of solitary lung lesions. An open thoracotomy is the most satisfactory means of obtaining adequate tissue for histologic examination, but there is a degree of morbidity, and even mortality, associated with this procedure. Percutaneous needle or drill biopsy of the lung also has limitations, for diseased lung tissue may be missed, and occasionally pneumothorax, hemothorax or pleural infection may occur.

Lung tissue has also been obtained through a bronchoscope by means of a long flexible forceps which is inserted into the diseased area under fluoroscopic control. Although the amount of tissue obtained is very small, many specimens may be obtained from different lobes.

An aspiration biopsy of a solitary lesion, under fluoroscopic control, may yield a cytologic or a bacteriologic diagnosis.

LYMPH NODE BIOPSY

Enlarged lymph nodes should be examined in order to establish whether they are due to granulomatous disease such as sarcoidosis, tuberculosis or a lymphoma, such as Hodgkin's disease or carcinoma. Even when a definitive diagnosis of bronchogenic carcinoma has been established, the lymph nodes should be examined to decide whether the lesion is surgically resectable. Although biopsy of the scalene nodes, which are situated in a pad of fat lying anterior to the scalenus anticus muscle in the neck, has been utilized, mediastinoscopy is

generally accepted as yielding the highest number of positive results. An oval illuminated tube (mediastinoscope) is inserted into
the superior mediastinum through an incision just above the suprasternal notch and is advanced along the anterior surface of the trachea. Blunt finger dissection of the pretracheal fascia allows entrance
into the mediastinum so that the lateral tracheal or parabronchial
lymph nodes can be visualized and removed for histologic as well
as bacteriologic examination.

PLEURAL BIOPSY

The etiology of a pleural effusion can be determined by clinical
assessment of the patient's illness or laboratory examination of the
fluid in the majority of cases, but the cause cannot be elicited in a
significant number of patients. By means of a pleural biopsy, it is
possible to prove that a high percentage of patients who suffer from
an acute serous pleurisy have tuberculosis. A specially designed
needle is used to aspirate the pleural effusion and to obtain a biopsy
from the parietal pleura. Since it is quite possible to biopsy a relatively normal area and miss a pathologic lesion, several pleural
biopsies should be taken at different sites.

In certain selective cases, particularly if a malignancy is suspected, it may be necessary to carry out an exploratory thoracotomy.
This enables the surgeon to visualize the pleura and thus to detect
a lesion which may have been overlooked by the needle biopsies.

DIAGNOSTIC SKIN TESTS

Skin tests are of value in the diagnosis of diseases which are
associated with the development of hypersensitivity to a specific
antigen, such as a foreign protein. There are three major important
types of reactions to the skin tests: the immediate reaction (Type 1),
the Arthus reaction (Type 3) and the delayed reaction (Type 4).
The Type 2 reaction, which is an antigen-antibody reaction, does
not occur in the skin.

THE IMMEDIATE OR TYPE 1 REACTION

As pointed out in Chapter 13, approximately 30 per cent of patients who suffer from bronchial asthma can be regarded as being
allergic, no matter whether the asthma began in childhood, ado-

lescence or early adult life. If the history of the episodes of bronchial asthma is strongly suggestive of being extrinsic in origin, skin tests are frequently used to discover the responsible allergens. Crude aqueous extracts of the common airborne antigens, such as pollen, household dust and animal fur, are injected intradermally or by means of either a prick or a scratch in the skin. Allergic bronchial asthma is associated with Type 1 or immediate hypersensitivity to an allergen. As described in Chapter 13, the allergic reaction is probably precipitated by the interaction of allergen with reaginic antibody on the mast cell; this leads to the release of histamine and slow-reacting substances. A positive skin reaction is indicated by the development of a pruritic, erythematous wheal within 15 to 20 minutes. However, approximately 25 per cent of healthy persons may develop a reaction to the intradermal injection of the common airborne antigens, and many allergic subjects react to a number of the injected antigens. For these reasons a positive skin reaction must be considered in conjunction with a thorough elucidation of the possible environmental factors and the history of each attack in arriving at the particular antigen responsible.

ARTHUS OR TYPE 3 REACTION

The repeated inhalation of organic dust particles which are small enough to reach the alveoli may result in the development of an allergic alveolitis (see Chapter 14). This is apparently mediated through precipitating heat-stable antibody, belonging at least in the IgG and IgM classes of immunoglobulins, which form microprecipitates in and around the small vessels and cause damage of the alveoli secondarily. Thus, in patients who present with pulmonary fibrosis a careful investigation should be carried out into occupation, hobbies and domestic pets, since more than a minor exposure to the pertinent allergen is required before extrinsic allergic alveolitis is produced. Determination of the etiologic agent responsible for extrinsic allergic alveolitis is especially important, for the disease is arrested on removal of the offending allergen from the patient's environment, and the amount of residual symptoms will depend upon the extent of the pulmonary fibrosis.

This skin reaction is characterized by two phases. There is an immediate Type 1 wheal which usually resolves completely within 1 to 2 hours and is followed 3 to 4 hours later by an itchy soft edematous swelling with ill-defined borders and little central induration. This reaction reaches its maximum at around 8 hours and subsides within 24 hours.

Many organic dusts may cause an allergic alveolitis and in each of these conditions the Arthus type reaction and specific precipitating antibodies or precipitins can be found in the patient's serum. Examples of such conditions are "farmer's lung," which is due to thermophilic actinomycetes; "bird fancier's lung," which is due to the antigen in avian excreta and serum; and "pituitary snuff-taker's lung," which is due to the inhalation of porcine and bovine posterior pituitary powder.

DELAYED OR TYPE 4 REACTION

Hypersensitivity which is not associated with the formation of antibodies but is mediated by specifically sensitized lymphocytes produces a delayed type of skin reaction which is usually manifest within 48 to 72 hours and occurs in association with mycobacterial infections and a few of the mycotic diseases.

MYCOBACTERIUM TUBERCULOSIS

A positive reaction to Old Tuberculin or its active principle, which is known as *purified protein derivative (PPD)*, is an example of the Type 4 hypersensitivity reaction and indicates that the patient has been infected previously with the tubercle bacillus. A positive skin reaction consists of an area of induration, the diameter of which should be measured, surrounded by a zone of erythema. Erythema alone, without induration, is not considered to be a positive reaction. The skin reaction should be interpreted 48 hours after the injection of the desired concentration of PPD (usually 5 TU), although occasionally a positive reaction may develop after 72 hours.

A positive tuberculin skin test of the delayed type indicates that the patient has been infected with some type of Mycobacterium, either recently or in the distant past. An induration between 5 and 9 mm. in diameter is considered to be a doubtful reaction and can be caused by atypical mycobacterial infection, but an induration greater than 10 mm. in diameter is indicative of a *Mycobacterium tuberculosis* infection.

In most circumstances, a tuberculin reaction remains positive throughout the patient's life, although it may wane with advancing age, decrease temporarily during severe illness, especially if associated with a high fever, or disappear completely if treatment is carried out during the early stages of infection. Certain diseases, such as sarcoidosis, Hodgkin's disease and measles, or the administration of the adrenal corticosteroids are often associated with a temporary loss of skin sensitivity to tuberculin.

ATYPICAL MYCOBACTERIA

Antigens of the nonphotochromogen Battey strain (PPD-B), the photochromogens (PPD-Y), and scotochromogens (PPD-G) are injected intradermally in a manner similar to PPD, and reactions are noted after 48 hours. An infection due to one of the atypical Mycobacteria results in an area of induration whose size exceeds that of standard tuberculin by at least 5 mm.

FUNGAL DISEASES

A fungal infection often results in the development of hypersensitivity of the tissues to the subsequent invasion by the fungus or proteins characteristic of it. A delayed Type 4 skin reaction may be seen in persons with fungal disease following the intradermal injection of the appropriate antigen. Three fungal antigens which are of diagnostic value are those produced by *Coccidioides immitis, Histoplasma capsulatum* and *Blastomyces dermatitidis* and are called *coccidioidin, histoplasmin* and *blastomycin,* respectively.

Fungal skin tests, particularly the histoplasmin skin test, should be performed after complement-fixation and precipitin tests are carried out, for the injection of antigen may have a "boosting effect" on the circulating antibodies. The test is carried out by injecting the antigen at a dilution of 1:100 intradermally. As with tuberculosis, a positive intradermal reaction only implies that there has been infection with a particular fungus, but it does not indicate whether this was recent or in the remote past, and it does not necessarily mean that the pulmonary disease under study is caused by that fungus. The skin reaction to blastomycin is rarely positive in a patient suffering from active blastomycosis, and conversely, a positive reaction may occur in patients who are infected with *Histoplasma capsulatum.* Histoplasmin may cross-react with blastomycin as well as coccidioidin, but the antigen of the fungus causing the disease generally produces the strongest reaction.

SARCOIDOSIS

The diagnosis of sarcoidosis, a systemic granulomatous disease of unknown etiology which primarily affects the reticuloendothelial system, is generally established by demonstration of a noncaseating epithelioid cell granuloma in lymph nodes, skin, liver, lung or conjunctiva. However, the skin test (*Kveim test*) is valuable in cases in which histological confirmation is not available. The intracutaneous injection of a crude, unstandardized sarcoid antigen prepared by emulsification of either lymph node or splenic tissue of patients with active sarcoidosis, results in a specific granulomatous skin reaction in patients who are suffering from an active form of the disease. Unfortunately, it requires 6 to 8 weeks or even longer before a positive reaction (a reddish papule) appears. After 8 weeks, the injection site should be excised and examined microscopically whether or not a papule develops.

HYDATID DISEASE

A positive response to an antigen consisting of fluid from an uncomplicated hydatid cyst which has been passed through a Berkefeld or Seitz filter for sterility (*Casoni skin test*) is positive in 90 per cent of infected patients and persists for a lifetime. A negative reaction generally means that the patient has not been infected by the Echinococcus.

There are two phases to a positive reaction: an immediate wheal which enlarges in size, develops pseudopodia and is surrounded by a zone of erythema, reaching its maximum within one-half hour; and a late response which occurs about 24 hours later and consists of an indurated area surrounded by an erythematous zone.

BIOCHEMICAL STUDIES

There are a number of biochemical estimations which contribute to the assessment of respiratory diseases. The tests will not be described in any detail here and will only be commented on briefly.

SWEAT CHLORIDES

Most patients suffering from cystic fibrosis show a marked elevation of sodium and chloride levels in the sweat due to an inability of the sweat glands to conserve salt. This electrolyte abnormality has been found also in untreated adrenal insufficiency, and it is being found with increasing frequency in patients who have bronchiectasis. Many patients with cystic fibrosis also have pancreatic insufficiency; an absence of trypsin, lipase and amylase in the duodenal contents; and an excess of fat and nitrogenous matter in the feces.

SERUM PROTEINS

The serum normally contains between 6.0 and 8.5 grams of protein per 100 ml. The principal components of the serum proteins are albumin, alpha globulins, and beta globulin, all of which are produced in the liver, and gamma globulin which is formed by the lymphocyte-plasma cell system. By means of immunoelectrophoresis the various globulins can be separated into groups which are antigenically distinct from each other.

The gamma globulins vary considerably in respiratory disease. Chronic infection and many connective tissue disorders, such as lupus erythematosus and rheumatoid disease, are usually associated with high levels of gamma globulin. Low levels of gamma globulin, either congenital or acquired in nature, or myelomatosis in which there are high levels of an abnormal nonfunctional globulin in the serum are associated with frequent bacterial infections or recurrent pneumonias. Hyperglobulinemia may be present in chronic diseases such as bronchiectasis, tuberculosis and sarcoidosis, as well as lupus erythematosus and periarteritis nodosa.

$ALPHA_1$-ANTITRYPSIN

A deficiency of alpha$_1$-antitrypsin in the serum, a defect which is genetically determined, has been described in a certain number of cases of panlobular emphysema. Alpha$_1$-antitrypsin is the major circulating proteolytic enzyme inhibitor in the body, and it forms the major component of the alpha$_1$-globulin fraction of the serum. Deficiency of this protein may be suggested by immunoelectrophoresis and then confirmed by further specific laboratory studies. Persons with an antitrypsin activity of less than 10 per cent (homozygotes) invariably exhibit panlobular emphysema. Those with alpha$_1$-antitrypsin activity of less than 60 per cent of normal (heterozygotes) may be more susceptible to the development of obstructive pulmonary disease, but this is still controversial.

LE CELL

The lupus erythematosus cell (LE cell) can only be demonstrated in special preparations of the blood and bone marrow. It is a polymorphonuclear leukocyte that contains a phagocytized, round, homogenous, structureless inclusion body. This inclusion body is apparently nuclear protein that has been altered by the LE factor in the serum, an immunoglobulin with specificity against nucleoprotein. The presence of LE cells on two or more occasions establishes the diagnosis of systemic lupus erythematosus, a collagen disease in which pleural involvement is frequent.

RHEUMATOID FACTOR

The serologic tests of rheumatoid factor, a term applied to a group of macroglobulins having a nonspecific antiglobulin activity directed against mammalian proteins, utilize suspensions of particles of either sheep red blood cells, latex or bentonite. With the latex fixation test, which is the most widely used procedure, titers above 1:160 are considered positive.

A high titer of rheumatoid factor is found commonly in rheumatoid arthritis, with or without an associated diffuse fibrosing alveolitis. Rheumatoid factor is also found in a variety of diseases characterized by prolonged antigenic stimulation, such as chronic parasitic and bacterial infections, or in patients who have undergone organ transplants. It has been suggested that apparently healthy persons with a high rheumatoid factor titer have a greater than average chance of developing rheumatoid arthritis.

ANTINUCLEAR FACTOR

This antinucleoprotein antibody may be found in the blood in patients suffering from lupus erythematosus, rheumatoid arthritis, scleroderma and drug hypersensitivity.

PRECIPITINS

Precipitating antibodies to specific antigens are present in the Type 3 hypersensitivity lung diseases, such as farmer's lung and bird fancier's disease. Using gel-diffusion techniques, a line of precipitate will form between specific antigens and the patient's serum if it contains antibody to the antigen.

Complement-fixation and precipitin tests on the serum may also be helpful in establishing the diagnosis of a mycotic infection. These tests only become positive after the development of a hypersensitivity reaction in the tissues. The complement-fixing antibodies appear later than the precipitins and persist for a longer time so that the precipitin test is of more value in the early phase of the disease. A negative reaction to either test, however, does not imply that a mycotic infection is not present.

The complement-fixation test is positive in about 75 per cent of cases of hydatid disease, but it may be negative if the cyst is well walled off or if the cysts are inactive.

SERUM ENZYMES

Certain tissues contain characteristic enzymes which enter the blood when the tissues are damaged or destroyed. Measurement of these serum enzymes can be of diagnostic value in respiratory disease. The level of lactic dehydrogenase in the serum can be elevated by damage to nearly any tissue. It was previously thought that an elevation of serum lactic dehydrogenase without a concomitant increase in glutamic oxalacetic and glutamic pyruvic transaminases was indicative of pulmonary embolism and infarction, but this may not be specific.

Elevation of the serum amylase ordinarily indicates pancreatic disease. In acute pancreatitis, absorption of the peritoneal fluid from the upper abdomen may result in a pleural effusion which characteristically contains a considerably higher amylase content than that in the serum.

OTHER BLOOD CHEMISTRY

The blood urea nitrogen may be elevated because of functional impairment of the kidneys in chronic nephritis. If diabetes mellitus is present, hyperglycemia is usually found, and hypercalcemia may be a feature of active sarcoidosis. Significant elevation of the serum acid phosphatase is indicative of prostatic carcinoma which has metastasized. Amyloidosis, a complication of long-standing suppuration, can be demonstrated by the intravenous injection of Congo red, a dye which has an affinity for amyloid tissue.

HEMATOLOGY

Anemia may result from the accelerated blood destruction which occurs in certain bacterial infections, particularly those caused by the hemolytic streptococcus. A chronic infection, such as tuberculosis, may produce anemia as a result of depression of the bone marrow. A neoplasm which has metastasized to the bone marrow may cause anemia by mechanical interference with blood formation. Secondary polycythemia may occur in diseases with associated chronic hypoxia.

A neutrophilic leukocytosis is generally present in acute infections produced by pyogenic organisms, such as *Staphylococcus aureus,* hemolytic streptococcus and pneumococcus. The degree of leukocytosis is governed by the resistance of the patient as well as the virulence and the number of the invading organisms. A severe leukocytosis, called a leukemoid reaction, may occasionally be seen in malignant pulmonary conditions, particularly those with associated infection and necrosis.

An eosinophilic leukocytosis most commonly occurs in allergic disease and is particularly severe in the migratory pulmonary infiltrations of Löffler's syndrome. It is a feature of parasitic infestations such as ascariasis, amebiasis and hydatid disease, as well as periarteritis nodosa and Hodgkin's disease.

A relative lymphocytosis may occasionally be seen in diseases with associated generalized lymphadenopathy, such as Hodgkin's disease and lymphosarcoma, and a high degree of relative lymphocytosis may be found in pertussis.

In contrast to the bacterial pneumonias, in which it is usually greater than 15,000, the leukocyte count is usually within normal limits and rarely greater than 15,000 per cu. mm. in viral and mycoplasmal pneumonias. Various degrees of neutropenia may be found in such viral diseases as measles and influenza as well as in some overwhelming bacterial infections, probably because of depression of the bone marrow by the organisms or their toxins.

The erythrocyte sedimentation rate frequently provides an indication of the activity of the disease process. An accelerated rate is an important finding, especially if it is known that the rate had been normal in the past. In acute infective processes, the sedimentation rate is accelerated in the early part of the disease and gradually falls to normal levels as recovery takes place.

URINE

The urine should be examined routinely, and if the disease is a chronic one, the examination should be repeated periodically. A small percentage of patients suffering from pulmonary tuberculosis develop genitourinary tuberculosis, particularly when the disease has apparently become inactive. Chronic suppurative diseases may become complicated by the development of renal amyloidosis. Carcinoma of the kidney may metastasize to the lungs or may produce a secondary polycythemia. Patients suffering from diabetes mellitus are more liable to develop pulmonary tuberculosis.

ELECTROCARDIOGRAPHY

The typical electrocardiographic changes of right ventricular hypertrophy and strain and "P pulmonale" may be found in patients suffering from chronic pulmonary diseases who have developed an increased pulmonary vascular resistance. Respiratory insufficiency is frequently associated with supraventricular and sometimes ventricular arrhythmias.

Section Four

The Patterns of Respiratory Disease

AIRWAY OBSTRUCTION

RESTRICTIVE LUNG PARENCHYMAL DISEASE

PULMONARY VASCULAR DISEASE

PLEURAL DISEASE

DISEASES OF THE CHEST WALL AND DIAPHRAGM

Chapter 13

Airway Obstruction

The bronchi are involved in most pulmonary diseases. In some diseases the bronchi are diffusely involved, but in others involvement is limited to a single bronchus or one of its subdivisions. Even when the disease process involves primarily the lung parenchyma, the lumen of the bronchus draining the diseased area may be narrowed by mucosal swelling or inflammatory exudate, and air movement into and out of the alveoli and drainage of secretions are impaired.

The term "airway obstruction" is relative, for the severity of the obstruction of an affected bronchus varies inversely with the diameter of its lumen. For instance, mucosal swelling does not produce the same degree of obstruction in the larger bronchi that it does in one of the finer bronchi. In the infant, in whom the diameters of all bronchi are small, inflammatory swelling of even the larger bronchi may have serious obstructive effects. Even in persons with normal lungs there may be some degree of airway narrowing under certain circumstances, particularly in the dependent lung regions, such as when breathing at a low residual volume with a fixed tidal volume or when obesity is present.

GENERAL FEATURES OF BRONCHIAL OBSTRUCTION

The three mechanisms by which a bronchial lumen may be narrowed are depicted in Figure 97. The cause may be *extramural,* in which case the narrowing of the bronchus is produced by external pressure, such as enlarged mediastinal lymph nodes occluding the right middle lobe bronchus. Bronchial obstruction may also be *mural,* the obstruction resulting from a pathological lesion within the confines of the bronchial wall, such as a bronchogenic carcinoma projecting into the lumen of the bronchus, or from mucosal edema. *Intraluminal* causes of bronchial obstruction include inhaled foreign bodies or thick bronchial secretions.

A bronchial obstruction may be either partial or complete. In a partial obstruction, airflow and drainage of secretions are impaired, but in a complete obstruction, both airflow and drainage of secretions can no longer occur.

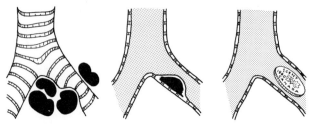

FIGURE 97. The causes of bronchial obstruction. *Left,* Extramural; *middle,* mural; *right,* intraluminal.

PARTIAL BRONCHIAL OBSTRUCTION

A partial bronchial obstruction always acts as either a *bypass valve* or a *check valve,* depending on both the degree of narrowing of the bronchial lumen and the nature of the pathological process producing it.

BYPASS BRONCHIAL OBSTRUCTION

A bypass type of partial obstruction is illustrated in Figure 98. The lumen of the bronchus is only slightly narrowed so that although airflow resistance is increased, air is still able to move in and out past the site of obstruction. A bypass bronchial obstruction often

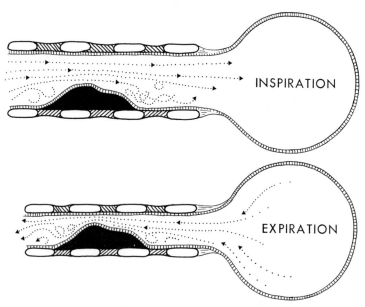

FIGURE 98. The bypass partial bronchial obstruction.

results in overdistention of the lung parenchyma distal to the obstruction because the airways narrow during expiration so that resistance to flow is higher than it is during inspiration. If the bypass obstruction is diffuse and involves much of the lungs, generalized overdistention occurs for several reasons. In the inspiratory position the airways are more widely open. In addition the increase in elastic retractive force associated with an increase in lung volume helps to overcome the increased resistance to airflow during expiration.

CHECK-VALVE BRONCHIAL OBSTRUCTION

This type of bronchial obstruction differs from a bypass obstruction in that the bronchial lumen is completely occluded during expiration so that the egress of air is prevented. This is illustrated in Figure 99. An endobronchial tumor attached to the bronchial wall by a pedicle can produce this type of obstruction. During inspiration, the bronchial lumen widens so that air is able to pass over the obstruction. However, expiratory narrowing of the bronchial lumen completely occludes the lumen; air is then trapped in the affected pulmonary segment, and the alveoli become overdistended.

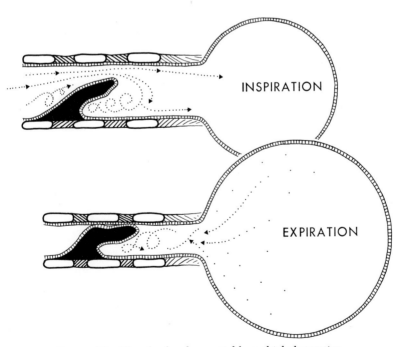

FIGURE 99. The check-valve partial bronchial obstruction.

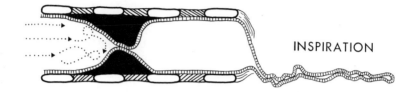

INSPIRATION

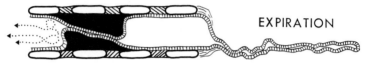

EXPIRATION

FIGURE 100. The complete bronchial obstruction.

COMPLETE BRONCHIAL OBSTRUCTION

In the complete or stop-valve type of obstruction, which is illustrated in Figure 100, the bronchus is completely occluded so that air cannot move in or out. The consequence of this type of obstruction is atelectasis of the affected portion of the lung (see section on Atelectasis, p. 307).

CLINICAL MANIFESTATIONS

The clinical manifestations depend on the type of bronchial obstruction as well as its location in the tracheobronchial tree. Complete obstruction of the trachea results in asphyxia and death. Partial obstruction of the trachea results in a forceful and prolonged inspiration, with visible indrawing over the sternal notch, the supraclavicular spaces, the intercostal spaces and the epigastrium. At the same time, a coarse low-pitched sound is heard during both inspiration and expiration and is called *stridor*.

If obstruction of a large bronchus develops gradually, there may be no symptoms, aside from a cough; whereas, if the obstruction develops abruptly, intense dyspnea is usually experienced. The extent of the symptoms resulting from obstruction of the finer bronchi or bronchioles depends on the number of bronchi involved. If the obstruction is localized to a few smaller bronchi, there may be no symptoms, but if there is diffuse involvement of the smaller bronchi, such as in asthma, intense dyspnea may be experienced.

A cough is almost always associated with all types of bronchial obstruction. As the degree of obstruction increases, so does the cough.

Interference with bronchial drainage is a frequent consequence of bronchial obstruction, and because bacteria grow very easily in retained secretions, infection frequently develops in the affected area of the lung. This creates a vicious circle, with the production of more secretions and more cough.

PARTIAL OBSTRUCTION

In a bypass obstruction eddies produced in the air currents at the site of the obstruction cause vibrations which result in a wheezing sound or rhonchus during expiration, particularly if the expiration is forceful and prolonged. These rhonchi may be heard over all areas of the chest cage, or they may be confined to a single area. Generalized rhonchi indicate diffuse involvement of the tracheobronchial tree, as in asthma or bronchitis; rhonchi confined to a single area indicate a localized partial bronchial obstruction. If the rhonchi are due to secretions, the wheeze may often disappear after a cough, but if the obstruction is immovable, the rhonchi persist even after vigorous coughing.

As pointed out previously, the affected segment frequently becomes overdistended when there is a partial obstruction. If a large portion of lung is involved, the mediastinum will be shifted toward the opposite side, movement will be diminished, the percussion note hyperresonant, and the intensity of the breath sounds will be reduced over the affected area.

COMPLETE OBSTRUCTION

Complete bronchial obstruction leads to absorption of gas and collapse of the distal alveoli. The clinical manifestations of complete bronchial obstruction vary with the size of the affected bronchus and the amount of lung tissue involved.

Atelectasis. The term "atelectasis" is derived from the Greek words "ateles," meaning imperfect, and "ektasis," meaning expansion. It is used synonymously with the term "pulmonary collapse," and it implies that the alveoli in the affected area of the lung have become airless and have collapsed.

If a bronchus is obstructed for any length of time, the alveolar gases are gradually absorbed into the pulmonary capillaries. Blood flow in the pulmonary capillaries is essential for atelectasis to develop; it will not take place if the pulmonary artery supplying the affected lobe is ligated before its bronchus is blocked. The alveolar gases are absorbed into the circulating blood because the total gas pressure in the alveolar air is higher than that in the mixed venous blood as shown in Table 12.

TABLE 12

THE PARTIAL PRESSURES OF GASES IN ALVEOLAR AIR AND MIXED VENOUS BLOOD

	ALVEOLAR AIR	MIXED VENOUS BLOOD
Oxygen	110	40
Carbon dioxide	40	46
Nitrogen	563	563
H_2O	47	47

Although all of the gaseous exchanges occur simultaneously, it is easier to describe the process of absorption of air from the alveoli as a sequence of exchanges of the individual gases. Initially, because of the partial pressure differences, oxygen moves from the alveolus into the pulmonary capillary while carbon dioxide moves in the opposite direction. As a result of the net diffusion of gas into the blood, the alveolar volume is reduced. The lung, by virtue of its elasticity, accommodates itself to this new volume, and compression continues until all the alveolar gases are absorbed and the alveoli are completely collapsed. This process takes several hours because there is little partial pressure difference between the alveoli and the blood of nitrogen, which is the major contributor to the total gas pressure. On the other hand, if the alveoli contain pure oxygen rather than nitrogen, complete atelectasis can occur within a few minutes because of the marked difference in total gas pressure.

Atelectasis may not develop when a bronchiole becomes obstructed because there may be collateral ventilation through minute apertures in the interalveolar septa between neighboring lobules. Thus, even though a terminal bronchiole becomes obstructed, the primary or secondary lobule may continue to contain air because it is supplied from the alveoli of neighboring lobules.

Atelectasis also occurs when there is air or fluid in the pleural cavity. In this situation, the atelectasis is usually thought to be due to compression of alveoli, leading to their complete emptying. It is also possible that compression of the lung leads to a reduction in volume to the point at which airway narrowing or even closure occurs, and gas is then absorbed, resulting in further emptying of alveoli. An increase in surface tension at the air-liquid interface in alveoli will also produce atelectasis since, as was pointed out in Section One, in the presence of an increased surface tension the transmural pressure necessary to maintain patent alveoli becomes markedly increased.

Provided the collapse has not been present for too long a time, the atelectatic lung usually re-expands when the bronchial obstruction is alleviated. Initial expansion of the collapsed area of lung may require a very high transpulmonary pressure in order to overcome resistance to expansion due to the forces of surface tension. This is analogous to inflation of the degassed lung under experimental conditions, as was described in Chapter 1.

It is usually impossible to detect an atelectasis of a segment or smaller areas of lung by physical examination, although it may be demonstrable on the chest roentgenogram. When the atelectasis involves a greater portion of the lung, the physical signs present are the consequence of a decreased size and increased density of the affected lung parenchyma.

The affected part of the chest may appear retracted, with the ribs closer together, and there may be inspiratory indrawing of the costal interspaces. The trachea and apex beat of the heart are shifted to the affected side, and chest movement is diminished, the percussion note dull, and vocal fremitus and breath sounds reduced or absent over the affected area. On the other hand, if the bronchus underlying the atelectasis is patent, sound transmission may be increased rather than reduced, vocal fremitus is increased and bronchial breathing may be present. If the bronchioles and collapsed alveoli should contain secretions or inflammatory exudate, fine, high-pitched rales may be heard during the terminal phase of inspiration.

ROENTGENOLOGIC MANIFESTATIONS

The roentgenologic changes brought about by bronchial obstruction depend on the degree and site of obstruction. If there is a localized check-valve obstruction, the affected portion of lung is hyperin-

FIGURE 101. Overinflation due to a check-valve obstruction.

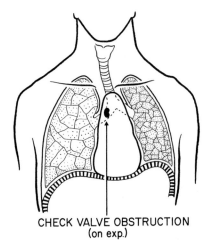

CHECK VALVE OBSTRUCTION
(on exp.)

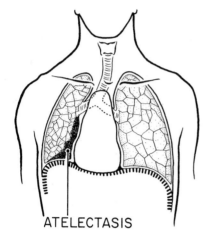

ATELECTASIS

FIGURE 102. Atelectasis of the right lower lobe.

flated. A check-valve obstruction may be particularly evident during expiration, and this can best be demonstrated during fluoroscopy or on inspiration-expiration chest roentgenograms (Fig. 101). In addition, the mediastinum may shift toward the unaffected side during expiration. With diffuse partial obstruction of the smaller bronchi, there is frequently generalized hyperinflation of the lungs.

The atelectasis following complete bronchial obstruction produces characteristic radiologic signs. The airless lobe tends to become wedge-shaped with concave borders, the apex being at the mediastinum and the base in apposition to the chest wall. Figure 102 illustrates the radiologic appearance of an atelectasis of the right lower lobe. If there is sufficient reduction in lung volume, the mediastinum will be obviously shifted to the affected side.

DISEASES WITH PREDOMINANT AIRWAY OBSTRUCTION

Airway obstruction may develop acutely as a result of the inhalation of foreign material into the tracheobronchial tree or because of acute or chronic inflammation.

ACUTE AIRWAY OBSTRUCTION

INHALATION OF FOREIGN MATERIAL

The inhalation of foreign material may produce local or diffuse airway obstruction. The commonest cause of diffuse acute airway obstruction is aspiration of gastric contents, which results in general-ized bronchitis. Localized acute airway obstruction is most commonly the result of aspiration of a foreign body and occurs frequently in children under 4 years of age. About 2 per cent of inhaled foreign bodies are spontaneously expelled by coughing, but the rest usually result in complications. Because the orifice of the right main stem bronchus is slightly wider than the left and lies in a more direct line with the trachea, 70 per cent of aspirated foreign bodies enter the right main stem bronchus, 25 per cent lodging in the left main stem bron-chus and 5 per cent in the trachea.

Clinical Manifestations. The first symptoms immediately following aspiration are choking, gagging, temporary aphonia, cough, respiratory distress and wheezing. Laryngospasm lasting a few seconds is common. Hoarseness or aphonia and a brassy cough are usually present if the object lodges in the larynx. If the foreign body lodges in the trachea, signs and symptoms similar to those of laryngeal lodgement may be produced, or there may be a relatively symptom-less period after the initial aspiration.

A foreign body which lodges in a major bronchus usually pro-duces unilateral signs. On the affected side, there may be a bypass obstruction with inspiratory and expiratory rhonchi, a check-valve obstruction with hyperinflation or complete obstruction with signs of atelectasis. Commonly, a partial obstruction progresses to complete obstruction because of mucosal swelling and edema. Because of its vegetable nature, an aspirated peanut is particularly dangerous, causing a marked local inflammatory reaction and mucosal edema. A common complication is infection distal to the obstruction which may lead to pneumonia, abscess or bronchiectasis.

Radiologic Manifestations. Since most foreign bodies are of vegetable or plastic origin they cannot be visualized in the chest roentgenogram. The radiologic manifestations depend on the type of obstruction present and have been discussed earlier in this section.

CROUP

Inflammation of the upper airway occurs in both children and adults, but it is particularly important in children, in whom it produces a clinical syndrome commonly called *croup*. This syndrome consists of inspiratory stridor, cough and hoarseness resulting from varying degrees of laryngeal obstruction. Most cases occur during the cold season of the year, at a time when there is an increased incidence of respiratory infection. A viral etiology has been implicated in 85 per cent of patients with this disease, the parainfluenza virus being the commonest agent isolated.

Haemophilus influenzae type B accounts for the majority of the remainder of patients, and it causes inflammation of the epiglottis, which becomes enlarged because of inflammatory edema. the infection commonly extends downward into the respiratory tract and involves the trachea and bronchi.

Clinical Manifestations. The cough associated with croup is characteristically brassy and barking in nature. Laryngeal obstruction of varying degrees gives rise to both inspiratory and expiratory stridor, and in severe obstruction marked supraclavicular, suprasternal, and subcostal retractions may be seen. The majority of patients with viral croup are between 3 months and 3 years of age. Infection of the upper respiratory passages is followed in 3 to 4 days by inflammation, edema and spasm of the true cords and subglottic structures. Croup resulting from *Haemophilus influenzae* type B infection is a serious disease, for it has a fulminant course over a few hours, and the inflammation may spread to involve the remainder of the supraglottic as well as the subglottic areas. Examination of the pharynx will reveal a fiery red, swollen, edematous epiglottis.

Diphtheritic croup is now a rare occurrence. In these cases there is usually a preceding respiratory tract infection of 3 to 4 days' duration before the onset of croup. The patients are quite toxic and ill. On physical examination there is frequently a serosanguinous nasal discharge, and a membrane may be present in the posterior pharynx. The symptoms of croup usually develop slowly, but signs of severe obstruction may occur suddenly if the membrane becomes dislodged and obstructs the laryngeal airway.

Radiologic Manifestations. The correlation between the clinical severity of the disease and the roentgenogram is usually poor, but the exact site of involvement is often seen on a lateral view of the neck. In the case of viral croup the subglottic area is swollen, and there is obliteration of the normal tracheal air shadow. In bacterial croup there is involvement of the supraglottic structures, including the arytenoepiglottic folds and epiglottis.

ACUTE BRONCHITIS

Bronchitis is a condition in which there is inflammation of the bronchial tree with the production of excessive mucus. The acute variety of bronchitis is moderately common, and it usually leads to little permanent disability. It may occur as a primary manifestation during the course of such infectious diseases as measles and typhoid fever or as a concomitant of an acute bacterial pneumonia such as a streptococcal lobular pneumonia. It develops most commonly as a consequence of a viral infection, such as influenza, and generally becomes complicated by secondary bacterial infection. Sometimes, especially in patients with chronic bronchitis, acute symptoms appear to be precipitated by irritative rather than infective factors, the most frequent irritant being a high concentration of atmospheric pollutants.

Clinical Manifestations. The onset of acute bronchitis is heralded by a substernal burning discomfort, which is due to an associated tracheitis, and a harassing, rasping, painful cough. Paroxysmal attacks of cough and wheezing are precipitated by the inhalation of irritants such as cigarette smoke or exposure to cold air. Initially, there is a scanty expectoration of mucus, which later may become more abundant and mucopurulent. Recovery from the illness is usually complete.

BRONCHIOLITIS

Inflammation of the bronchioles occurs in both adults and children and is probably usually due to a viral infection. Since flow resistance is inversely related to the fourth power of the radius of the airways involved, bronchiolitis is particularly serious in children under 2 years of age whose airways are relatively small.

Bronchiolitis is most commonly associated with respiratory syncytial virus (RSV) infection. Bronchiolar obstruction results because of edema and lymphocytic infiltration of the bronchiolar walls as well as obstruction of the lumen with mucus and cellular debris. A check-valve obstruction results in hyperinflation of the lung distal to the site of obstruction; a complete obstruction results in atelectasis.

The mortality rate with RSV infection is low (about 1 per cent), but adenovirus infection has been associated with a severe fulminating disease. In its most severe form the adenovirus may cause widespread necrotizing lesions of the mucosa of the entire respiratory tract and destruction of the walls of bronchi and bronchioles.

Clinical Manifestations. The first sign of illness in the infant is coryza, which may last for several days or may rapidly progress to paroxysmal cough, an audible expiratory wheeze and occasionally an expiratory grunt. In the more severe cases the respiratory rate may be as high as 80 per minute, and cyanosis may be evident. The anteroposterior diameter of the chest is increased, and there are subcostal, intercostal and suprasternal retractions. The chest is hyperresonant to percussion, and on auscultation, breath sounds are diminished bilaterally, and expiration is prolonged. There may be widespread fine inspiratory and expiratory rales as well as high-pitched rhonchi, particularly near the end of expiration.

Radiologic Manifestations. Hyperinflation with depressed and flat diaphragms, an increased anteroposterior diameter of the thorax, abnormally translucent lung fields and an increase in the size of the retrosternal air shadow is always present. The thickened bronchioles are often visible as abnormal linear shadows, and frank infiltrates or areas of linear atelectasis may also be present.

Functional Manifestations. Both inspiratory and expiratory flow resistance may be elevated with a resultant increase in the work of breathing. Since the peripheral airways are primarily affected, the standard measurements of airflow resistance may be relatively unaffected, so that the functional disturbances may not be obvious. However, the disturbance of the peripheral airways will result in an unequal distribution of time constants within the lungs so that the dynamic compliance will be frequency dependent, and the distribution of gas is often impaired. The A-a PO_2 difference will be increased in the majority of patients, and the arterial PO_2 will be low because of a mismatching of ventilation and perfusion. In severe cases carbon dioxide retention may be associated with the hypoxia.

CHRONIC AIRWAY OBSTRUCTION

It has been estimated that there are currently more than 15 million persons in North America suffering from some degree of chronic airway obstruction. The mortality rate has been doubling every five years and is now more than 35,000 deaths annually.

The common clinical entities in which chronic airway obstruction is the predominant feature are chronic bronchitis, emphysema, bronchiectasis, asthma and cystic fibrosis.

CHRONIC BRONCHITIS

Chronic bronchitis is characterized by a chronic cough with excessive production of sputum, which is not due to known specific causes such as bronchiectasis or tuberculosis and which persists for more than three months of the year for two or more successive years. It is commoner in males (more than 20 per cent of adult males) and outranks all other respiratory diseases as a crippler and a killer.

In a well-established case there is hypertrophy of the bronchial mucous glands and the goblet cells. In the absence of an acute infection the cilia are usually intact, although if many goblet cells are discharging, the effective ciliary area may be reduced or the cilia may become inefficient so that drainage is impaired. The finding of a high bronchial gland/bronchial wall ratio (Reid index) is very suggestive of the diagnosis of chronic bronchitis, but the correlation between clinical bronchitis and the amount of mucous gland hyperplasia is not good, and there is considerable overlap of the Reid index between bronchitics and nonbronchitics.

The factors involved in the etiology of chronic bronchitis have undergone considerable scrutiny, but the picture is still not completely understood. Irritation of the tracheobronchial tree is common to all cases of bronchitis, and it would appear that cigarette smoking is the single most important determinant. However, not all cigarette smokers develop bronchitis, and it is possible that immunologic or familial susceptibility may play an important part in some persons.

All epidemiological studies have uniformly shown that the prevalence of cough and phlegm is higher in smokers than in nonsmokers. Heavy smokers are more seriously affected than light smokers, and the longer the history of cigarette smoking, the worse the symptoms are.

It has been shown that the majority of particulate matter in cigarette smoke is deposited on the bronchial mucus blanket. Ciliary activity is inhibited by tobacco smoke so that movement of the bronchial mucus blanket is diminished considerably, and the irritating effect on the underlying bronchial epithelium is enhanced. The mucous glands and goblet cells are stimulated to produce more mucus, and this, together with the altered ciliary activity, leads to the development of chronic cough and expectoration. The bronchial mucus secreted in chronic bronchitis is apparently biochemically no different from normal bronchial mucus. The hypersecretion of mucus increases the liability to infection and delays the tendency to recovery; as a result a vicious circle of hypersecretion, infection, and more hypersecretion results.

Another important effect of inhaled cigarette smoke is bronchoconstriction, which is presumably due to irritation of nerve endings in the bronchial tree and occurs in both smokers and nonsmokers whether or not they are suffering from cardiopulmonary disease. Airway resistance may double following a cigarette, and this may persist for as long as 30 minutes. The inhalation of an aerosol of carbon particles produces a similar effect, but an aerosol of nicotine does not.

Another important source of bronchial irritation is the upper respiratory tract. Although it is often difficult to sort out which comes first, infection in the upper respiratory tract and postnasal discharge are common concomitants of bronchitis.

Although many bacteria which normally inhabit the mouth and nasopharynx are probably inhaled during respiration, they usually adhere to the tracheobronchial mucus blanket and are removed by ciliary activity or coughing so that the lower respiratory tract is essentially sterile. In patients with chronic bronchitis, however, many of these organisms can be isolated in variable proportions from the sputum. There is considerable controversy regarding the relationship of these organisms to acute exacerbations of the disease. Many of the acute episodes of bronchitis which develop in patients with chronic airway obstruction are probably caused by a virus infection, but the resulting damage to the bronchial mucosa may encourage the growth of bacteria. *Haemophilus influenzae* and the *Diplococcus pneumoniae* seem to be the important organisms, although occasionally the *Staphylococcus aureus* and the Friedländer's bacillus may have pathogenic significance.

It is difficult to assess the role of occupation in the etiology of bronchitis. The prevalence of this disease is highest in industrial areas, particularly among men who work in dusty occupations, such as coal miners, but no close relationship with the duration of exposure to dust has been demonstrated. It is interesting that the incidence of bronchitis among the wives of these workers is also high, suggesting that an environmental cause—i,e., atmospheric pollution—might be implicated.

There is no doubt that air pollution aggravates and may influence the progression of bronchopulmonary disease, but whether this, per se, can actually cause bronchitis has not been established. In the major cities there appears to be a significant correlation between the day-to-day condition of patients suffering from bronchitis and the average concentration of sulfur dioxide in the atmosphere. Large particles of pollution, such as droplets in wet fog, are usually trapped in the nose and pharynx, and medium-sized particles are generally trapped in the upper bronchial tree, but the smaller particles penetrate deep into the bronchial tree. It has been shown that the inhalation of inert dust particles or a very low concentration of sulfur dioxide causes a twofold increase in the airway resistance, even in healthy human subjects.

Clinical Manifestations.   The onset of the disease is generally insidious, a chronic cough often being attributed to smoking. Respiratory difficulty may only become clinically apparent to the patient after about 30 years of smoking. It is important to understand that the so-called "cigarette cough" is not a normal event but is an early manifestation of bronchitis. It may disappear if cigarette smoking is given up early enough. Often there is an underlying chronic rhinitis or sinusitis, which also improves if one stops smoking.

Some patients develop recurrent bronchitis during the winter months with variable degrees of disability but remain relatively well during the warmer months. Many patients trace the onset of symptoms to some acute infective episodes, such as pneumonia. The clinical condition may vary day to day, the symptoms being aggravated by irritants and cold, damp or foggy weather and are punctuated by recrudescence of infection. In many persons it progresses further to become a year round affliction, with intercurrent acute exacerbations. Death due to bronchopneumonia, respiratory insufficiency, and right-sided heart failure may occur 20 to 35 years after the onset of symptoms.

The sputum is usually mucoid and difficult to expectorate, but it becomes more copious and purulent during acute infections. Exertional dyspnea is usually noted 5 to 10 years later, and it may remain fairly stationary, but usually the breathlessness is aggravated during the episode of acute bronchitis and progressively increases in severity. Wheezing may be present, particularly during acute exacerbations or on exertion. Cough, wheezing and breathlessness may awaken the patient, thus mimicking an attack of paroxysmal nocturnal dyspnea, but in this case the symptoms are generally relieved by the expectoration of sputum.

The serious complications of chronic bronchitis are intercurrent bronchopulmonary infection, emphysema, and right ventricular heart failure. The link between chronic bronchitis and emphysema is probably the associated bronchiolitis, which may lead to obliteration of bronchioles as well as weakening and dilatation of their walls, with the resultant development of centrilobular emphysema, which is described later. When hypoxia and acidemia are present pulmonary hypertension develops, particularly if there is associated emphysema which has reduced the effective pulmonary capillary bed. As a result of the increased pulmonary vascular resistance the work of the right ventricle increases, and its wall hypertrophies. Later, the right ventricle may fail, and then the full-blown picture of right ventricular failure will develop.

The physical signs will depend on the degree of airway obstruction. Respiratory distress may be evident with minor activities or even while talking. In the advanced stages, the patient may have a florid appearance and cyanosis of the mucous membranes. The chest cage is often in an inspiratory position, and this, together with a kyphosis of the dorsal spine, increases the anteroposterior diameter of the chest, producing a barrel-like shape. The accessory muscles are used excessively during breathing, and the chest cage moves "en bloc," the so called "thoracic heave," with inspiratory indrawing of the lower intercostal spaces. The percussion note may be hyperresonant and the breath sounds faint. Medium-pitched rhonchi are usually present, and high-pitched sibilant rhonchi may be heard if the disease involves the smaller bronchi and the bronchioles. Quite often these sibilant rhonchi may only be elicited by having the patient expire forcibly for as long as possible.

A systolic heave in the left parasternal area of the precordium, together with an accentuated second pulmonic sound, suggests the presence of pulmonary hypertension and right ventricular hypertrophy. If this has progressed to congestive heart failure, than there will be distention of the external jugular veins, an enlarged tender liver and dependent edema.

Radiologic Manifestations. If bronchitis affects only the major bronchi, there may be no roentgenologic abnormality. If the more peripheral bronchi are involved, the lungs may be hyperinflated and the diaphragm depressed. Other features are parallel shadows or "tram lines" and prominence of the lung markings, particularly at the bases.

Bronchograms often demonstrate small spike-like protrusions which project outward from the major or segmental bronchi and are probably collections of radiopaque media in the ducts of the enlarged mucous glands. The caliber of the bronchi is often slightly narrowed, and irregularities of the bronchial lumen result from a mixture of stenosis and dilatation. Occasionally a circular pool is seen at the abrupt ending of a long, narrow branch, giving it a beaded appearance; this probably represents a dilated bronchiole or an area of centrilobular emphysema.

Fluoroscopic examination usually reveals a depressed diaphragm with restricted movements, poor aeration of some areas of the lungs during inspiration and evidence of check-valve obstruction with failure to deflate during expiration.

Functional Manifestations.   The pattern of altered pulmonary function in chronic bronchitis is quite variable. As long as the elastic recoil of the lungs is normal, the presence of mild to moderate bronchitis and bronchiolitis may not materially affect standard tests of ventilatory function or flow resistance. As has been pointed out previously, the peripheral airway resistance must be increased considerably before total resistance is significantly increased, but disease in small airways, such as mucous plugging or inflammation, may lead to a fall in dynamic lung compliance with increasing respiratory frequency or mismatching of ventilation and perfusion distribution so that the A-aPO_2 difference will be increased.

In established but uncomplicated chronic bronchitis, airflow resistance is increased, but there is little alteration in lung distensibility. There is evidence of lung overinflation with an enlarged residual volume and functional residual capacity, the total lung capacity being either slightly increased or normal. The vital capacity is either normal or low, depending on the relative size of the residual volume. The rate at which the forced vital capacity (FEV) is expired is considerably delayed in time, and the $FEV_{1.0}$, the maximal midexpiratory flow rate and airflow at 50 per cent of the vital capacity are considerably reduced.

Each acute exacerbation of infection leaves behind it a legacy of further deterioration in function. As the disease progresses, mismatching of ventilation and perfusion is greater and hypoxia increases. Carbon dioxide retention does not develop as long as the perfused areas of lung are capable of being hyperventilated. However, the alveolar ventilation may become inadequate to cope with the carbon dioxide which is being produced in the body (particularly if the work of breathing is high), and therefore carbon dioxide retention develops along with the hypoxia.

EMPHYSEMA

Emphysema, the Greek word meaning overinflation, is a pathological process consisting of permanent overdistention of the respiratory portion of the lung beyond the terminal bronchioles, with attenuation and loss of pulmonary septal tissues. Two major forms of emphysema have been described.

Centrilobular emphysema (CLE) involves predominantly the respiratory bronchioles, which are enlarged, destroyed and become confluent, so that punched out areas are separated by normal lung parenchyma. Centrilobular emphysema occurs most commonly in the upper zones of the lungs, is much commoner in males and is often associated with chronic bronchitis; it rarely occurs in nonsmokers.

Panlobular emphysema (PLE) involves the acinus almost uniformly with enlarged alveoli which are not easily distinguished from the ducts and show abnormal fenestrations in their walls. With progression, there is loss of parenchyma until all that may remain are thin strands of tissue around blood vessels. Panlobular emphysema occurs somewhat randomly throughout the lung but tends to involve the lower zones of the lungs; it is as common in women as in men and is not usually associated with bronchitis. PLE may occur together with CLE, in which case it is associated with chronic bronchitis and a history of cigarette smoking. It has also been found in association with familial alpha$_1$-antitrypsin deficiency.

The incidence of emphysema in the general population has not yet been fully elucidated. In the postmortem examination there is well-defined centrilobular and/or panlobular emphysema in about two-thirds of lungs from adult males and about one-quarter of females. The incidence rises sharply in the fifth decade and then tends to level off.

There is still considerable controversy about the etiology and the mechanism of development of emphysema. Laennec, a pioneer in the study of emphysema, thought that the disease could be entirely explained by mechanical factors and claimed that it begins as a catarrh of the bronchi, which leads to partial bronchial obstruction during both inspiration and expiration. Current thinking has hardly improved on this concept. The disease probably develops as a result of partial or complete bronchiolar obstruction due to inflammation, infection, secretions, bronchial muscular constriction or mucosal congestion, all of which increase resistance to airflow and lead to air-trapping. Repeated inflammatory episodes cause obliteration of bronchioles and greater air-trapping so that more and more lung tissue becomes disrupted until finally the clinical picture of emphysema becomes fully developed.

The failure of the emphysematous lung to collapse when the chest is opened during the postmortem examination, the appearance of atrophied stroma and the fact that the pleural pressure fluctuates in the neighborhood of atmospheric pressure indicate that the elastic retractive force is diminished. However, the relationship between alveolar distention and loss of elasticity is not necessarily one of cause and effect. It is possible that alveolar distention over a long period of time hastens the loss of elasticity, but it is also true that a primary loss of elasticity may lead to alveolar distention. In other words, each may be the cause or the effect of the other, and the loss of elasticity in emphysema may be the basic defect or may be a secondary development.

It has also been shown that obstruction of large numbers of pulmonary blood vessels or the inhalation of papain in animals produces a pathological picture similar to that found in human emphysema.

The relationship between pulmonary emphysema and bronchial asthma is also controversial. Evidence of emphysema is rarely found in the postmortem examination of the lungs of patients suffering from asthma, although episodes of dyspnea and wheezing may precede the clinical picture of emphysema. It is not necessary to implicate asthma, for it is more likely that these episodes of dyspnea are due to acute bronchial obstruction as a result of secretions. On the other hand, there would appear to be no doubt about a relationship between chronic bronchitis and emphysema. Emphysema is more common in bronchitics than in nonbronchitics, and clinical chronic bronchitis and a high Reid index are usual in patients with severe emphysema. Many clinicians believe that emphysema always occurs as a sequel to chronic bronchitis, but there is a definite group of patients in whom emphysema is heralded by the onset of dyspnea with no preceding chronic cough. Even in these patients, however, pathological evidence of bronchiolitis is frequently found in the postmortem examination. There also appears to be a relationship between bronchiectasis and emphysema, particularly when the bronchiectasis is extensive. In addition, there appears to be a high incidence of emphysema in other chronic inflammatory diseases of the lung, particularly when both lungs are diffusely involved.

Clinical Manifestations. Although emphysema, once severe, has characteristic clinical features, the diagnosis of emphysema on purely clinical grounds is extremely difficult.

The chief symptom of emphysema is dyspnea which usually begins slowly and is characteristically brought on by exertion. It is aggravated by exposure to cold air and therefore is much more severe during the winter months. Severe episodes of dyspnea associated with wheezing are usually precipitated by an upper respiratory infection and are accompanied by an increased production of sputum. Conversely, failure to expectorate sputum may in itself precipitate an attack of severe dyspnea because of the accumulation of secretions and the increased airway obstruction. The dyspnea usually progressively increases in severity so that ordinary daily activities such as walking even short distances may induce severe breathlessness.

Coughing may be absent or inconspicuous during the early stages, but in most patients, cough is present for 15 to 25 years before the onset of dyspnea. The severity of the cough is frequently out of proportion to the amount of expectoration produced. Sooner or later, however, defective drainage is followed by infection and the production of mucoid or purulent sputum, and ultimately there may be profuse expectoration. At this stage the condition may resemble bronchiectasis, and indeed, bronchiectasis may finally supervene as a consequence of the frequent attacks of pneumonitis or lobular pneumonia and subsequent fibrosis.

General nourishment is usually below normal, and weight loss is common. Occasionally the weight loss may be so rapid that a neoplasm may be suspected.

Clubbing of the digits does not occur in emphysema; its presence usually indicates an associated or complicating septic condition or new growth.

The incidence of peptic ulcer is increased in patients suffering from emphysema. The reason for this is uncertain, but it has been suggested that ulceration is due to the effect of hypoxia and acidosis on the gastric and duodenal mucosa.

The chest is in a position of hyperinflation, and the diaphragm is depressed, often with inspiratory indrawing, particularly in the areas overlying the insertions of the diaphragm. Movement of the chest cage is noticeably diminished but is equal bilaterally. There is excessive use of the accessory muscles of respiration, particularly the pectoral muscles, which raise the anterior part of the chest cage in a "heaving" manner. Since the ratio of air-containing tissue to solid tissue is increased, tactile and auditory fremitus are reduced and the percussion note is hyperresonant. The breath sounds are distant, especially at the bases of the lungs, and in the late stages the lungs may become so silent as to suggest a pneumothorax. The expiratory breath sound is prolonged because of the increased airflow resistance. Rhonchi may not be detected during ordinary breathing, but extremely high-pitched sibilant rhonchi can frequently be elicited during the late phase of a forced and prolonged expiration.

The heart sounds are often inaudible or heard very faintly at the apex, although they are usually easily detected in the epigastrium. If pulmonary hypertension has developed, the pulmonic second sound becomes accentuated, and it may not be split during inspiration.

The most serious threat to the life of the patient suffering from emphysema is an increase in hypoxia and hypercapnia, which is usually precipitated by an acute infection. The severe hypoxia and acidosis further increase the pulmonary vascular resistance, leading to extreme pulmonary hypertension and often acute right ventricular failure. In the late stages of the disease, chronic right-sided heart failure is common and is manifested by cardiac enlargement, an elevated venous pressure, hepatomegaly and edema. In addition, as pointed out earlier, hypercapnia, per se, may be responsible for further fluid retention.

Radiologic Manifestations. Roentgenograms are usually not helpful in establishing the diagnosis of emphysema when the condition is mild. On the posteroanterior roentgenogram the lungs are usually hyperlucent, with involvement of both lungs equally or only one or more lobes. In the lateral projection, the retrosternal space is seen to be abnormally increased and translucent. The diaphragm is usually depressed and flat, and the thoracic contour may be altered, the ribs running in a more horizontal direction, especially in the upper half of the chest. The peripheral segmental vascular markings may taper rapidly as they proceed distally or they may be very sparse, particularly in panlobular emphysema. The diminution in vascular markings may be localized, as in $alpha_1$-antitrypsin deficiency, in which the lower lobes of the lungs are usually involved. Conversely, the lung markings may be increased in size and more numerous peripherally in centrilobular emphysema.

The heart is usually long and narrow, having been drawn downward by the descending diaphragm. In the later stages, there may be evidence of hypertrophy of the right ventricle with an increase in cardiac size, prominence of the main pulmonary artery segment and enlargement of the hilar pulmonary arteries.

It must be stressed that, in the absence of heart failure, the roentgenologic appearance of emphysema may be no different from the overinflation due to other causes of diffuse bronchial obstruction, such as chronic bronchitis or asthma. It has been suggested that an x-ray film taken in a sagittal plane in approximately the central portion of the chest (full-chest tomogram) may help to substantiate the presence of emphysema. In a patient without emphysema the vessels are usually prominent and can be followed out toward the periphery of the lung. In emphysema, on the other hand, because there has been destruction of the alveolar walls and obliteration of the capillaries, the peripheral pulmonary vasculature is not seen in the full-chest tomogram.

During fluoroscopy, the lungs are seen to be hyperinflated, characteristically deflating poorly during expiration. The diaphragm is low and relatively immobile, but it may move upward paradoxically during inspiration.

Functional Manifestations. The identification and understanding of the alterations in pulmonary function have led to considerable progress in the management of this disease. Since it is extremely serious and widespread, the physiologic disturbances will be dealt with in some detail.

MECHANICS OF BREATHING. The resistance to airflow is high in patients suffering from emphysema, particularly during expiration. Loss of lung elasticity may contribute to the high expiratory resistance because the intrapleural pressure may rise to a point at which the bronchi are compressed. If some of the increased resistance to airflow is reversible, the administration of bronchodilating agents will reduce the nonelastic resistance and decrease the work of breathing.

Although the compliance of the lungs is greater than normal (diminished elasticity), it may be normal or low during resting breathing when the respiratory rate is rapid. This is because the time constants are unequally distributed throughout the lung, and during inspiration the air primarily enters areas of lungs in which the time constants are low so that these areas become overdistended. When the respiratory frequency is slow, the air is distributed relatively equally to most areas of the lung so that the calculated value for the compliance of the lung may be high. The principle has already been illustrated in Figure 25.

As is illustrated in Figure 103, the oxygen consumption of the respiratory muscles is considerably increased in these patients. In addition, it has been suggested that the efficiency of the respiratory muscles is low.

LUNG VOLUMES. As a result of the chronic hyperinflation of the lung, the total lung capacity is often greater than normal, the most striking features being an increased residual volume and functional residual capacity. Although these findings are a reflection of the characteristic inability of the emphysematous lungs to empty, they are in no way diagnostic of this disease, for this pattern may be found in other diseases with diffuse airway obstruction. Great variations in the functional residual capacity can occur in the same patient within a short period of time, especially when there have been exacerbations of bronchospasm or bronchitis. In addition, blebs, bullae and air cysts which communicate poorly or not at all with the tracheobronchial tree are inaccessible to physiologic measurement so that in some cases the estimated total lung capacity is reduced despite an obviously hyperinflated chest.

The vital capacity may be nearly normal in size, or it may be

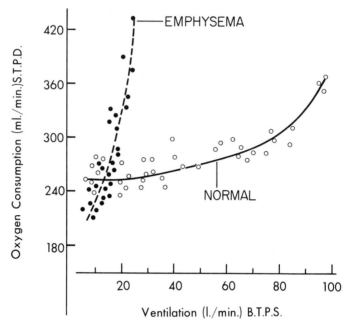

FIGURE 103.   The changes in O_2 consumption with increasing ventilation in a normal subject (O), and in a patient with emphysema (●).

reduced because of the hyperinflation and increased residual volume. There is considerable obstruction to airflow so that the $FEV_{1.0}$, the maximal midexpiratory flow rate and maximal breathing capacity are reduced.

DISTRIBUTION OF AIR AND BLOOD AND GAS EXCHANGE.   Because the loss of lung elasticity and increased flow resistance are not equal in all parts of the lung, the inspired air is unequally distributed, as is the distribution of blood flow, and gross mismatching of ventilation and perfusion is a characteristic feature.

Some alveoli with relatively little perfusion may be relatively overventilated; the physiological effect of this situation is similar to that of an increase in the dead space. The blood perfusing these alveoli becomes fully oxygenated and probably excessively depleted of carbon dioxide, but the quantity of blood flow is so small that the total gas exchange in these alveoli is slight, and a greater than normal burden falls on the other alveoli.

Perfusion of poorly ventilated alveoli results in arterial hypoxia and a tendency toward carbon dioxide retention because not enough oxygen is added to, or carbon dioxide removed from, these alveoli. The physiological effect of this situation is similar to that of a shunt from the venous to the arterial blood. Carbon dioxide retention may not occur if there is sufficient hyperventilation of the remaining well-ventilated, well-perfused alveoli, but this will not correct the hypoxia to any significant degree.

The diffusing capacity of the lungs is reduced in this condition, particularly in the later stages, probably because of the marked mismatching of blood and gas distribution, and the reduction in the size of the pulmonary vascular bed.

In advanced disease, particularly when associated with bronchitis, the carbon dioxide tension of the arterial blood is frequently elevated, even at rest, because the alveolar ventilation is inadequate to cope with the carbon dioxide production.

REGULATION OF RESPIRATION. Because of the hypercapnia and a diminished ventilatory response to inhaled CO_2, it is thought that the sensitivity of the respiratory center is diminished. However, as pointed out earlier, these findings are at least partially the result of the mechanical difficulty in ventilating the lungs. Nevertheless, when the ventilatory response to excessive levels of carbon dioxide is diminished, the peripheral chemoreceptors may become the principal regulators of the respiratory drive, and hypoxia the prime stimulus—a factor which becomes extremely important when oxygen therapy is considered.

PULMONARY CIRCULATION. Because of obliteration of the pulmonary capillaries, the presence of hypoxia and, in some cases, acidosis, all of which constrict the pulmonary vasculature, the pulmonary vascular resistance is frequently elevated, even at rest, and may rise considerably during exercise. The increased pulmonary vascular resistance imposes a heavy load on the right ventricle so that it eventually hypertrophies and may even fail, producing the clinical picture of cor pulmonale.

BRONCHIECTASIS

The term "bronchiectasis" is derived from the Greek words "bronchos," meaning windpipe and "ektasis," meaning extension and is applied to a disease characterized by permanent abnormal dilatation and distortion of either the bronchi or bronchioles or both. This condition develops when the bronchial walls are weakened by chronic inflammatory changes involving the bronchial mucosa, submucosa and the muscular coat. Smoking is not a significant etiologic factor, and women are as commonly affected as men. Patients with bronchiectasis often date their symptoms to childhood, and if they develop severe cardiorespiratory failure, they do so at a relatively early age.

Pathogenesis. The many theories which have been advanced to explain the pathogenesis of bronchiectasis include congenital or developmental defects, distention of the bronchi by cough, destruction of the bronchial wall by necrotizing inflammation, obstruction, atelectasis and fibrous retraction. It is now generally considered that bronchiectasis develops following an airway obstruction or atelectasis because the high intrathoracic pressure required to overcome the increased elastic resistance of an atelectatic lung pulls on the walls of the crowded bronchi. The degree of bronchial dilatation depends on the size of the bronchi affected. A large bronchus with cartilaginous rings does not dilate as readily as the more muscular medium-sized or smaller bronchi. If the bronchial obstruction has been prolonged, secondary infection inevitably supervenes, resulting in destruction of the bronchial walls and dilatation of the bronchi. The consequent reparative laying down of fibrous tissue further increases the traction on the bronchi, leading to still greater distortion. If a bronchial obstruction is relieved before infection has had a chance to develop, the bronchi may return to their normal caliber when the atelectatic area re-expands. This may explain the cases of dilated bronchi demonstrated after pneumonia which return to a normal size later (the so-called "reversible bronchiectasis").

Any lesion which narrows a bronchial lumen, be it extramural, mural or intraluminal, may produce bronchiectasis distal to the obstruction. It has been reported that localized bronchiectasis is found in 27 per cent of patients with cor pulmonale due to bronchitis and emphysema. Bronchiectasis rarely occurs as a congenital defect. Certain pulmonary infections, such as tuberculosis, adenovirus infection, or the pneumonias complicating measles, pertussis and influenza, are more liable to be followed by bronchiectasis.

Bronchiectasis is usually localized to a lobe or a segment, and the lower lobes, particularly that of the left lung, are most commonly involved. Fresh areas of bronchiectasis may subsequently develop in other parts of the same lung, but they are usually associated with a fresh bronchial obstruction. In many cases of bronchiectasis, the bronchial arteries tend to enlarge, often reaching the size of the pulmonary arteries at the same level. The bronchial and pulmonary systems frequently anastomose freely with each other. It has been postulated that the high bronchial artery pressure is transmitted to the pulmonary arterioles through the anastomoses, thereby causing unoxygenated blood to be shunted away from diseased portions of lung to healthy areas where the pulmonary vascular resistance is lower.

Clinical Manifestations. Cough and phlegm are usually the predominant symptoms in bronchiectasis. In most patients there are no symptoms except during periods of acute infection, when a cough with expectoration of purulent sputum and occasionally a fever are present. In some cases, the diseased, dilated bronchi may be insensitive and ciliary activity may be diminished or absent due to the inflammatory changes. In such cases, cough and expectoration of purulent material may be induced only after a change in posture results in movement of secretions into the larger bronchi, in which the mucosa is normal.

The amount of purulent secretions varies. There may be a non-productive cough (so-called "dry bronchiectasis"), small quantities of mucopurulent sputum, or large quantities of purulent sputum, depending on the size of the bronchiectatic cavities, their location and the organisms involved. Bronchiectasis affecting the upper lobes, which is usually secondary to arrested pulmonary tuberculosis, may be relatively asymptomatic because the upper lobes drain effectively in the erect position.

The expectorated material usually separates into three layers if left standing: an upper, frothy, watery layer; a middle, turbid, muco-purulent layer; and a lower, opaque purulent layer. The purulent layer may contain collections of small dirty-white or yellowish masses, known as Dittrich's plugs, or bits of elastic fibers if lung tissue has been destroyed.

A large proportion of patients with suppurative bronchiectasis also have chronic upper respiratory tract infection. Acute exacerbations of sinusitis which may mask the lower respiratory tract symptoms are frequent. The causal relationship between upper and lower respiratory tract infection is debatable, but it is generally assumed that the sinuses become secondarily infected by sprays of purulent sputum during paroxysms of coughing. Nevertheless, chronic upper respiratory tract infection, leading to constant drainage of purulent secretion into the tracheobronchial tree, may lead to bronchial obstruction and to sepsis.

Although not a usual feature of bronchiectasis, breathlessness may become a distressing symptom if both lungs are extensively involved, and particularly when fibrosis develops. Secretions in the bronchi and distortion of the bronchial tree may increase the resistance to airflow and cause wheezing.

Constitutional symptoms ordinarily are not present unless there is extensive chronic suppurative disease or an acute pneumonic infection has developed. Under these circumstances, the patient may complain of undue fatigability, weight loss, profuse night sweats, anorexia and vague abdominal discomfort.

The physical signs depend on the degree of bronchiectasis, its location and the extent of pulmonary involvement. A solitary bron-chiectatic segment may occasionally be detected by an astute clinical observer through the presence of rales, but many cases are discovered only by special radiologic means. More extensive disease always produces physical signs. The physical findings are often similar to those found in atelectasis. Using the left lower lobe as an example, the trachea and apex beat of the heart will be deviated to the left, the diaphragm is higher on the left, and the movement of the chest cage is diminished over the lower lobe. Since the density of the affected lung is increased, the percussion note will vary from dull to flat. The vocal fremitus and type of breath sounds found on examination will depend on the patency of the involved bronchus. If the broncus is still occluded, vocal fremitus and breath sounds will be absent, but if it is patent, vocal fremitus may be greater than normal, and the breath sounds bronchovesicular or bronchial, depending on the amount of the underlying disease present. If the area of lung is solid, whispering pectoriloquy and egophony will be elicited. Clearly, these physical findings are dependent upon the extent of atelectasis, pulmonary consolidation or fibrosis present and bear no relationship to the bronchiectasis. The extent of bronchial involvement can be determined only from the adventitious sounds which may be heard. Coarse, low-pitched rales during the initial third of inspiration are thought to be produced by secretions in the larger bronchi, medium-pitched rales during the middle third of the inspiration by secretions in the smaller bronchi, and fine, high-pitched rales during the final third of inspiration by exudate within the airless, collapsed surrounding alveoli. The rales heard during the initial and middle thirds of inspiration usually disappear if the patient coughs vigorously, but those in the final third usually persist. Expiratory rhonchi, whose pitch depends on the caliber of the bronchi involved, may be produced by an inflamed swollen mucosa, bronchospasm and secretions. Rhonchi detectable over both lungs, particularly during a forced expiration, are most likely due to an associated bronchitis.

Clubbing of the digits may develop, particularly when there is extensive suppuration, and if this is severe enough, the clubbing may progress to the stage of hypertrophic pulmonary osteoarthropathy. However, the development of digital clubbing does not appear to be related to either the duration or the extent of the disease. Another complication of extensive suppurative bronchiectasis may be secondary amyloidosis.

Radiologic Manifestations.   Dilated bronchi do not cast a roentgenologic shadow so that a normal posteroanterior and lateral x-ray of the chest do not exclude the diagnosis of bronchiectasis. However, chest roentgenograms frequently demonstrate abnormal radiographic opacities due to complications of the bronchiectasis. The extent and nature of the roentgenographic abnormality depend on the extent and severity of bronchiectasis. Peribronchial fibrosis may show up as irregular dense strands radiating downward and outward from the hilum. Occasionally, the dilated bronchi appear as thin-walled, translucent spaces, which may have a fluid level. Vascular markings are often increased, but they are often crowded together, indicating loss of volume of the affected region. Considerable loss of volume, amounting to almost complete collapse, may occur in severe bronchiectasis, and the uninvolved lung may undergo compensatory overinflation.

These radiographic abnormalities are suggestive but not diagnostic of the presence of bronchiectasis. Special films called "bronchograms," in which the lumen of the tracheobronchial tree is outlined with radiopaque, iodine-containing medium, will establish the diagnosis. The radiopaque contrast medium easily fills the dilated bronchi, provided they are patent.

Functional Manifestations. The alterations in pulmonary function in bronchiectasis depend upon the number of bronchi involved as well as the associated parenchymal disease. With minimal bronchiectasis involving one bronchopulmonary segment there is little effect on pulmonary function.

The vital capacity may be little altered unless there is much pooling of secretions or the elastic resistance is increased because of atelectasis or fibrosis. Usually, the nonelastic resistance is mildly increased because of an excess of secretions due to either the bronchiectasis or chronic bronchitis. The $FEV_{1.0}$, maximal midexpiratory flow rate and maximal breathing capacity are reduced, residual volume is increased and distribution of the inspired gas is impaired.

Even if the disease is mild, hypoxia may be present because of perfusion of poorly ventilated areas of lung, particularly if atelectasis or pneumonitis is also present. Hyperventilation of the uninvolved portions of the lung helps to maintain a normal or slightly lowered arterial carbon dioxide tension. When there is diffuse disease, there may be gross maldistribution of blood and gases, and the work of breathing may be so great that alveolar hypoventilation with consequent hypoxia and hypercapnia may develop.

ASTHMA

"Asthma" literally means difficult breathing. Asthma may be defined as recurrent generalized airway obstruction which, in the early stages, is paroxysmal and reversible and is accompanied by eosinophilia of the blood and sputum.

The cause of asthma is not known. Certain factors such as allergy, infection, and psychological and nonspecific irritants such as thermal changes, dust of any kind and emotional upsets may precipitate attacks of bronchospasm. Often there is a personal or family history of an allergic condition.

Because many physicians consider wheezing to be synonymous

with asthma, this disease may be too frequently misdiagnosed. The young patient with no bronchitis who has a family history of allergy can probably be diagnosed as having asthma, but in the middle-aged patient the diagnosis is difficult. Those who are middle-aged often have little evidence of allergy as indicated by the history, skin tests, or serum levels of IgE immunoglobulin. It is obvious from the previous discussion of bronchial obstruction that, although all patients suffering from asthma are subject to wheezing, all patients who wheeze do not necessarily have asthma.

Allergy is an important precipitating cause which should be investigated in all cases. It may be possible to remove the offending allergen from the patient's environment, thereby bringing about considerable improvement and even cure. In circumstances in which removal is not possible, hyposensitization with increasing dosage of the allergen is worthwhile in the case of pollens, animal danders and possibly some molds.

In allergic patients the clinical manifestations of asthma are considered to be precipitated by pharmacologically active substances released on combination of the allergen in question with the corresponding antibodies which are fixed to the mast cells in the tissues or the basophils in the peripheral blood of the patient. These antibodies, known as reagins or skin-sensitizing antibodies, are produced by the lymphoid system of the allergic patient on exposure to a specific antigen.

An antigen is a foreign substance which stimulates the formation of an antibody within an animal or a man and which is capable of reacting with that antibody. A specific antigen does not produce a unique clinical picture; the allergic manifestation depends on the shock organ. The same antigen may produce bronchial asthma in one person, rhinitis in another, urticaria in a third, purpura in a fourth, and even different symptom complexes in the same person at different times.

An antibody is a protein (an immunoglobulin) which is formed in response to an antigenic stimulus and is capable of combining specifically with the corresponding antigen. Antibodies are formed by specialized lymphocytes and plasma cells located in different compartments of the lymphoid system. The reagins responsible for asthma and other atopic sensitivities such as hay fever have been recently shown to belong to a distinct class of immunoglobulins known as IgE or γ_E. Increased amounts of IgE are found in most patients with allergic rhinitis and asthma. As stated earlier, IgE antibodies must be attached to a cell surface in order to cause its damage and thus trigger the allergic reactions.

Once sensitization is established, the antibodies may be widely distributed in the body. Nevertheless, certain "shock organs" show a greater degree of reactivity to contact with the antigen, presumably because of greater concentration of cells coated with reaginic antibodies in these areas. In bronchial asthma, reaginic antibodies are presumably heavily concentrated in the bronchial mucosa so that the bronchial tree becomes the shock organ. The reaction of the inhaled allergen with its specific antibody on the sensitized mast cells within the bronchial mucosa results in degranulation of these cells and the release of histamine and slow-reacting substance of anaphylaxis. Various kinins and serotonin and acetylcholine have been implicated as well. The mechanism by which the antigen-antibody reaction causes the release or activation of histamine is still not adequately elucidated, but it is presumed to occur by a series of enzymatic reactions. The consequences are dilatation of the blood vessels, excessive production of mucus, development of edema and contraction of smooth muscle. The lumina of the smaller bronchi become greatly narrowed by swelling of the mucosa and spasm of the bronchial muscle, and the secretion of thick, tenacious mucus by the bronchial glands further obstructs the bronchioli.

There are many allergens which cause bronchial asthma, the most important ones being inhaled pollens, mold spores, animal danders, feathers and common house dust. Recent evidence suggests that allergy to house dust may be due to the common household mite, of the *Dermatophagoides species,* which has been detected in most house dust samples, particularly in mattress dust. The occurrence of bronchial asthma during the spring and summer months suggests that a pollen or one of the mold spores may be the offending allergen. Attacks in the spring are usually due to tree pollens; grass pollens are usually responsible for attacks in the early part of the summner, and weed pollens for those occurring in the late summer. The occupational history may be important, for certain occupations involve exposure to particular allergens, such as enzymes in detergents. Practically any food may be a cause of asthma, particularly in children, and even drugs, such as morphine or aspirin, may precipitate attacks. Reaction may also occur to very unusual antigens, such as odors of cosmetic agents or hair spray. In addition, it is exceedingly important to realize that in most patients any irritant such as dust, smoke or drainage from an upper respiratory tract infection, physical agents such as extremes of temperature or exercise and even emotional upsets are capable of "triggering" an attack of bronchospasm in an already hyperirritable bronchial tree.

Psychic factors may precipitate attacks of bronchial asthma and also may influence the severity of symptoms, particularly in highly emotional persons with an underlying bronchial hypersensitivity. It has been suggested that an emotional crisis in a susceptible person induces hyperventilation, which in itself may precipitate an attack of bronchospasm. Heredity appears to play an important role in bronchial asthma. Although the hereditary background cannot be demonstrated in every case, allergic diseases tend to occur in certain families. The property that is inherited is probably not the specific allergy, but rather a tendency to develop a sensitivity to any of the antigens to which the person may become exposed and to which a normal person's immune system is tolerant.

Since most allergic reactions involve blood vessels and smooth muscle, which are innervated by the autonomic nervous system, some physicians have tended to incriminate these nerves in the pathogenesis of asthma. The vagus nerves carry efferent fibers which innervate the bronchial smooth muscle and possibly also the mucous glands of the bronchial passages. In the experimental animal, stimulation of the distal end of a cut vagus leads to bronchoconstriction and mucus production. Although it is tempting to postulate that the bronchospasm and excess mucus seen in asthma are the result of overactivity of these fibers, atropine has no significant therapeutic value in the human, whereas epinephrine and related sympathomimetic drugs are particularly effective. Nerves from the stellate and adjacent thoracic sympathetic ganglia contain fibers which are capable of influencing the bronchi, but various surgical procedures designed to resect the nerve supply to the bronchi have had little or no effect in patients with asthma.

Blockade of the β-adrenergic system in asthma has received prominence in recent years. It has been suggested that blockade of beta$_2$ subtype receptors may reduce cyclic AMP levels in bronchial smooth muscle and may foster bronchoconstriction. This theory provides an attractive unifying concept for the causation of asthma.

Chronic bronchitis may be associated with asthma, for recurrent bronchial infection is a common manifestation. As pointed out earlier, however, it is unlikely that asthma ever leads to the development of emphysema. Examination of the lungs of patients dying from status asthmaticus reveals massive air-trapping due to occlusion of bronchi and bronchioles by thick tenacious mucous plugs which contain shed mucosal epithelium arranged in whorls. There is a heavy infiltrate of eosinophilic granulocytes in bronchial and bronchiolar walls, up to the preterminal or terminal bronchioles. Bronchiolar muscle is prominent and the epithelial basement membrane is greatly thickened.

Clinical Manifestations.   Asthma is characterized by recurrent, paroxysmal attacks of difficult breathing, accompanied by wheezing, due to excessive turbulent resistance to airflow in the tracheobronchial tree, which may be seasonal or may occur at any time of the year. The attacks may be precipitated by direct exposure to a specific allergen, an unusual exertion, a sudden change in temperature, some emotional stress or infection of the upper or lower respiratory tract. The attack of breathlessness and wheezing may last for hours and often ends spontaneously. On the other hand, some patients may remain in a state of continuous respiratory distress for days, a condition known as "status asthmaticus."

Paroxysmal attacks of coughing due to diffuse bronchial obstruction are another frequent manifestation of asthma. Thick gelatinous mucus, produced by the glands in the bronchial wall, is frequently present but exceedingly difficult to expectorate.

A patient with uncomplicated asthma often has no symptoms between the paroxysms of wheezing. In about one-quarter of the cases beginning in childhood, the attacks may cease spontaneously after adolescence. A considerable number of patients, however, remain in a chronic state of mild asthma, with symptoms particularly noticeable during periods of exertion or emotional excitement.

The physical signs are characteristically those of partial airway obstruction. Since the lungs are frequently hyperinflated because of the airway obstruction, a hyperresonant note is obtained on percussion, and the breath sounds are distant. Expiration is prolonged and high-pitched rhonchi may be present throughout both lungs.

Radiologic Manifestations. There are no characteristic roentgenologic changes in the lungs in asthma. The bronchial markings may be more prominent and the lungs hyperinflated, just as in other cases of diffuse obstruction of the airways. The degree of overinflation is variable, depending on the severity of the airway obstruction. In contrast to the lack of peripheral vascularity noted in emphysema on the "full-chest tomogram," there is preservation of the normal caliber and tapering of the pulmonary vasculature; the pulmonary vessels extending to the periphery of the lung in asthma.

Functional Manifestations. Although a patient may appear to be clinically free of airway obstruction between attacks, an increased resistance to airflow is usually demonstrable as well as a nonuniform distribution of the inspired gas and a fall in lung compliance with increasing respiratory frequency. This may mean that mucous plugging of small airways is present even when the patient is relatively free of symptoms.

During an acute attack of asthma the airway resistance is markedly increased so that the $FEV_{1.0}$, maximal midexpiratory flow rate and maximal breathing capacity are all reduced. The volume of the vital capacity is also often considerably reduced, either because some bronchioles are completely obstructed or because of the marked overinflation. Frequently there is hypoxia present, but hypercapnia does not usually occur because there is compensatory hyperventilation of well-ventilated alveoli. When severe obstruction develops, extreme hypoxia and hypercapnia may be present; when this occurs in asthma it is indicative of a serious and grave situation.

CYSTIC FIBROSIS

Cystic fibrosis, a disease which is inherited as an autosomal recessive disorder, involves the exocrine glands of the body and is manifested clinically as a triad of chronic pulmonary disease with abnormally viscid secretions, pancreatic deficiency and high sweat electrolyte concentration. When it was first described in 1936 it was considered to be a rare fatal pancreatic disorder of small infants. Because of this early focus on the pancreas, several eponyms are used to describe the disorder, including *fibrocystic disease of the pancreas* and *mucoviscidosis.* However, the disease is not limited to the pancreas, and 90 per cent of the morbidity and mortality associated with the disease is due to involvement of the respiratory tract.

Cystic fibrosis is a frequent cause of chronic pulmonary disease in childhood. It occurs in approximately 1 out of 2000 live births in the Caucasian race, but is rare in the Negro, Eskimo, Indian and Asian populations. It has been estimated that from 3 to 6 per cent of the Caucasian populations are carriers (heterozygotes) of the gene. Although cystic fibrosis accounts for about 3 per cent of the post-mortem examinations performed in children's hospitals, improved treatment has resulted in a decreased mortality and many patients now reach adulthood.

Pathogenesis. Although the precise etiology of this disorder has not been elucidated, a generalized inborn error of metabolism, whose precise nature is not known, has been implicated. All of the clinical manifestations of the disease are a result of abnormal secretions of sweat glands, bronchial glands, mucosal glands of the small intestine, the pancreas and bile ducts of the liver. Four major theories have been proposed to explain the increased viscosity of secretions.

An increased fucose and decreased sialic acid concentration of the glycoprotein fraction of the secretions has been demonstrated. This glycoprotein abnormality is also seen in the fibroblasts and white blood cells cultured from patients with cystic fibrosis as well as heterozygotes.

An increase in parasympathomimetic activity at the neuroglandular junction has also been suggested. This seems logical, since exocrine secretions are controlled by the autonomic nervous system. Indeed, the sweat of patients with cystic fibrosis contains an increased concentration of acetylcholine. Furthermore, parasympathetic stimulation of the submaxillary gland of normal children results in abnormal secretions similar to those found in patients with cystic fibrosis.

A humoral abnormality has been implicated because serum from patients with cystic fibrosis has been found to disorganize ciliary activity of oyster gills. The serum factor which has been identified as a macroglobulin has also been found in low concentrations in the parents of children with cystic fibrosis.

A defect in ion transport (sodium reabsorption) has been demonstrated by micropuncture of sweat gland ducts of patients with cystic fibrosis. Saliva or sweat from cystic fibrosis patients will inhibit sodium reabsorption in rat parotid glands, presumably because of an as yet unidentified polypeptide.

SWEAT GLANDS. Although the sweat rate, the concentration of precursor solution produced in the coil of the sweat gland, and water reabsorption in the excretory duct are normal, reabsorption of sodium and chloride are diminished in patients with cystic fibrosis. As a result there is a high concentration of these electrolytes in sweat, and this forms the basis of the most reliable diagnostic test for this disease. The sweat chloride concentration is markedly elevated in 98 per cent of patients with cystic fibrosis and a concentration greater than 60 mEq./l. is considered to be diagnostic of this disease. The defect in reabsorption is also present in salivary glands.

RESPIRATORY TRACT. Pulmonary involvement occurs in over 98 per cent of cystic fibrosis patients, but the amount of disease is quite variable. At birth the bronchial gland size is normal, but bronchial gland hypertrophy and hypersecretion develop rapidly. Production of thick, tenacious mucus results in obstruction of small bronchi and bronchioles and impairment of the normal mucociliary clearing mechanism of the bronchial tree. Expiratory check-valve obstruction leads to overinflation of the lungs, and complete obstruction causes focal atelectasis. The stagnant mucus serves as an excellent culture media for bacteria, particularly *Staphylococcus aureus* and *Pseudomonas aeruginosa.* The resulting infection further increases mucus production and interferes with the clearance mechanism of the lung so that a vicious cycle is set up. Progression of the disease results in a chronic suppurative bronchitis with destruction of the normal ciliated epithelium and squamous metaplasia, with resultant cylindrical and saccular bronchiolectasis, peribronchial fibrosis, pneumonitis and multiple abscesses. With further progression there is often progressive respiratory failure with marked hypercapnia and hypoxemia and pulmonary hypertension which leads to right-sided heart failure.

The upper respiratory tract is frequently affected, and chronic sinusitis is usually present. Nasal polyps are found frequently and may appear as early as 3 years of age. Multiple, bilateral nasal polyps are found in 10 per cent of patients over 10 years of age.

PANCREAS. The pathological changes in the pancreas are variable, but 80 per cent of the patients with cystic fibrosis suffer from pancreatic insufficiency because of the secretion of a low volume, highly viscous fluid, whose enzyme content may be normal or nil, depending on the extent of pancreatic involvement. As a result, steatorrhea is present, and there is a failure to grow and develop normally. Even in the neonatal period the pancreas demonstrates increased fibrous stroma, mild dilation of acini, flattening of the lining cells and eosinophilic secretions and casts in acini and ducts. With time, replacement of the pancreas with fibrous and adipose tissue becomes more marked and cysts of dilated acini are seen. In the older patient involvement of the islets of Langerhans may be associated with the onset of diabetes mellitus.

INTESTINE. Involvement of the mucosal glands of the small intestine is one of the earliest lesions and occurs in about 10 per cent of newborn infants with cystic fibrosis. A homogeneous, acidophilic secretion accumulates within the mucous glands, and the meconium is tarry and extremely viscid. The commonest site of the obstruction is in the terminal ileum, and complications such as perforation, with meconium peritonitis, volvulus or secondary atresia may occur.

LIVER. The basic lesion in the liver is similar to that seen in the pancreas. Bile-containing mucous plugs produce focal obstructive lesions which result in cell atrophy, fatty metamorphosis, periportal fibrosis and proliferation of the bile ducts. Adjacent to the areas of proliferation are bile ducts with dilated obstructed lumens. Focal lesions of this nature are seen in about 20 per cent of cystic fibrosis patients at autopsy. In 5 per cent of patients there is more diffuse involvement leading to biliary cirrhosis, which is occasionally associated with portal hypertension.

Clinical Manifestations. As has already been mentioned, the clinical manifestations of this condition are variable and depend upon the degree of involvement of the various organ systems. Meconium ileus is the earliest manifestation of the disease and should be strongly suspected in the newborn infant who presents with abdominal distention and has not passed meconium within 12 hours after birth. A positive family history of cystic fibrosis is helpful in making the diagnosis.

After the newborn period most of the early manifestations of the disease are the result of pancreatic insufficiency or pulmonary involvement. Most infants have a good appetite, but weight gain and growth is poor. Typically, the abdomen is protuberant, and 3 to 5 bulky, foul smelling, often loose and pale stools are passed daily. Clinical evidence of deficiency of the fat-soluble vitamins A, D and E are unusual, but vitamin K deficiency, especially in early infancy, may cause easy bruising and bleeding secondary to hypoprothrombinemia.

Approximately 40 per cent of patients suffering from cystic fibrosis with manifest respiratory involvement are diagnosed before the age of 1 year. By 2 years of age, 75 per cent of children have respiratory tract involvement. The earliest pulmonary symptom is a dry, hacking cough which develops during the first few months of life. This usually progresses to frequent paroxysmal, coughing spells which are loose, deep and productive sounding. Fever is not a frequent manifestation, although acute febrile respiratory illnesses may initiate flareups of cough and phlegm.

In hot climates, the excessive loss of sodium and chloride in the sweat may lead to "heat stroke," and this may be the initial presentation. It is for this reason that additional salt intake must be given to patients with cystic fibrosis who live in hot climates.

Other symptoms and signs include tachypnea, easy fatiguability, decreased exercise tolerance, irritability and occasionally cyanosis during crying spells. Auscultatory findings may be normal in the early stages and may not be striking, even with advanced pulmonary disease. There may be prolonged expiration, localized or generalized rales, high-pitched rhonchi or areas of decreased breath sounds. With advanced pulmonary involvement the anteroposterior diameter of the chest is increased, and there is hyperresonance on percussion and diminished diaphragmatic movement. With severe involvement, pigeon breast, costal flaring and intercostal retractions, cyanosis at rest or during exercise, and severe clubbing of the fingers and toes may be present. A short stature and delayed skeletal maturation with thin extremities as well as decreased muscle mass and subcutaneous tissue may be evident. In the older child, delayed maturation and failure of the secondary sexual changes may be marked.

Radiologic Manifestations. The roentgenologic changes depend on the degree of involvement. In the small infant, the chest x-ray may only show some increased perihilar markings or scattered infiltrates associated with mild overinflation of the lung. If the child is over 1 year of age, however, signs of diffuse bronchial disease with abnormal densities radiating out from the hilum and along the blood vessels, as well as hyperinflation become more evident. Bronchi seen end-on show markedly thickened walls because of the inflammatory reaction in and around these structures. Rounded densities in the periphery represent secretions within airways, and lobular or lobar atelectasis may be present. Prominence of the pulmonary artery and enlargement of the heart reflects the onset of cor pulmonale.

Functional Manifestations. The earliest abnormalities in pulmonary function are an increase in residual volume and functional residual capacity and in airway resistance. The total lung capacity usually remains within normal limits so that the ratio of RV/TLC increases markedly. With progression of the disease the vital capacity decreases further, reflecting the presence of a restrictive component due to fibrosis, infiltration and congestion. The airway obstruction is manifest in a low $FEV_{1.0}$ and a decrease in the maximal midexpiratory flow rate.

There is gross mismatching of blood and gas within the lung as evidenced by an increase in the physiologic dead space, impaired gas distribution and an increase in the alveolar-arterial oxygen gradient. The ventilation-perfusion abnormality results in hypoxemia, and in severe disease there may be right-to-left shunting which is not corrected by breathing 100 per cent oxygen. With acute infection, the hypoxemia increases, and hypercapnia and a compensated respiratory acidosis develop. Progression of the disease can lead to severe pulmonary hypertension and congestive heart failure as a terminal event.

Chapter 14

Restrictive Lung Parenchymal Disease

As discussed in Chapter 8, the healthy lung remains sterile because of an efficient pulmonary clearance system which protects it against infection due to bacteria, viruses and other pathogens or the aspiration of foreign materials. Alteration of the mucociliary system or the cough reflex allows microorganisms which normally inhabit the healthy upper respiratory tract to enter the lower respiratory tract where they may propagate and invade the lung parenchyma. During acute or chronic infections of the upper respiratory tract, postnasal mucus or inflammatory exudate may be aspirated into the tracheobronchial tree and may cause obstruction of some of the smaller bronchi and bronchioles with resultant atelectasis. Infected material will produce an inflammatory reaction; sterile material may not.

In addition to infectious agents, aspiration of irritating substances can set up severe inflammatory reactions in the lung parenchyma. Thus, pneumonia may follow the aspiration of such substances as water or particulate matter in cases of drowning, vomitus in comatose or anesthetized patients, or regurgitated food in patients with esophageal obstruction. The inhalation of liquid lipid substances causes damage to the lung parenchyma and produces a "lipid" pneumonia. Until their manufacture was discontinued, the repeated instillation of oily nose drops was the commonest cause of this condition. The use of mineral oil for constipation, particularly if it is taken at bedtime, may also cause lipid pneumonia. The oily substance tends to adhere to the posterior pharyngeal wall and is aspirated into the lungs during sleep.

Accidental inhalation of irritating gases, such as nitrogen dioxide which may be present in silos or sulphur dioxide which occasionally occurs in underground mine explosions, may lead to an inflammatory reaction of the lung parenchyma. Severe, acute parenchymal inflammation can also develop following the inhalation of the fumes of such toxic substances as cadmium, beryllium and mercury. All these factors

339

lead to local conditions in the lung which favor the multiplication and spread of bacteria.

PULMONARY CONSOLIDATION

Consolidation, which implies that a portion of the normally soft, spongy lung parenchyma has become firm or solid, is the result of a pathologic process in which the air within the alveolar spaces has been replaced by cellular material. This is most commonly due to an inflammatory process, but it can also result from infiltration of the alveolar spaces by malignant cells. A consolidation may have a lobular distribution or may involve a pulmonary segment, part of one or more lobes, or the whole lung.

An inflammatory disease of the lung parenchyma is commonly referred to as "pneumonia" or "pneumonitis." However, these terms are not synonymous; "pneumonia" is often used to refer to the inflammatory diseases in which the etiologic agent can be identified, and "pneumonitis" is commonly applied to the nonspecific types of pulmonary inflammation in which the etiology cannot be ascertained.

A pneumonia may be primary when it is the presenting illness and may be due to viral, bacterial or mycoplasmal infection, or it may develop secondarily as a complication of a preceding nonrespiratory illness, in which case it is generally bacterial in origin.

Localized disease of the tracheobronchial tree often predisposes to infection and pneumonia. Thus, bronchial obstruction, such as occurs with bronchogenic carcinoma or bronchial adenoma, may lead to atelectasis, retention of secretions and infection. If a middle-aged or elderly person is subject to recurrent attacks of pneumonia and if the recurrence is in the same area of the lung or the pneumonia has an atypical course, the possibility of an underlying malignancy must be considered. In the young patient the possibility of an underlying bronchiectasis should be seriously considered.

It is now generally accepted that the majority of the acute pneumonias are viral in origin, but because the majority of these infections are mild, they frequently remain undiagnosed. Although bacterial pneumonias account for only approximately one-third of the acute infections of the lower respiratory tract, they are much more serious in nature and are, therefore, most frequently seen in the hospitals.

Bacterial pneumonia is often preceded by a viral infection of the respiratory tract. A viral infection apparently causes destruction of the ciliated epithelial cells lining the tracheobronchial tree and an increased production of mucus in these areas. These factors interfere with normal mucociliary clearance so that there is multiplication of bacteria in the lower respiratory tract, and a bacterial pneumonia may develop.

BACTERIAL AGENTS

GRAM-POSITIVE COCCI

The *Pneumococcus (Diplococcus pneumoniae)* is by far the most frequent and the most important of the bacterial agents capable of producing pneumonia. Pneumococcus infection results in an extensive consolidation of the lung parenchyma which involves the whole or part of a lobe and may be complicated by empyema, bacteremia or meningitis.

Staphylococcus aureus is most commonly responsible for a secondary pneumonia. It usually produces a lobular consolidation which tends to involve adjacent areas and frequently breaks down into a necrotic abscess which may spread to the pleura and produce an empyema, or a bronchopleural fistula and pyopneumothorax. Although still less frequent than pneumococcal pneumonia, the incidence of staphylococcal pneumonia has risen considerably in recent years. This is due to superinfection of patients suffering from viral pneumonia or who are being treated in hospitals for nonrespiratory conditions. Bacteremia is a serious complication, for it can result in widely disseminated metastatic abscesses, involving such organs as the brain, the liver, the bones and the kidneys.

Streptococcus pyogenes, once a very frequent cause of secondary pneumonia, is now relatively infrequent. This organism also tends to produce a lobular type of consolidation. It may be responsible for suppurative complications similar to those caused by the pneumococcus or for certain nonsuppurative complications, such as rheumatic fever and acute glomerulonephritis.

GRAM-NEGATIVE BACILLI

The incidence of pneumonia due to gram-negative bacilli is small in comparison with those produced by the gram-positive organisms. The *Klebsiella bacillus,* which is responsible for Friedländer's pneumonia, is the most common; others, in order of decreasing frequency, are *Aerobacter, Pseudomonas, Bacterioides, Proteus, Haemophilus* and *Achromobacter.* Pneumonias due to these organisms are most common in alcoholics or elderly, debilitated persons who are suffering from some chronic disease, such as diabetes. These pneumonias produce suppuration and destruction of lung parenchyma. A serious and often fatal complication is gram-negative bacteremia, which may result in an acute vascular collapse.

MYCOBACTERIAL AGENTS

The tubercle bacillus, *Mycobacterium tuberculosis,* which causes pulmonary tuberculosis, is a member of a group of acid-fast bacilli. The majority of the others are nonpathogenic and are common contaminants in nature, being found in sewage and tap water as well as in the gastric contents of humans. There is, however, a small heterogeneous group of acid-fast mycobacteria which are known as "atypical mycobacteria" and are capable of producing disease in man. It has been suggested that these atypical mycobacteria are saprophytes which have become pathogenic because of heavy colonization which has enabled them to invade tissue already affected by a disease process. In contrast to the *Mycobacterium tuberculosis,* atypical mycobacteria have never been shown to cause a contagious disease.

Of all the mycobacteria, the most common, most serious and most contagious disease is that produced by *Mycobacterium tuberculosis.* Tuberculosis in man can be produced by several strains of the *Mycobacterium tuberculosis,* but the human type is the commonest and most important cause. The bovine type, which is responsible for intra-abdominal and bone disease, has been fairly well eradicated, and the avian type is relatively uncommon.

Pulmonary Tuberculosis.   The initial, or primary, tuberculous infection results from the inhalation of mycobacteria into the respiratory tract, the result depending on the size of the infecting dose and the resistance of the patient. Invasion of pulmonary tissue by the tubercle bacillus produces a granulomatous reaction, resulting in a pneumonic consolidation with a lobular distribution. The infection spreads by way of the lymphatics to involve the draining lymph nodes in the hilum. In the majority of patients there is a mild, short-lived illness, which usually resolves by fibrosis and the deposition of calcium. The "primary lesion" or the "Ghon focus" develops approximately 6 weeks after the initial infection, coincident with the development of a positive skin reaction to tuberculin and occasionally with the occurrence of erythema nodosum. Organisms lodged in the subpleural areas may cause a serous pleural effusion within 12 months or longer after the initial infection. If there has been massive infection by virulent organisms, the disease process may erode into a pulmonary vessel so that caseous material is discharged into the blood stream and may result in miliary tuberculosis and tuberculous meningitis.

It has been suggested that there is a bacteremia between the initial infection and the development of the immune reaction and that when the immune response does take place, the organisms circulating in the blood stream are trapped in various organs of the body, where they may lie dormant for years. Later in life, these trapped organisms may propagate and produce tuberculous disease in such organs as the lung, kidney or bone.

The usual site of reactivation of the disease is in the apex of the lungs. This adult form of the disease is usually subacute or chronic and generally develops insidiously with a low-grade fever, slight cough and the expectoration of a scanty amount of mucoid sputum.

Cavitation commonly develops as the disease progresses with expectoration of purulent sputum, blood or blood-stained sputum. Frequently, the patient is awakened from his sleep by excessive sweating
which has soaked his nightclothes, the so-called "slumber sweats."

In the early stages of the disease, physical examination of the
lungs may reveal no abnormality, the disease only being apparent on
roentgenologic examination. In more extensive disease, the physical
signs are those of a consolidation, most commonly affecting the posterior segment of the upper lobe. Often there are rales, and occasionally there is bronchial breathing, especially if cavitation has taken
place.

Atypical Mycobacterial Infection.   The atypical mycobacteria
have been classified into four major groups on the basis of their speed
of growth and the color of their cultures.

The foremost group consists of the *photochromogens,* of which
the *Mycobacterium kansasii* has the greatest potential for disease
production in the human. The cultures of this group are characterized
by nonpigmented colonies which turn yellow when exposed to the
light.

The group II organisms, the *scotochromogens,* are a heterogeneous group consisting of many strains. Their colonies develop a yellow-
orange pigment when grown in the dark. These organisms are often
recovered from the sputum and gastric contents of healthy people
as well as from tap water.

The group III organisms, the *nonphotochromogens,* produce no
pigment whether grown in the dark or light. The Battey bacillus,
which is the most important member, is frequently isolated from
throat swabs of healthy people.

The group IV organisms, the *rapid growers,* also have no pigment
on culture but are characterized by the fact that their cultures grow
in a matter of days; the other atypical mycobacteria take weeks.

Both the *Mycobacterium kansasii* and *Mycobacterium Battey* are
capable of producing pulmonary disease which is indistinguishable
from that produced by the *Mycobacterium tuberculosis* by either the
clinical, radiologic or pathological examination, the differentiation
requiring cultural techniques. The group II organisms may occasionally be found in association with cervical adenitis or chronic
pulmonary diseases such as chronic bronchitis and bronchiectasis.
Clinical disease due to group IV organisms has not been reported.

MYCOPLASMA AND VIRAL AGENTS

MYCOPLASMAL INFECTION

Mycoplasma pneumoniae is the most frequent cause of non-
bacterial pneumonia in the civilian population. This organism shares

both viral and bacterial characteristics; its particle size is similar to that of viruses, but its enzyme systems are similar to those of bacteria. Mycoplasmal infection is usually endemic and occurs throughout the year.

VIRAL INFECTION

Despite considerable advances in techniques for the isolation of viruses, they are only identified in about 50 per cent of the non-bacterial pneumonias. Viral pneumonias due to *influenza A* and *B* are the most frequent cause of epidemics. Other viruses causing pneumonia are the respiratory syncytial virus, which has a pre-dilection for children, as well as advenoviruses 4 and 7 and parainfluenza 3.

Characteristically the radiologic opacities are much larger than indicated on clinical examination. The consolidation is usually lobular in distribution and may affect one or both lungs. Aside from epidemics in which a specific viral agent is identified, an etiological diagnosis in a sporadic case based on clinical grounds alone is virtually impossible.

PSITTACOSIS AGENT

Psittacosis is an infectious disease which may affect any member of the bird family and can be transmitted to humans. The responsible organism, which resembles a large virus but has characteristics similar to those of bacteria, is present in the excreta of birds suffering from this disease and is inhaled by humans. The human disease closely resembles the pneumonia which is produced by a viral infection. Constitutional symptoms with a high fever, generalized myalgia and severe headache predominate, and a dry, hacking, usually nonproductive cough is often present. Once again a lobular consolidation is more prominent radiologically than on clinical examination.

RICKETTSIAL AGENTS

Rickettsial microorganisms are intracellular parasites which are the size of bacteria and are readily visible by light microscopy. They are responsible for causing a variety of acute, self-limiting, infectious diseases, such as typhus, Rocky Mountain spotted fever and Q fever. Of these, Q fever is the only one commonly associated with a pneumonia, which is lobular in character, but it tends to be confined to a portion of a lobe. As in viral pneumonia, fever and constitutional symptoms predominate, mild respiratory symptoms only developing several days later.

FUNGAL AGENTS

Although much less frequent than other infectious agents, the possibility of fungal infection must be considered in any case of pneumonia which runs an atypical or complicated course. Fungi are most frequently secondary invaders of the lung, generally developing in association with some pre-existing bronchopulmonary disease, such as bronchiectasis, lung abscess and bronchogenic carcinoma. They are less frequently the primary and sole cause of the pulmonary lesion.

The prolonged use of antibiotics may alter the bacterial flora in the human body and allow fungi, which are normally unable to grow, to propagate and become invasive. This may also occur in patients who have altered immune mechanisms or have been treated for long periods with immunosuppresive drugs or corticosteroids.

Fungal pneumonias produce no characteristic symptoms or signs, but certain features may assist one in arriving at a possible etiological diagnosis. Some fungal infections, such as actimomycosis, moniliasis and cryptococcosis, are endogenous and occur in any part of the world with no regard to climate or the social status. All of the other fungal infections in man are exogenous and result from the inhalation of airborne spores. The majority of these organisms have been isolated from the soil; their prevalence is higher amongst certain occupations, such as farming.

Some fungal infections have a fixed geographic distribution. Coccidioidomycosis is found only in persons who have been in the arid deserts of the southwestern United States and northern Mexico. Histoplasmosis occurs in the valleys of great rivers, such as the Mississippi, the Ohio and the St. Lawrence rivers. North American blastomycosis is confined, as the name implies, to the North American continent.

A fungal pneumonia is generally characterized by necrosis and suppuration. It has been suggested that this is due to either the liberation of toxin by the fungi or hypersensitivity of the host to either the fungi or their breakdown products.

PROTOZOAL AGENTS

Toxoplasmosis is a disease caused by the protozoa *Toxoplasma gondii.* Serological studies have shown that infection by this organism is widespread among the general population throughout the world in a subclinical form. Pneumonia is a feature in the acquired disease in which the illness resembles that of virus pneumonia. In the congenital form of the disease, in which the fetus is infected by the diseased mother through the placenta, the central nervous system is chiefly affected.

"Interstitial plasma cell pneumonia" is caused by the protozoa *Pneumocystis carinii.* This organism produces extensive diffuse lobular opacities and affects chiefly debilitated and premature infants, but the infection also occurs in adults suffering from diseases of the reticuloendothelial system, such as Hodgkin's disease and lymphosarcoma, and particularly those being treated with cytotoxic agents, irradiation or corticosteroids.

CLINICAL MANIFESTATIONS

The symptoms of the pneumonias vary considerably, depending on the specific type present. Each has its own characteristic history and clinical course.

Pneumonococcal pneumonia is frequently preceded by an acute upper respiratory tract infection. The onset of the pneumonia is usually heralded by violent shaking chills which are followed by a rapidly mounting fever, a severe paroxysmal cough with expectoration of tenacious, rusty colored sputum, severe dyspnea and evident cyanosis.

In staphylococcal pneumonia, which is a very severe infection with a high mortality rate, the onset is usually gradual with a progressive, increasingly severe cough and purulent sputum, a high swinging temperature, shaking chills and often a pleuritic type of chest pain. In infants and children the disease is more acute and fulminating, and empyema is a common complication.

Primary streptococcal pneumonia is rare; it is more commonly seen as a secondary complication of a viral infection, such as influenza or measles. It usually begins insidiously, severe bronchitis being the prominent feature and empyema often developing at the height of the illness.

Pneumonia due to a gram-negative bacillus generally begins abruptly, without preceding upper respiratory symptoms. A high temperature, shaking chills and a severe cough, with the expectoration of thick, tenacious, jelly-like, purulent sputum which is frequently blood-stained are present. Because necrosis and abscesses are common complications, frank blood is frequently expectorated, particularly in pneumonias due to Klebsiella or Proteus.

Viral and mycoplasmal pneumonias present with strikingly similar clinical features. Constitutional symptoms predominate, and feverishness, generalized aches and pains and a severe headache are usually associated with a watery nasal discharge and a severe sore throat. This is then followed by substernal soreness due to acute tracheobronchitis, a paroxysmal cough and a scanty amount of mucoid sputum.

Although certain fungal diseases such as histoplasmosis and coccidioidomycosis may present as an acute pneumonia, the majority of the mycotic pneumonias usually develop in a more protracted form. Increasing fatigability, progressive weight loss, general malaise, profuse slumber sweats, cough and the expectoration of purulent sputum are all features of these diseases.

It is thus clear that certain general clinical features enable the examiner to distinguish whether an acute pneumonia is bacterial, viral or mycoplasmal in origin. Cough and purulent sputum at the onset of the disease are presenting features in a bacterial pneumonia. In viral and mycoplasmal pneumonia, cough is usually a late feature and is usually nonproductive. Sputum, when it does develop, is scanty and mucoid in character but may later become purulent because of secondary bacterial infection. Blood-stained sputum is also a feature of bacterial pneumonia but is extremely uncommon in viral pneumonia. In bacterial pneumonias, the administration of the appropriate antibiotic, i.e., one based on identification of the offending organism and its sensitivity, usually results in a prompt improvement in the patient's illness; however, a viral infection runs its course of fever for a period of 5 to 6 days before the temperature finally subsides by lysis despite the administration of antibiotics.

The abnormal physical findings in pneumonia depend upon the amount of parenchymal tissue involved and are naturally more distinctive when the consolidation involves a lobe than when patchy areas are involved. When there is lobar involvement, movement of the chest cage over the affected area is restricted, since the alveoli, which are filled with exudate, offer an increased resistance to distention. The trachea and the apex beat of the heart are not displaced because the volume of the alveoli is unaltered. Percussion over the affected area produces a high-pitched note because the ratio of solid tissue to air-containing tissue is increased. The lung parenchyma loses its "selective transmitter" property, and as a result, the high-frequency vibrations of breathing or the spoken voice are transmitted to the chest wall and overshadow the low frequency vibrations so that the breath sounds are bronchial. The voice sounds have a bleating, nasal quality, which is known as "egophony." In addition, whispering pectoriloquy is present. The whispered voice can be heard distinctly over the consolidated area.

A lobular consolidation may be difficult to detect on physical examination. The affected areas are patchy and scattered and usually and surrounded by healthy lung parenchyma so that the percussion note may still be resonant, and there may be no obvious diminution in chest movement. However, by careful auscultation, it may be possible to recognize localized areas of bronchial or bronchovesicular breath sounds, whispering pectoriloquy and end-inspiratory high-pitched rales.

Rales which are produced by cellular exudate in the alveolar spaces or bronchi are frequently present over a consolidated area of lung. They are generally high-pitched and tend to occur predominantly during the terminal phase of inspiration. The rales become more coarse and low-pitched during resolution of the consolidation. If secretions are present in the draining bronchi, rhonchi may become evident, and if the inflammatory process involves the visceral pleura, a pleural rub may be detected.

RADIOLOGIC MANIFESTATIONS

A consolidation appears radiologically as an opacification of the affected area of the lung. This may be evident in one or more segments of a lobe or it may involve several lobes. The important point to be noted is that the mediastinum occupies its normal midline position (Fig. 104).

If the pneumonia has a lobular distribution, the consolidated lobules may present as scattered, poorly outlined patchy opacities, although several of these may coalesce to involve a few segments or even an entire lobe. The shadows are irregular in shape, vary in size and frequently are seen in the lung bases. With resolution the radiologic opacities lose their homogeneity and become streaky and web-like, finally disappearing completely.

Occasionally, areas of translucency may develop within the radiologic opacities. Although these may be cavities, they actually may represent re-aeration of the consolidated lung tissue during the process of healing. Pneumatoceles are a common feature of acute staphylococcal pneumonia, particularly in young children. These air-con-

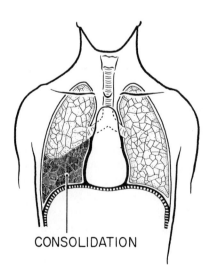

FIGURE 104. Consolidation of the right lower lobe.

CONSOLIDATION

taining cysts, which possess smooth, thin walls, are tension cavities caused by a check-valve obstruction.

Pneumonias caused by *E. coli,* Bacterioides and Pseudomonas usually produce patchy, lobular infiltrates involving the lower lobes, and are frequently associated with large empyemas. Pneumonias due to Proteus and the Klebsiella-Aerobacter group are usually associated with dense infiltrates involving the upper lobes, and empyema is an infrequent occurrence.

FUNCTIONAL MANIFESTATIONS

The degree of disturbance in pulmonary function that occurs in pneumonic consolidation depends on the extent of the disease process. There is an increase in the elastic resistance to distention, and therefore the vital capacity is reduced. Unless secretions are present in the airways, there is no increase in the nonelastic resistance, the $FEV_{1.0}$ and MMF remain essentially normal and the maximal breathing capacity is only slightly reduced. Because of the local alteration in elastic resistance, the distribution of inhaled air may be uneven. Hypoxia results because of continued perfusion of the consolidated nonventilated lung. The arterial carbon dioxide tension is frequently lower than normal because of the hyperpnea induced by the hypoxia.

PULMONARY ABSCESS AND CAVITATION

A pulmonary abscess is a collection of pus within the substance of the lung resulting from suppurative necrosis due to either bacteria or fungi. It must be distinguished from other collections of purulent material, such as bronchiectasis. Through long usage, a chronic tuberculous abscess is generally called a "cavity," but the term "abscess" is applied to a wide variety of suppurative diseases of the lung. However, there is no difference between the lung excavation which follows the discharge of tuberculous caseous material and that which follows the evacuation of purulent material of a suppurative pneumonia. Both are abscess cavities, the only difference being the etiologic agent.

A pulmonary abscess is not a distinct entity in itself, nor is it ever a primary condition. It is a pathologic process which develops during the course of any number of inflammatory conditions of the lung and is caused by a combination of suppuration and necrosis of lung tissue. The more chronic an abscess, the more thickened and putrid its contents. The abscess may rupture into a bronchus so that some or all of its contents are evacuated, depending on the size of the lumen of the involved bronchus.

PATHOGENESIS

A pulmonary abscess develops most commonly following aspiration of infected or foreign material, but it may also occur following obstruction of the bronchial tree, a primary suppurative pneumonia, an infected embolus, a pulmonary infarct, a congenital cyst or an emphysematous bulla.

In the normal course of events, the bronchial defenses are able to deal adequately with nasopharyngeal and oral secretions which may be aspirated into the trachea during sleep. During surgical anesthesia, the postoperative state, alcoholic stupor, traumatic shock or cerebral accidents with coma these defenses are seriously impaired. In addition, if the aspirated secretions are thick, tenacious, mucopurulent or contain clotted blood, the ciliary activity is impaired and the aspirated secretions may penetrate into the finer bronchioles, where they may produce a segmental atelectasis and an inflammatory reaction which may break down parenchymal tissue. The severity of the inflammatory reaction depends on the virulence of the infection and the resistance of the patient. Aspiration of a large quantity of irritant fluid, such as vomitus, usually results in a diffuse lobular pneumonia with multiple abscesses; whereas solid matter, such as a piece of a tooth, usually causes a localized abscess.

The site of development of an aspiration abscess depends on the force of gravity as well as the posture of the patient during aspiration. Aspirated material tends to lodge in the most dependent bronchus so that if the patient was lying on his back the superior segment of the lower lobe is usually involved. If he was lying on his side, the most likely site is the upper lobe, and if he was upright, such as during a dental extraction, the lower lobes are most likely to be affected.

An abscess cavity may occasionally develop within the substance of a pulmonary neoplasm, whether primary or secondary, and is most frequent in squamous carcinoma. This may be due to a deficient blood supply, leading to aseptic necrosis of the rapidly developing tumor tissue, retention of secretions, infection and suppuration beyond the obstruction, or hemorrhagic infarction following thrombosis of a pulmonary vessel in the region of the growth. In contrast to a pyogenic abscess, which is generally smooth and round, a malignant cavity characteristically has a thick wall with a shaggy, irregular appearance.

Abscess formation only rarely complicates primary pneumococcal and streptococcal pneumonias, except in infancy or debilitation, but occurs frequently in pneumonia caused by the staphylococci, Friedländer's bacilli, tubercle bacilli and certain fungal infections, such as blastomycosis.

As long as it is in communication with a patent bronchus, a pulmonary cavity always contains air, either alone or in association with fluid. The abscess is generally spherical in shape because of the pull of the surrounding healthy elastic lung parenchyma, much like the effect of stretching a thin elastic sheet in which small, irregular holes have been burned; when stretched taut, the irregularly shaped holes assume a perfectly round shape.

Occasionally a tension cavity may develop as a result of a check-valve obstruction with trapping of inspired air so that the cavity enlarges and the intracavity pressure becomes higher than atmospheric. Tension cavities can develop fairly rapidly over a period of weeks or even days. Elimination of the obstruction leads to their disappearance almost as quickly, with re-aeration of the compressed parenchyma surrounding the cavity.

Complete occlusion of an affected bronchus may lead to gradual absorption of air from an abscess cavity in a manner similar to that described in atelectasis. The rate of absorption depends on the permeability of the wall of the abscess as well as the amount of pulmonary blood flow in the surrounding parenchyma. If the wall is thin and the surrounding parenchyma little affected by disease, absorption of gas is rapid and complete so that the cavity collapses and resolves. If its wall is thick and fibrotic or has become calcified, it will not collapse because no absorption of air can take place.

CLINICAL MANIFESTATIONS

The symptoms and clinical course of a pulmonary abscess depend on the etiology and type of pre-existing pulmonary disease, the size and progression of the cavity and the presence of complications, such as empyema. Usually the clinical picture is dominated by the underlying pulmonary disease, the abscess frequently only being discovered by roentgenography.

A pulmonary abscess should be suspected if a febrile respiratory illness develops in a patient who has recently undergone a surgical procedure, particularly if it involved the mouth, nose or throat. This is also true of a patient who has been unconscious from any cause or who has had a sudden choking spell while swallowing food.

The onset may be sudden, accompanied by high fever and severe constitutional symptoms. Initially there is a nonproductive cough or expectoration of scanty, mucoid and odorless sputum. An associated pleuritis may cause a localized pleuritic pain over the corresponding area of the chest wall.

Rupture of an abscess into a bronchus frequently occurs about 10 to 14 days after the onset of the illness and is indicated by the sudden expectoration of a large quantity of purulent sputum. The sputum is green or brown, may be mixed with blood and often has a very offensive odor. Large quantities of purulent sputum continue to be expectorated daily, especially in association with sudden changes in position. The temperature frequently returns to normal levels, the constitutional symptoms disappear and a sense of well-being returns. If the abscess should persist, however, low-grade constitutional symptoms continue, and acute exacerbations alternate with periods of relatively good health.

The abnormal physical signs depend on the degree of the surrounding pneumonitis, the size of the abscess cavity, and its distance from the chest wall. Usually the findings are related to the suppurative pneumonia with the associated atelectasis and fibrosis. There is a shift of the mediastinum to the affected side, with restricted movement of the chest wall, an impaired percussion note, bronchial breath sounds of diminished intensity, and coarse rales during the second and third phases of inspiration over the affected area of the lung.

Distinctive signs may be present if an abscess cavity is large, comparatively empty of secretions, surrounded by a relatively narrow zone of consolidated parenchyma, and in communication with a patent bronchus. Under such circumstances, a particularly loud, hollow-sounding form of bronchial breathing, known as "amphoric breath sounds," can be detected. Most often, however, this type of breath sound is not heard and the breath sounds are diminished or absent because either the communicating bronchus is partially obstructed or the cavity is some distance from the chest wall.

Digital clubbing frequently occurs in the early stages of this disease and often progresses to hypertrophic pulmonary osteoarthropathy. This condition rapidly regresses when the abscess heals.

RADIOLOGIC MANIFESTATIONS

An abscess cavity can only be definitely diagnosed by roentgenologic examination of the chest. Lateral and oblique views, as well as the standard posteroanterior one, are usually required to localize its position. An abscess can generally be recognized by its radiotranslucent circular shadow; the thickness of its border depends on the extent of involvement of the surrounding parenchyma. The most definite diagnostic feature of an abscess is the presence of a fluid level within the confines of its cavity. Owing to the presence of air, the fluid level is recognized by a straight horizontal upper border which moves if the patient changes position. The radiologic opacity which is produced by the surrounding pneumonitis may be so dense as to obscure the abscess cavity on the standard film. Tomography will often demonstrate the abscess cavity under these circumstances.

FUNCTIONAL MANIFESTATIONS

Since an abscess cavity is essentially a localized process and the majority of the lung tissue is healthy, little disturbance in pulmonary function occurs. Nevertheless, if sufficient tissue is involved in the reparative process, then the elastic resistance to distention may be increased so that the vital capacity is reduced and the distribution of inspired air impaired. As a result of alterations of ventilation-perfusion ratios, minimal hypoxia may be present.

CYSTS OF THE LUNG

In cystic disease of the lungs, whether congenital or acquired, the continuity of the lung parenchyma is interrupted by thin-walled, sharply defined, open spaces which contain either fluid or air and often both. These may occur singly, or there may be many in one or both lungs. They vary in size from a space so small as to be barely visible to the naked eye to one that is so large that it occupies a whole lung. A solitary cyst may result from the coalescence of several smaller cysts. Multiple cysts may be confined to a segment, a lobe or an entire lung, or both lungs may be riddled with small cysts, giving the involved tissue a honeycombed or spongy appearance.

PATHOGENESIS

The pathogenesis of cystic disease of the lungs has been a matter of debate for many years, and the etiology is still in doubt. For many years, it was considered that the presence of epithelialization of the cyst wall, particularly by stratified columnar epithelium, pointed conclusively to a congenital origin. It is now known that this type of epithelium can be present on the wall of an acquired cyst and that the development of infection within a congenital cyst may destroy its epithelial lining. It is generally impossible, then, to determine the origin of cystic disease of the lungs unless the cysts are found in the lung of a fetus or a newborn infant.

CONGENITAL CYSTS

Congenital cystic disease is not as uncommon as was formerly thought, and a large number of cases are being diagnosed by surgical excision. They are frequently associated with other congenital abnormalities, and there appears to be a familial tendency. Although there is a difference of opinion as to the exact embryological fault which leads to congenital cystic disease, it is generally agreed that the cysts arise during fetal lung development by separation of a fragment from the main bronchial buds or their derivatives, the forerunners of the bronchi. If only one bronchial bud is involved, a solitary cyst is formed; if many bronchial buds are affected, multiple cysts develop.

The structure of the cyst walls varies considerably and may contain tissues resembling those of bronchi, bronchioles or alveoli. They may be lined with ciliated, columnar or cuboidal epithelium, and they may contain muscle fibers, elastic tissue and cartilage. The cyst may be filled with air or fluid which is usually clear and watery in consistency. Occasionally it may be viscid or purulent and foul-smelling if it has become infected. However, since the lungs are normally sterile, these cysts rarely become infected.

Occasionally, particularly in childhood, an air-filled cyst may enlarge if its cyst wall compresses the draining bronchus, and a check-valve type of obstruction occurs. Such a ballooning cyst may crowd the mediastinum and compress the opposite lung. Although this may produce dyspnea on exertion, symptoms are frequently completely absent until a complication such as a spontaneous pneumothorax or infection supervenes. Thus, the condition may remain undiagnosed unless a routine roentgenogram of the chest is carried out, or a complication has occurred.

BRONCHOPULMONARY SEQUESTRATION

Sequestration of a lobe or a bronchopulmonary segment which is frequently cystic and often becomes infected occurs in a lower lobe. This condition is characterized by its failure to communicate with the bronchial tree and also by its vascular supply which is derived from an aberrant artery from one of the branches of the aorta.

CYSTIC BRONCHIECTASIS

There is little doubt that the majority of cases of bronchiectasis, even those which develop soon after birth, are acquired. There is, however, a rare form, due to maldevelopment of the bronchi, which can simulate the acquired form of the disease, both clinically and radiologically. The origin of the congenital variety is similar to that of congenital cystic disease of the lungs, except that the bronchial sacculations probably develop from an outgrowth of bronchial tissue rather than from pinched-off bronchial buds.

ACQUIRED CYSTS

Blebs are collections of air which lie in the interlobular connective tissue just beneath the pleura. They are formed by ruptured alveoli, the escaped air tracking along the tissue planes of the lungs and finally becoming localized in the subpleural areas. The bleb may persist, or it may rupture through the visceral pleura, producing a spontaneous pneumothorax. On rare occasions, the air may track medially and rupture into the mediastinum. The actual cause of the alveolar rupture is unknown, although it has been suggested that it is caused by a localized check-valve bronchiolar obstruction which produces alveolar overdistention.

Bullae are air spaces within the lung parenchyma which are generally encountered in lungs severely affected by panlobular or centrilobular emphysema. They generally develop because of a check-valve bronchiolar obstruction, leading to alveolar overdistention and coalescence of several alveoli because of fragmentation of the interalveolar elastic tissue and subsequent rupture of the attentuated interalveolar septae. In emphysema there may be a single bulla or many which may or may not communicate with each other.

Pneumatocele, a fairly frequent complication of staphylococcal pneumonia in infants, is an acutely hyperinflated cavity deep within the substance of the lung parenchyma. It always contains air, but it may also contain inflammatory exudate. Its development is also associated with a check-valve obstruction in the bronchiole draining the inflamed lung parenchyma. A pneumatocele does not usually persist, and it often subsides spontaneously with resolution of the pneumonia.

Honeycombing is diffuse cystic involvement of the lungs. In "honeycomb lungs" the lung parenchyma is replaced by numerous thin-walled cysts which may affect a portion of lung, an entire lung or both lungs diffusely so that the lungs have the appearance of a sponge or a honeycomb. The cysts, which are approximately 1 cm. in diameter, possess thin walls and contain air; a few may contain small amounts of fluid. There is minimal inflammatory reaction in the surrounding lung parenchyma and connective tissue.

The pathogenesis of this condition is not clear. Although honeycomb lungs are rarely found in either embryos or infants, it has been suggested that a defect in development of the terminal elements of the bronchial tree results in a failure of alveolar formation and that isolated segments of small bronchi and bronchioles then grow out in the form of cysts. However, this kind of lesion is undoubtedly acquired as well and is seen particularly as an end-stage of generalized pulmonary fibrosis or with generalized systemic infiltrative diseases, such as the xanthomatoses, tuberous sclerosis and collagen diseases.

CLINICAL MANIFESTATIONS

Cysts usually produce no symptoms until some complication arises and are frequently only discovered during a routine roentgenologic examination of the chest. The symptoms depend on the amount of lung tissue that is replaced and the degree of pulmonary compression which occurs when the cysts expand in size.

If a cyst containing fluid is not in communication with the bronchial tree, there are generally no symptoms until it ruptures into a bronchus, at which time the patient generally coughs up varying amounts of mucoid material. In cystic bronchiectasis, hemoptysis occurs relatively frequently, even in the absence of any superimposed infection. Since the blood is derived from dilated bronchial arteries, the hemoptysis may be profuse.

In general, pulmonary cysts are difficult to detect on physical examination. Symptoms and signs may develop as a result of complications such as infection or pneumothorax. When either of these occur, the typical findings associated with the condition are then detected. A large tension cyst may produce signs which simulate those of a pneumothorax; therefore, it may not be possible to distinguish between these two conditions on clinical grounds.

RADIOLOGIC MANIFESTATIONS

Cystic disease of the lungs is usually diagnosed radiologically rather than clinically. The number and the size of the cysts, as well as the presence of air or fluid, can be determined by means of the standard posteroanterior and lateral views of the chest. A cyst which is filled with fluid appears as a round or oval opacity with a sharply defined border. An air-filled cyst is translucent, has a thin, sharply defined wall and occasionally shows a fluid level. An opaque cyst may become translucent, indicating that a bronchial communication has opened, or an air-filled cyst may become opaque, indicating that it has filled with fluid, which is generally of an inflammatory nature. An infected cyst is generally surrounded by a hazy opacity which is due to the associated pneumonitis, and because of this the outline of the cyst may be obscured. The cyst may progressively increase in size, indicating a check-valve type of obstruction. A tension cyst may become so large that it is impossible to distinguish from a pneumothorax.

Pneumatoceles or cysts superficially resemble pulmonary abscesses, but their walls are thin and the surrounding lung parenchyma is healthy. A distinguishing feature of a pneumatocele is that it often varies in size from day to day.

The presence of multiple diffuse small cysts, particularly if both lungs are involved, indicates the diagnosis of "honeycomb lung." If only a small area of lung is affected, particularly the upper lobe, it may be obscured by overlying healthy lung tissue so that the irregular mottled appearance may be mistaken for tuberculosis.

FUNCTIONAL MANIFESTATIONS

The disturbances in pulmonary function depend largely on the extent of the disease. A solitary cyst occupying little space usually causes no alteration in function. If multiple cysts are present, the distensibility may be reduced so that the vital capacity is diminished. No increase in nonelastic resistance occurs unless the airways are compressed or there is an associated bronchitis. Ventilation-perfusion ratios are usually altered so that hypoxia frequently occurs. Carbon dioxide retention does not usually develop, except in the later stages when alveolar hypoventilation and an increase in the work of breathing may occur.

PULMONARY FIBROSIS

The term fibrosis implies the presence of an excessive amount of connective tissue in the whole or part of an organ. It is a method of tissue repair which follows any disease process that produces inflammation or necrosis of lung tissue.

PATHOGENESIS

The deposition of excess fibrous tissue in the lungs is not indicative of any one disease but is usually a sequel to a variety of diseases. The distribution of the fibrous tissue in the lungs varies in different disease processes, and the resulting scar tissue may be confined to a small segment of lung parenchyma, a lobe, or a lung or may involve both lungs diffusely.

A localized fibrotic area of the lung is the commonest type of pulmonary fibrosis encountered clinically. This is the usual consequence of a localized area of tissue necrosis, such as may follow a suppurative pneumonitis, a pulmonary abscess or tuberculous caseation. A similar type of fibrosis may be produced by repeated irradiation of the lung, such as is administered after surgery for carcinoma of the breast, or inflammation and necrosis following the aspiration of irritating substances, such as vomitus, oily nose drops or liquid paraffin.

The generalized form of pulmonary fibrosis, in which both lungs are diffusely involved, usually follows either some widespread pulmonary infection or the inhalation of organic or inorganic irritating dusts or noxious fumes. Prolonged exposure to dusts containing minute particles of irritating inorganic chemicals such as silicon dioxide, silicates or asbestos frequently causes an extensive form of pulmonary fibrosis which is known as pneumoconiosis. The accidental inhalation of high concentrations of irritant gases such as mustard gas or ammonia produces a diffuse, bilateral inflammatory reaction, which also generally heals by fibrosis. Similarly, the inhalation of organic antigens may produce an allergic alveolitis and fibrosis. Extensive fibrosis may also develop in certain types of noncavitating granulomatous diseases, such as sarcoidosis, or in collagen diseases, such as scleroderma.

Parenchymal fibrosis occurs as a result of an allergic or an inflammatory process involving the lung parenchyma, so that its extent will vary. The inhalation of an organic dust antigen may produce bronchiolar and alveolar reactions of a Type 3, Arthus type, and the condition has been called "extrinsic allergic alveolitis." It is possible that this may be the mechanism underlying many cases of so-called "diffuse interstitial fibrosis." The exposure to a particular allergen such as the spores of the thermophilic actinomycete, *Micropolyspora faeni,* which probably causes farmer's lung, or the protein in pidgeon or budgerigar droppings, which probably causes bird-fancier's disease, may sensitize some persons to the specific allergen and produce precipitins against it. Classically, attacks of cough, dyspnea, fever, malaise, and generalized aches and pains begin hours after exposure to the specific allergen. In some patients who are exposed to smaller concentrations of allergen over a prolonged period, the disease may develop insidiously without the characteristic attacks. In these conditions, precipitating antibody in the presence of moderate antigen excess forms antigen-antibody aggregates to which the enzymatically activated $\beta_1 C$ component of complement is fixed. These are phagocytosed by neutrophil cells and destroyed, liberating lysosomal enzymes which, in turn, cause extracellular digestion and tissue damage.

Examination of lung biopsies in early cases demonstrates infiltration of the alveolar walls and peribronchiolar tissue, mainly with lymphocytes; mononuclear and plasma cells and epithelioid cell granulomata are seen later. Fibrotic changes occur in areas of inflammatory cellular infiltration, and organizing endobronchial exudates, bronchiolitis obliterans and acute vasculitis of the alveolar capillaries are also seen. Fibrinoid necrosis of the vessel walls with the formation of hyaline thrombi and hemorrhage results.

Fibrosis obliterates the alveolar spaces and is frequently associated with bronchiolar and interstitial fibrosis as well. In localized fibrosis the neighboring alveoli are frequently hyperinflated, or if the fibrosis is very extensive in one lung, the opposite normal lung may become hyperinflated.

CLINICAL MANIFESTATIONS

The severity of the symptoms which may be caused by pulmonary fibrosis are related not as much to the extent of the fibrosis as to the pattern of the distribution of the scar tissue. There may be no symptoms even when there is gross shrinkage of a lung in a case of long-standing localized pulmonary fibrosis. The primary symptom associated with fibrosis is dyspnea on exertion, the degree depending on the extent of the fibrosis. The dyspnea may be masked by other symptoms resulting from the pulmonary conditions which are frequently associated with fibrosis, such as bronchiectasis or bronchopneumonia.

As pointed out earlier, diffuse interstitial fibrosis may be the final result of repeated exposure to some organic allergenic dust so that a history of repeated attacks of fever, cough and dyspnea on exposure to a particular occupation may be elicited. The parenchymal type of fibrosing alveolitis often produces little in the way of abnormal physical signs except for bilateral basal rales.

When the fibrosis is localized, such as may be seen in the upper lobe following tuberculosis, the size of the affected lung is reduced. The trachea and the apex of the heart are shifted to that side, the chest wall over the diseased area is retracted, and its movement is restricted. The percussion note is dull or flat, depending on the degree of parenchymal involvement. The breath sounds are usually bronchovesicular, although they may be loud and bronchial in extensive fibrosis. Even in the absence of an underlying infective process, one can often hear rales or dry, interrupted, creaky sounds which extend throughout both the inspiratory and expiratory phases of respiration. These adventitious sounds, which are considered to be produced by the extension and retraction of the fibrous tissue, may be the only abnormal findings in an uncomplicated case of bilateral diffuse fibrosis of the parenchymal type.

If pulmonary hypertension develops, the degree of dyspnea increases. There is accentuation of the pulmonic second sound and evidence of right ventricular hypertrophy. Later, the manifestations of right-sided heart failure may become evident.

RADIOLOGIC MANIFESTATIONS

The radiologic appearance of the localized type of pulmonary fibrosis is usually that of an opacity with hard linear strands of fibrous tissue and crowded pulmonary vessels. An example of localized fibrosis involving the right lower lobe is illustrated in Figure 105. The walls of the bronchi may be visible as narrow, hard lines. The pleura overlying the fibrotic area may be thickened. Because the size of the lobe is decreased, the fissure which forms its boundary is usually displaced. The mediastinal structures are shifted to the affected side, and the ribs over the fibrotic area are drawn closer together. The diaphragm is elevated and often irregular because of pleural adhesions.

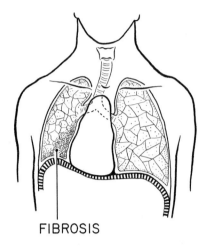

FIBROSIS

FIGURE 105.   Localized pulmonary fibrosis involving the right lower lobe.

In the diffuse form of parenchymal fibrosis, bilateral, coarse linear strands are visible throughout both lungs, and the mediastinum is not displaced from its midline position. In extrinsic allergic alveolitis, the upper lobes are predominantly involved, and in fibrosing alveolitis the lower lobes are predominantly affected. Multiple small, thin-walled cysts or honeycombing, which is a late manifestation of fibrosis, may be present throughout both lung fields.

FUNCTIONAL MANIFESTATIONS

The disturbances of pulmonary function in pulmonary fibrosis depend upon the extent of the fibrosis as well as the pattern of its distribution. Whenever there is fibrosis of the lung parenchyma or the pleura, the distensibility of the lung is diminished, and the vital capacity becomes reduced; the extent of the reduction depends upon the amount of fibrosis. There is usually no measurable increase in nonelastic resistance so that indices of airflow resistance are little altered. On the other hand, since there is considerable alteration of ventilation-perfusion ratios, the A-a Do_2 is elevated and the arterial Po_2 is low. Because of the increased ventilation induced by the hypoxia, the arterial carbon dioxide tension is frequently lower than normal.

HYALINE MEMBRANE DISEASE

Hyaline membrane disease (idiopathic respiratory distress syndrome) is a restrictive lung disorder in which the primary pattern is that of diffuse atelectasis, secondary to a deficiency of pulmonary surfactant. This disease principally affects the preterm infant (i.e., less than 37 weeks of gestation completed) and accounts for about 40 per cent of the deaths of these infants. It has been estimated that on the North American continent alone the disease causes some 30,000 deaths per year, and it is therefore not surprising that a great deal of investigation has been undertaken to elucidate its pathogenesis.

PATHOGENESIS

The disease is world-wide, affecting all races, and males more often than females. Aside from gestational age, a number of other situations appear to enhance the risk of developing hyaline membrane disease. These are: cesarian section, particularly when associated with a history of maternal hemorrhage; a diabetic mother; history of a previous child with respiratory distress; and signs of fetal or perinatal asphyxia. The second-born of twins is at greater risk than the first-born, perhaps because of this last factor.

The lungs in this disorder are known to contain a deficiency of the phospholipid which lines alveoli at the air-alveolar membrane interface, i.e., the alveolar lining layer or surfactant (see Chapter 1). Numerous theories explaining this deficiency have been proposed, but based on recent investigations, two theories seem to be most appealing. The first states that hyaline membrane disease is a consequence of immaturity, the alveolar type II cells responsible for surfactant production being immature and failing to produce sufficient surfactant to prevent atelectasis. The association of this disease with prematurity supports this hypothesis. The second postulate is that the disease is a result of an ischemic insult to the lungs either while the fetus is in utero or during the time of delivery. Since the fetal pulmonary vasculature is exquisitely sensitive to hypoxia and acidosis, it is believed that an asphyxial insult around the time of birth produces ischemia of the lungs, resulting in failure to produce sufficient surfactant for normal pulmonary function. This theory would explain the association between perinatal asphyxia and the high incidence of the disease.

Whatever the precise mechanism for the deficiency of surfactant, extracts of the lung of such infants studied in postmortem examinations exhibit an elevated surface tension. The elevation of surface tension of the alveolar lining layer in vivo would result in poor distention of the lung during inspiration and a marked propensity toward atelectasis during expiration. Indeed, the lungs at postmortem examination are completely atelectatic and resemble liver in their consistency and color (red-purple). On histological examination, atelectasis is interspersed with areas of overdistended terminal bronchioles and alveolar ducts, producing the so-called "Swiss cheese" appearance. Eosinophilic, refractile membranes, from whence the name of the disease is derived, line the aerated portions of lung. The hyaline ("glassy") membranes are now known to be derived from substances within the circulation and are not exogenous in origin. The membrane is not a unique feature of this disease, since it may be found in the lungs of patients dying from a number of other causes, including viral pneumonia and radiation pneumonitis. Indeed, a hyaline membrane is rarely present in those infants who live less than a few hours, a fact which supports the view that the cardinal feature of the disease is atelectasis secondary to surfactant deficiency.

CLINICAL MANIFESTATIONS

The high incidence of this disease in preterm infants and in those suffering from perinatal asphyxia has already been noted. Most infants who eventually die from this disease are in fair to poor condition from birth and have a low Apgar score at 1 minute of age (see Chapter 6).

The disease is characterized by the onset of respiratory difficulty at or within two hours of delivery. Tachypnea (i.e., a respiratory rate above 60 breaths per min.) is present in all patients. The respiratory rate is usually between 70 and 100 but may be as high as 120 breaths per min.

Since the chest wall of the preterm infant is very compliant, there is retraction of the chest cage. Intercostal and subcostal retractions may be mild to marked, depending on the severity of the disease. In severe disease, the lower portion of the sternum is markedly retracted during inspiration, and indeed the entire sternum may remain depressed during expiration so that the upper chest appears overinflated. The abdomen may protrude in a sort of "seesaw" pattern with respect to the chest during inspiration.

Because of the wide transmission of sounds, percussion of the chest is of little help in preterm infants, and auscultatory findings are variable. With mild disease the inspiratory breath sounds are harsh, and usually there are fine rales in the terminal phase of inspiration. With severe disease breath sounds may be markedly diminished or even absent. An expiratory grunt may be heard with the stethoscope, or it may be loud enough to be audible with the naked ear. Like purse-lipped breathing in emphysema patients, the grunt is believed to be beneficial, but in this case, it creates a positive pressure in the airways during expiration, thereby tending to prevent alveolar collapse and enhance gas exchange. The grunt often disappears with oxygen therapy.

TABLE 13

SOME CAUSES OF RESPIRATORY DISTRESS IN THE NEONATAL PERIOD

1. *Congenital Malformations*
    Choanal atresia
    Laryngeal webs or clefts
    Tracheal or bronchostenosis
    Cysts
        Bronchogenic
        Solitary or loculated in parenchyma
        Cystic adenomatoid malformation
    Lobar emphysema
    Hypoplasia or agenesis
    Accessory or sequestered lobes
    Tracheoesophageal fistula

2. *Trauma*
    Pneumothorax (spontaneous or iatrogenic)
    Phrenic nerve palsy (Erbs)
    Fractured clavicle or ribs

3. *Aspiration Syndromes*
    Aspirated meconium, squames, thick mucous from amniotic fluid,
        gastric contents
    Transient pharyngeal incoordination
    Vocal cord paralysis

4. *Immaturity*
    Hyaline membrane disease (idiopathic respiratory distress
        syndrome or IRDS)
    Pulmonary hemorrhage

5. *Disorders in Other Systems*
    Hypoventilation from CNS depression
    Airway compression from aberrant vessels
    Pulmonary edema

6. *Delayed Physiologic Adjustments at Birth*
    Transient tachypnea of newborn
    Persistent fetal circulatory pathways

7. *Toxic*
    Salicylates
    Reserpine
    NH_4Cl

8. *Infection*
    A. Transplacental
       Cytomegalic inclusion disease
       Rubella
       Coxsackie
       Syphilis
       Tuberculosis
       Toxoplasmosis
    B. Retrograde (intrauterine)
       E. coli, Staphylococcus, Streptococcus
    C. Postnatal (acquired)
       Chiefly gram-negative bacilli
       Pneumocystis carinii

363

The severely ill infant continues to grunt loudly, and deep retractions persist for several days. Cyanosis is always present in severe disease and progressive cyanosis despite oxygen therapy is a grave prognostic sign. During the second 24 hours of life respiratory failure may begin to be apparent, and the respiratory rate may fall with physical exhaustion of the baby. Irregular respirations may be followed by periods of apnea, bradycardia and ashen cyanosis. The infant may look pale and dusky with pooling of blood in dependent areas. Systemic hypotension and poor peripheral circulation are also features of severe disease. Although peripheral edema is often present in preterm infants, it is more severe in those with hyaline membrane disease. Death will occur if ventilatory assistance is not provided.

The mildly ill baby usually continues to have a rapid respiratory rate for 36 to 72 hours. Although cyanosis may not be recognized while breathing room air, arterial hypoxemia is present, and the baby requires moderately elevated inspired oxygen concentrations. A diuresis will frequently occur on the second or third day. The respiratory rate gradually slows, and the infants become more alert as they improve.

A variety of complications may alter the clinical picture and course of the disease. Severe hypoxemia may be associated with cerebral hemorrhage and the sudden onset of apnea. Preterm infants are subject to hypothermia, hypocalcemia and hyperbilirubinemia. Other complications may be the result of therapy, and these include fibrosis of the lungs or retrolental fibroplasia.

It should be pointed out that the clinical signs and course, which have been described, are not pathognomonic of this disease and that a wide variety of diseases may cause respiratory difficulty in the immediate neonatal period (Table 13).

RADIOLOGIC MANIFESTATIONS

The chest film is the single, most helpful diagnostic procedure used to differentiate various causes of respiratory distress in the newborn infant. In hyaline membrane disease the x-ray findings consist of uniform, minute reticulogranular densities distributed evenly throughout both lung fields. These minute opacities probably represent groups of atelectatic alveoli. Marked reticulogranularity or even solid lung fields are found in very severe disease, and this finding is associated with a poor prognosis. Air-filled bronchi may be seen in relief against the opacified peripheral areas, producing a so-called "air-bronchogram." The lateral view may show an increased convexity of the upper thorax and retraction of the lower sternum.

FUNCTIONAL MANIFESTATIONS

Despite uncertainty as to the precise etiology of hyaline membrane disease, a high surface tension of lung extracts and a relative deficiency of pulmonary surfactant has been well documented. The elevation in surface tension at the air-liquid interface in the lung results in an increase in the retractive force of the lung on deflation, leading to atelectasis. There is a decrease in lung compliance, functional residual capacity and vital capacity in association with a normal airway resistance, indicative of a restrictive lung disorder. The transpulmonary pressure required to produce a tidal volume is markedly increased, explaining the severe retractions of the very compliant chest wall. Tidal volume is decreased so that, despite the marked tachypnea, minute ventilation remains normal or slightly decreased. However, the mechanical alterations result in as much as a sixfold increase in the work of breathing and an associated increase in oxygen requirement and carbon dioxide production.

The pulmonary vascular resistance is markedly increased and the proportion of pulmonary blood flow which undergoes gas exchange in the alveoli is reduced. Marked ventilation-perfusion abnormalities are present; areas of lung are overventilated in relationship to their blood flow, and the physiologic dead space may be as much as 75 per cent to 80 per cent of the tidal volume; other areas of lung are underventilated in relation to their blood flow, resulting in arterial hypoxemia.

The true right-to-left shunt may be calculated to amount to as much as 70 per cent of the cardiac output in severe disease. About three-quarters of the calculated shunt is due to continued blood flow through areas of the lung which are not ventilated. It has been estimated that 20 per cent of the right-to-left shunt occurs through the foramen ovale, and about 5 per cent at the ductus arteriosus as a result of the elevated right atrial pressure due to increased pulmonary vascular resistance. This shunt increases for the first 36 to 48 hours in severe disease and then begins to decrease if the infant is going to recover.

Because of the marked ventilation-perfusion abnormality and right-to-left shunt, hypoxemia is always present and may not be reversed, even by the administration of high concentrations of oxygen. The severe hypoxemia interferes with aerobic metabolism, and there is a resultant accumulation of lactic acid so that a metabolic acidosis is found in this situation. As the disease worsens, respiratory failure occurs and is accompanied by a gradual rise in the arterial Pco_2. Analysis of the arterial blood will reveal a combined metabolic and respiratory acidosis.

The prognosis of this condition has been related to the severity of the arterial blood gas changes. It is relatively good in those infants who achieve an arterial oxygen tension of over 100 mm Hg. while breathing 100 per cent oxygen within 10 hours of birth; however, it is poor in those infants in whom the arterial oxygen tension does not rise to 100 mm Hg. while breathing 100 per cent oxygen and in whom the arterial pH is below 7.20.

Chapter 15

Pulmonary
Vascular Disease

The lungs are one of two organs of the body with a double supply of blood, the other being the liver. One blood supply comes from the right ventricle through the pulmonary circulation, the other from the left ventricle through the bronchial circulation. The major portion of the circulation of the lung comes from the pulmonary arteries to the pulmonary veins, the bronchial arteries normally carrying only about 1 per cent of the blood. Although anastomoses have been demonstrated between the bronchial and pulmonary arteries, these have never been shown to function in normal lungs. In diseased lungs, however, these anastomoses dilate and the bronchial arteries may contribute a considerable part of the pulmonary circulation.

THE PULMONARY CIRCULATION

ANATOMY

The pulmonary trunk and the large pulmonary arteries are elastic arteries whose media consist predominantly of elastic tissue; histologically, they resemble the aorta fairly closely. In each pulmonary artery the media is composed of smooth muscle fibers bounded by internal and external elastic laminae. These correspond to systemic vessels, such as the femoral and brachial arteries, but are very much smaller (0.1 to 1.0 mm. diameter) and have much thinner walls than the muscular arteries of the systemic circulation. The muscular pulmonary arteries lie close to the bronchioles, respiratory bronchioles and alveolar ducts. The walls of the pulmonary arterioles, the diameter of which is less than 0.1 mm. (100μ), consist of an endothelial lining, a single elastic lamina with no muscular or other media and virtually no adventitia. The structure of pulmonary venules is the same as the arterioles so that the pulmonary circulation does not contain any vessels corresponding to the muscular arterioles of the systemic circulation.

367

The pulmonary blood vessels derive their nerve supply from both the sympathetic and parasympathetic nervous systems, and afferent and efferent fibers of each system are present. The nerve supply is less abundant than that of systemic arteries and even of the bronchial arteries.

PULMONARY BLOOD VOLUME

The pulmonary circulation constitutes a distensible reservoir which is situated between the right and left ventricles. Normally about 10 per cent of the total circulating blood volume is in the lungs. About 30 per cent of the pulmonary blood volume is found in the arteries, 60 per cent in the veins and 10 per cent in the pulmonary capillaries. The resting pulmonary capillary blood volume has been estimated to vary between 75 and 100 ml., depending on the size of the lung. Although this seems small, the surface area of the capillaries necessary to contain this volume of blood is 70 square meters.

The distribution of blood between the pulmonary and systemic vascular beds varies normally with posture, the state of contraction of the smooth muscles of these beds, and other factors which influence the pressure difference between the thorax and the abdomen. The pulmonary capillary blood volume is increased in certain conditions, such as in congestive heart failure, and is reduced in others, such as in pulmonary fibrosis.

PULMONARY BLOOD PRESSURE AND FLOW

The perfusing blood pressure in the pulmonary blood vessels is less than 15 per cent of that in the peripheral circulation, and the drop in pressure from the main pulmonary artery to the left atrium is about 10 per cent of that between the aorta and the right atrium.

In a normal person who is breathing quietly, the systolic and diastolic pressures in the pulmonary artery are approximately 23 and 8 mm. Hg, the mean pressure being about 14 mm. Hg. Pulmonary blood flow has been shown to be pulsatile. In the basal state, the rate of pulmonary blood flow is very stable, averaging 3.0 liters per minute per square meter of body surface area. Pulmonary blood pressure, blood flow and blood volume are influenced by respiration, increasing during inspiration and decreasing during expiration. These changes are related chiefly to variations in the venous return to the right side of the heart; these variations in turn are associated with changes in the intrathoracic pressure. Not all the pulmonary capillaries are open at rest, and the pulmonary capillary blood volume has been estimated to increase by 60 to 90 ml. during exercise, presumably because of opening of previously closed capillaries.

During exercise the pulmonary arterial pressure does not rise appreciably until the blood flow increases three- to fourfold. Thus, the pulmonary arteriolar resistance falls during exercise.

As has been pointed out in Chapter 2, the pulmonary circulation may be influenced by several different factors. The major portion of the pulmonary vasculature is surrounded by a pressure which is less than atmospheric. The pulmonary arteries and veins are exposed to the pleural pressure, but the capillaries surrounding the alveoli are exposed to the alveolar pressure, which varies above and below atmospheric. As was pointed out earlier, the pulmonary blood flow in any part of the lung depends on the relationship between the arterial, capillary, venous and extravascular pressures as well as on the state of contraction of the vascular smooth muscles. Thus, the blood flow through the lung is lower at the apex than at the base when one is upright because of the effect of gravity. During exercise, blood flow at the apex of the lung increases more than at the base, although there is still a gradient down the lung. This greater increase at the apices probably accounts for the fall in physiologic dead space which normally occurs during exercise.

Hypoxemia due to respiratory disease or a reduction in the oxygen tension of the inspired air causes constriction of pulmonary blood vessels so that the resistance and the pressure in the pulmonary artery are raised. Vasoconstriction probably involves both the pre- and postcapillary vessels. It has been suggested that this effect is particularly important because it causes the blood to be shunted away from the poorly ventilated areas of the lung toward better ventilated regions.

Mild increases in the concentration of carbon dioxide in the inspired air do not appear to affect the pulmonary circulation in normal subjects. The inspiration of high concentrations of carbon dioxide increases the pulmonary vascular resistance, presumably because of the resultant acidemia. In patients with respiratory disease the presence of acidemia increases the pulmonary vascular resistance and pressure. The additive effects of hypoxia and acidemia can cause a marked increase in pulmonary vascular resistance, and this, of course, has important implications in the management of patients with severe cardiopulmonary insufficiency.

Certain pharmacologic preparations affect the pulmonary circulation. Epinephrine produces a transient vasoconstriction of the pulmonary arterioles as well as a slight rise in the pulmonary artery pressure. Histamine, norepinephrine and serotonin appear to be potent pulmonary vasoconstrictors as well. On the other hand, the injection of a small dose of acetylcholine into the pulmonary artery of a patient suffering from hypoxia and pulmonary hypertension causes a transient fall in the pulmonary artery pressure. The role of these substances in the development of pulmonary hypertension, however, is not clear.

THE BRONCHIAL CIRCULATION

In man, the bronchial arteries usually arise from either the proximal portion of the thoracic aorta or one of the first two intercostal arteries. Each lung possesses at least one bronchial artery. These vessels follow the course of the bronchial tree into the lung parenchyma, where they branch elaborately and rejoin to form plexuses around the bronchi and in the bronchial submucosa. The bronchial arteries are nutrient arteries which deliver oxygenated blood to the walls of the tracheobronchial tree and to the tissues of the pulmonary arteries and veins. The bronchial arteries supply the lower part of the trachea, the bronchi as far as the respiratory bronchioles, and the visceral pleura. By means of anastomoses with numerous other vessels, they also supply the vasa vasorum of the pulmonary artery and vein, the vagi and the mediastinal structures—particularly the pericardium—and the tracheobronchial lymph nodes.

In the healthy person, blood brought to the lungs via the bronchial arteries may follow one of two courses during its return to the heart. In the proximal part of the major bronchi, some of this blood is carried via the bronchial veins into the azygos veins and then to the right atrium. More distally, the venous drainage enters into the pulmonary veins. The pulmonary veins therefore normally carry small amounts of unoxygenated blood. Although there have been numerous attempts to measure the bronchial arterial blood flow, it is too small to be measured by the indirect techniques which have been utilized.

BRONCHOPULMONARY ANASTOMOSES

Extensive microscopic vascular connections at the capillary level and precapillary connections have been demonstrated between the pulmonary and the bronchial arterial systems in the normal lung. These shunts are located in the lobular subdivisions of the bronchopulmonary segments as well as in the pleura.

When the vascular capillary bed is reduced by disease, the pulmonary artery may become thickened and even thrombosed. The lumina of the peripheral bronchial arteries frequently enlarge, often reaching the size of the pulmonary artery at the same level. The most striking changes are found in bronchiectasis, in which the bronchial arteries usually form a dense plexus of thick-walled, large-lumened channels. Their anastomoses with the pulmonary artery which are situated distally in the walls of bronchiectatic sacs may have a diameter as large as 2 mm. These plexuses of collateral arterial vessels may become very extensive, and conspicuous dilatation of the bronchial veins often takes place in such conditions as pulmonary embolism with infarction, abscess of the lung, tuberculosis, primary tumors of the lung and certain forms of congenital heart disease.

The burden of this collateral circulation must fall on the left side of the heart, for the blood is brought to the lung from the aorta and then returned to the left atrium principally by means of the pulmonary veins. In other words, there is a shunt between the aorta and the left atrium. The added work load on the left side of the heart may lead to the development of left-sided heart failure, and it may also account for the left ventricular hypertrophy which is occasionally observed in cases of cor pulmonale. Conversely, blood shunted into the pulmonary arteries by way of these bronchial anastomotic channels tends to elevate the pressure within the lesser circulation, increasing the work of the right side of the heart and thereby predisposing to right-sided heart failure or cor pulmonale.

In patients with massive disease of one lung, there may be only slight desaturation of the systemic arterial blood. It has been postulated that the high pressure in the bronchial arterial system is propagated through bronchopulmonary anastomoses to the pulmonary circulation, thereby preventing the flow of unoxygenated pulmonary arterial blood into the diseased portions of the lung and diverting it to normal areas. In this way, a fairly normal oxygen saturation is maintained in the efferent pulmonary veins. The large arterial vessels containing blood under systemic pressure are often situated superficially within the lamina propria of the bronchi, so that any ulceration may easily rupture them; this may account for the pulmonary hemorrhages which occur in bronchiectasis or other chronic pulmonary diseases. The bleeding may be massive and may consist of obviously oxygenated, bright red blood.

PULMONARY HYPERTENSION

In a healthy person there is undoubtedly a large pulmonary vascular reserve because the pulmonary artery pressure does not rise appreciably during exercise until there is a greater than three- or fourfold increase in pulmonary blood flow. The total pulmonary vascular resistance decreases, most likely because of the opening up of new vessels, thereby increasing the size of the pulmonary vascular bed. When there is a greater than threefold increase in pulmonary blood flow, the pulmonary artery pressure rises almost proportionately with the increase in blood flow.

As a result of alterations in the pulmonary vascular bed, the resistance within the pulmonary vessels frequently increases, causing an elevation of the pulmonary artery pressure. When the systolic pulmonary blood pressure is above 30 mm. Hg and the diastolic pressure is above 15 mm. Hg, pulmonary hypertension exists. This may occur for a number of reasons, such as an appreciable elevation of the left atrial pressure, an increase in the pulmonary blood flow, obstruction or obliteration of the pulmonary vascular bed, or active pulmonary vasoconstriction. Except in the case of left-to-right cardiac shunts, in which the pressure in the pulmonary artery is elevated but the vascular resistance is normal, when pulmonary hypertension develops in respiratory disease the resistance to blood flow is nearly always increased.

The pulmonary vascular resistance is determined from the following formula:

$$\text{Resistance (R)} = \frac{\text{Pressure gradient}}{\text{Flow}}$$

$$\text{Thus, R} = \frac{\text{Pulmonary artery pressure} - \text{Left atrial pressure}}{\text{Pulmonary blood flow}}$$

This resistance is often expressed in units of force. Pressures in mm. Hg are converted to dynes per square meter; flows in liters per minute are converted to milliliters per second. The normal gradient between the pulmonary artery and the left atrium is about 8 to 12 mm. Hg, and the pulmonary vascular resistance is about 80 to 160 dynes/sec./sq. cm.

ELEVATION OF LEFT ATRIAL PRESSURE

Impairment of pulmonary circulatory outflow (i.e., elevation of left atrial pressure) due to an obstruction (e.g., stenosis of the mitral valve) or failure of the left ventricular pump will cause a rise in pressure behind the impediment. Left ventricular failure may be due to aortic valve disease, systemic hypertension, ischemic heart disease or cardiomyopathy. Although the raised pressure has certain advantages in terms of maintaining a higher level of flow across the obstruction than would otherwise be the case, this is bought at a price. As pulmonary venous pressure rises, the pulmonary capillary pressure may reach levels in excess of the plasma oncotic pressure (25 to 30 mm. Hg). Pulmonary interstitial edema may develop in the perivascular spaces and later in the alveolar septa, and if the transmural pressure is very high or lymphatic drainage inadequate, it may progress to alveolar edema. Time is a factor, and levels of pulmonary capillary pressure which may cause severe pulmonary edema in acute situations may be well tolerated in chronic cases. The difference in the two situations is probably related to the development of a more capacious and efficient lymphatic system in the latter case.

In pulmonary venous hypertension transudation will be maximal in the lower lung zones because the venous pressure is higher there, and lymphatic engorgement will also be seen in the lower zones. There is a redistribution of pulmonary blood flow, with more going to the upper zones so that the ratio of upper to lower zone flow in the erect position may be 1:1 or greater.

INCREASED PULMONARY BLOOD FLOW

When a large communication exists between the right and left ventricles, as in a ventricular septal defect, or between the aorta and the pulmonary artery, as in a patent ductus arteriosus, the pulmonary blood flow is increased. The left ventricular pressure (in the former situation) or the aortic systolic pressure (in the latter) is transmitted to the pulmonary arterial system so that pulmonary hypertension develops.

OBSTRUCTION OF THE PULMONARY VASCULATURE

The pulmonary vascular resistance rises if the caliber of the pulmonary vessels is decreased or the number of vessels is reduced. Acute obstruction of one pulmonary artery by means of an inflatable balloon produces variable results, although usually it produces only a transient rise in the pulmonary artery pressure. This suggests that the vascular bed of the opposite lung, to which the blood has been diverted, is expansile. This procedure has been used as a prognostic test before a pneumonectomy is performed; if the pressure rises, the surgeon can anticipate that the pulmonary artery pressure and right ventricular pressure will remain elevated.

In contrast to the experimental acute occlusion of a main pulmonary artery, acute occlusion of a pulmonary vessel by an embolus raises the pulmonary artery pressure. It has been suggested that this rise in pressure is caused by reflex vasoconstriction which is induced by occlusion of small pulmonary arteries but which does not occur when the main pulmonary arteries are obstructed. Another hypothesis is that the vasoconstriction is caused by the release of 5-hydroxytryptamine, or serotonin, from the blood clot.

OBLITERATION OF THE PULMONARY VASCULATURE

In such respiratory diseases as fibrosis, emphysema and kypho-scoliosis the pulmonary capillaries may be obliterated or compressed so that the effective bed available for perfusion is reduced and the pulmonary vascular resistance is elevated.

VASOCONSTRICTION OF THE PULMONARY VASCULATURE

Active vasoconstriction is probably associated with many of the forms of pulmonary hypertension which have been described. Most investigators believe that the pulmonary blood vessels possess tone and, therefore, that the tone can be altered. Hypoxia and often acidemia occur in most cases of respiratory insufficiency and are probably instrumental in causing vasoconstriction and pulmonary hypertension. A number of observers have suggested that the pulmonary vasoconstriction is mediated through the sympathetic fibers. The intense vasoconstriction after pulmonary embolism may be forestalled by a sympathectomy, an anatomic block or the use of adrenergic-blocking and ganglion-blocking agents. When pulmonary hypertension is present, the infusion of acetylcholine into the pulmonary circulation may produce a fall in the pulmonary artery pressure, suggesting active dilatation of the pulmonary vessels. The reversal of an elevated pulmonary vascular resistance complicating congenital heart disease or mitral valve disease which may follow successful surgery further suggests that a vasomotor element may be involved. It would seem that, provided the intimal changes have not progressed beyond a certain point, removal of the vasoconstrictor stimulus causes regression of the hypertrophy of the vascular walls.

PRIMARY PULMONARY HYPERTENSION

Primary pulmonary hypertension is a condition in which there is neither intrinsic cardiac nor pulmonary disease. An increase in vascular tone has been implicated, although it is possible that there have been multiple small pulmonary emboli. The incidence of this condition appears to be slightly greater in females, and the majority of cases are found to occur in persons between the ages of 20 and 40. The structural changes are confined mainly to the small pulmonary arterial branches and result in a progressive increase in pulmonary vascular resistance and pulmonary hypertension.

CLINICAL MANIFESTATIONS

The salient symptoms are those of exertional dyspnea and muscular weakness, both of which are probably related to a low cardiac output. Palpitation, exertional substernal and left-sided chest pain and syncopal attacks are present in about one-quarter of the cases. The syncope has been explained on the basis of acute elevations of the pulmonary vascular resistance so that the left ventricular output falls. Hemoptysis occurs occasionally; however, the mechanism of its production is not clear (but the possibility of pulmonary emboli must be considered). The terminal manifestations are characterized by the development of right-sided heart failure, and often there is a sudden demise.

The positive physical signs are usually limited to the heart and those organs which are affected by right ventricular failure. The second pulmonic sound is accentuated and fails to split during inspiration. There is evidence of right ventricular hypertrophy which is accompanied by distention of the neck veins, hepatomegaly and, later, peripheral edema.

RADIOLOGIC MANIFESTATIONS

An x-ray of the chest demonstrates the right ventricular hypertrophy—a bulging pulmonary artery segment and prominent hilar vessels. These findings are associated with normal or diminished intrapulmonary vascular markings.

FUNCTIONAL MANIFESTATIONS

Ventilatory function studies are all within normal limits. Ventilation-perfusion ratios are altered so that the A-a DO_2 is increased and mild hypoxemia may be present. Hemodynamic studies performed during cardiac catheterization reveal an elevated pulmonary artery pressure and an increased arteriovenous oxygen difference in the presence of a normal systemic blood pressure and a low cardiac output.

PULMONARY EMBOLISM AND INFARCTION

Pulmonary embolism and infarction are major circulatory emergencies. Unfortunately, they are often unsuspected clinically, frequently only being discovered at postmortem examination. Recently, however, it has become apparent that pulmonary embolism is one of the most important causes of morbidity and mortality, exceeding pneumonia in some centers.

PATHOGENESIS

Most pulmonary emboli originate as detached portions of venous thrombi located in the deep veins of the lower extremities. Occasionally, the thrombi may be in the right side of the heart, the veins of the pelvic area or the upper extremities. Nonthrombotic materials, such as amniotic fluid, fat, air, bone spicules and fragments of organs, comprise a very small percentage of pulmonary emboli.

Venous thrombosis and pulmonary embolism occur predominantly in bedridden patients. Contrary to previously held views, most cases occur in nonsurgical patients, cardiac disease with congestive heart failure being the most important single condition predisposing to venous thrombosis. The postoperative state is next in importance, especially that following abdominal or pelvic surgery in which there may be injury to the iliac veins. Pulmonary emboli are also common following operations of long duration or of such magnitude that there has been considerable injury to the tissues. Other factors which may predispose to venous thrombosis are trauma to the lower extremities, pregnancy, varicose veins, carcinoma, obesity, polycythemia vera and other blood diseases, particularly when any of these conditions are associated with prolonged bed rest.

The mechanism responsible for the intravascular formation of blood clots is poorly understood. The factors which facilitate the production of intravascular clotting are retardation of the venous circulation, damage to the vessel walls and conditions favoring the coagulation of blood. Venous stasis is promoted by the combination of immobilization, shallow breathing and hypotension. Thrombi may develop in the cardiac chambers, particularly if there is pooling of blood in the atrial appendage or damage to the endocardium. This situation develops when there is cardiac dilatation due to heart failure, myocardial infarction, atrial fibrillation or endocarditis.

Venous thrombosis occurs frequently in polycythemia vera as well as in other hematologic abnormalities such as sickle-cell anemia and the sickle state. The increase in blood viscosity in these conditions, combined with the mechanical consequences of an increased number of erythrocytes or the presence of sickled cells, predisposes to vascular stasis and thrombosis. Thrombosis in situ due to a primary alteration in the clotting mechanism has been produced experimentally in animals by the infusion of small quantities of certain serum factors, the only necessary adjuvant factor being venous stasis.

Once a clot fragment loses its anchorage in a peripheral vein or in the right atrium, it is swept rapidly into the pulmonary arteries. Very large thrombi do not progress beyond the larger arteries, but smaller emboli pass into the narrower lobar arteries of the lungs. Emboli lodge in the vessels of the lower lobes, particularly the right lower lobe, more frequently than the upper lobes. The posterior basal segments are most commonly involved, perhaps because these areas lie in the more direct axial stream of the pulmonary arteries.

Much has been learned from animal experimentation about the effects of pulmonary embolism. Embolization of the lungs with particulate matter invokes severe pulmonary hypertension, a fall in the systemic pressure, distention of the right cardiac chambers, engorgement of the peripheral veins and often death. It is probable that most of these effects are largely mechanical. Nevertheless, when the lungs of the animals are denervated at the height of the embolic reaction, the pulmonary hypertension gradually subsides, the left ventricular output increases and the animals survive, suggesting that embolization produces a widespread pulmonary vascular constriction, which is mediated through sympathetic impulses. The vascular constriction might also result from either the local or reflex effects of 5-hydroxytryptamine, or serotonin, which is known to provoke constriction of the pulmonary vasculature. It has been postulated that the serotonin liberated from platelets in the process of blood clotting produces reflex pulmonary vasoconstriction, with a resultant increase in the right ventricular pressure, bradycardia, hypotension and apnea.

PULMONARY INFARCTION

A pulmonary infarct may develop if the embolus is large enough to obstruct either a lobar or a lobular branch of the pulmonary arteries. It has been estimated that only about 25 per cent of pulmonary emboli result in infarction. It is less likely to occur when the lungs are healthy and apparently only develops when embolic obstruction of a pulmonary artery is attended simultaneously by some additional factor which retards blood flow through the lungs, such as passive congestion due to congestive heart failure, a previous pulmonary vascular obstruction and the hypostatic influences of posture. A pulmonary embolus is also more likely to lead to infarction of the lung if alveolar hypoventilation or an infection, such as pneumonia, is present.

A pulmonary infarct is usually sterile, and secondary infection is an uncommon feature. Rarely an abscess may develop from an infected embolus or from necrosis or infection secondarily of a bland infarct. Since this type of abscess extends to the pleura, empyema may be an added complication.

CLINICAL MANIFESTATIONS

The diagnosis of pulmonary embolism with or without infarction is based chiefly on the symptoms and only partly on abnormal physical signs. Pulmonary embolism should be suspected in every elderly bedridden patient who develops a chest pain which is either anginal or pleuritic in character, acute dyspnea, unexplained vascular collapse, syncope, unexplained fever, refractory congestive heart failure or edema of one of the lower extremities. A knowledge of the predisposing factors is of prime importance. In an average case, a slightly elevated temperature and a mild tachycardia for a few days prior to the event may be the only indications that a focus of phlebitis and venous thrombosis is developing.

Embolic occlusion of the main pulmonary arteries is usually rapidly fatal. The manifestations of smaller single or multiple thromboemboli or embolic episodes are exceedingly varied, and changing symptom patterns are frequent. Although most symptoms and signs of pulmonary embolism are manifest in the respiratory system, they may also be suggestive of a cardiac, neurological or intra-abdominal disease; in other instances, there may be no symptoms at all. When present, the symptoms may be short-lived or may persist for weeks, months or even years.

Pulmonary embolism most often presents itself with sudden chest pain which may be of two types: one which is due to pleural reaction over the site of the infarction and another severe one which is retrosternal and indistinguishable from the pain of myocardial ischemia. This second type of pain may be due to a fall in the coronary blood flow or to distention of the pulmonary artery. As a general rule, the pain is pleuritic, being exaggerated by deep breathing, and is most likely caused by pleuritis in the region of the infarct. Because most infarcts develop in the lower lobes of the lungs, the diaphragm may be involved in the pleuritis so that the pain may be referred to the neck and shoulder. There is usually an associated splinting of chest movement as well as difficulty in breathing. On rare occasions there may be severe upper abdominal pain and muscle guarding which may be due to irritation of the lateral portion of the diaphragm or distention of the liver capsule (if the pulmonary embolism has resulted in acute right-sided heart failure).

An irritating cough may develop on the second or third day following the infarction. Hemoptysis is present in only a few cases, but the sputum may be bloody during the early period of an infarction, and dark blood may be expectorated during the healing process.

Dyspnea often begins suddenly; it may be mild and hardly noticeable or progress rapidly to gasping respirations which may be out of

proportion to the amount of lung tissue involved. The difficult breathing has been attributed to many factors—notably bronchospasm,
immobility or diminished excursion of the diaphragm; atelectasis;
hypoxia; stimulation of receptors in the pulmonary artery, the right
side of the heart and the superior vena cava; and possibly increased
Hering-Breuer reflexes. The hyperpnea may be accentuated if fever
is present because this increases the rate of tissue oxidation. The
hyperpyrexia is related to the extent of the infarction and the development of a secondary pneumonitis as well as to the presence or absence of phlebitis.

Only a few cases demonstrate the classic syndrome of a pulmonary embolism, which has been described to consist of a sudden
pleuritic type of chest pain, dyspnea, hemoptysis and fever, with
signs of consolidation, a pleural rub and evident venous thrombosis.
In many subjects, pulmonary embolism is promptly followed by signs
of circulatory collapse, a rapid and feeble pulse and hypotension
because so little blood passes the blockade in the pulmonary circulation that the left ventricle does not fill adequately and the cardiac
output falls. This may result in manifestations of cerebral ischemia
such as restlessness, apprehension, syncope and coma. Occasionally,
a transient episode of unconsciousness is present, and in elderly
patients, hemiplegia and convulsive phenomena may be the chief
signs of pulmonary embolism.

The physical signs of pulmonary infarction are rarely distinctive,
and the physical examination is entirely negative more often than not.
Tenderness in the plantar veins of the foot or the muscles of the
calves is an early sign of venous thrombosis. Tenderness along the
course of the great veins along the inner aspect of the thighs, swollen
and tender inguinal lymph nodes and pitting edema are later de-
velopments. However, in many instances, embolism occurs in the
absence of any signs or symptoms of peripheral venous thrombosis.

In most instances the physical signs found are those due to pulmonary hypertension. Pulmonary hypertension and acute dilatation
of the right ventricle are indicated by the presence of a loud pulmonic second sound, with narrowing of the normal physiologic
splitting; prominent pulsation along the right border of the sternum;
and an increased presystolic pulsation or "a" wave of the jugular
venous pulse. An early systolic click may develop, and there is often
a short pulmonary ejection murmur. In late cases a murmur of pulmonary incompetence may be heard at the left sternal edge. Obstruction of the pulmonary vasculature by multiple pulmonary emboli
may recur over a long period of time so that right ventricular hypertrophy and heart failure develop gradually. The minute emboli themselves appear to be innocuous, and it is not until there are numerous

episodes of vascular obstruction that the function of the right ventricle deteriorates. When the right ventricle begins to fail a third heart sound may be heard at the lower sternal edge. Later tricuspid incompetence may develop so that a parasystolic murmur which increases during inspiration may be heard. Jugular venous distention is common, and in the late stages, the liver enlarges and peripheral edema develops.

When respiratory signs are present, they are similar to those found in association with pneumonia or atelectasis. Diminished chest expansion on the side of the lesion, dullness to percussion, diminished breath sounds or bronchial breathing, and rales are often present over the affected area so that a consolidation due to pneumonia may be suspected. A pleural friction rub may develop on the second or third day. If a pleural effusion develops, both the breath sounds and the vocal fremitus may be diminished. A localized exquisitely tender area at the site of chest pain is a valuable diagnostic sign. It occurs most frequently in association with a small peripheral pulmonary infarction and may be due to spasm of the intercostal muscles secondary to inflammation of the underlying pleura.

Tachycardia is observed in most patients. Arrhythmias are often present and may be responsible for the embolic episode in patients with heart failure. Paroxysmal cardiac arrhythmias, atrial fibrillation, atrial flutter and supraventricular tachycardia are possibly related to the stimulation of the autonomic nervous system which occurs in conjunction with pre-existing myocardial disease or as the result of the hypoxia and cardiac strain engendered by the embolus.

Very minimal icterus may occasionally be noted. It is presumed that the hemolysis of erythrocytes in the hemorrhagic lung infarct is the source of the increased serum bilirubin, although it has also been suggested that it may be related to hepatic dysfunction resulting from congestive heart failure.

RADIOLOGIC MANIFESTATIONS

The clinician relies too often on the presence of a radiologic opacity in order to diagnose pulmonary embolism, even though it appears in only a minority of cases. Nevertheless, the chest roentgenogram may offer some valuable clues. For instance, there may be accentuation of the hilar shadows and elevation of the diaphragm on the side of the embolus. Plate-like atelectasis may develop as a result of poor ventilation of the affected area. Occlusion of the larger branches of a pulmonary artery may occasionally be recognized by the abrupt termination and dilatation of a large pulmonary arterial shadow and a wedge of increased radiotranslucency which is most likely due to avascularity in the portion of the lung field beyond it. Pulmonary embolism is frequently accompanied by small pleural effusions which are often bilateral, but a large effusion, usually unilateral, is also common.

Angiographic examination of the pulmonary vasculature will confirm the dilated major pulmonary artery branches and may reveal complete obstruction of segmental or lobar branches of the pulmonary arteries or irregular filling defects which presumably represent adherent, retracted partially lyzed emboli or thrombi along the walls of the larger arteries. In some cases only retardation of blood flow to one or more segments may be demonstrated. A follow-up angiogram later often reveals complete disappearance of these findings.

The intravenous injection of macroaggregated human serum albumin with either I^{131} or Cr^{51} also permits evaluation of the lung perfusion. This technique demonstrates the distribution of the capillary perfusion of the lung and is particularly valuable in acutely ill patients.

It must be pointed out that if there is a parenchymal infiltration on the chest x-ray, one cannot say whether the decreased blood flow in the pulmonary arterial system demonstrated by radioactive techniques is due to an infarction or some other pulmonary disease. However, if the x-ray is clear, and particularly if there is an increased radiolucency, one should be highly suspicious of pulmonary thrombo-embolism. The simplicity of this technique makes it more readily available for the assessment of patients and permits serial determinations.

The radiologic appearance of a pulmonary infarction may at times suggest minimal or massive collapse of the lung. Although the opacity frequently has a conical shape, with its apex toward the hilum and its base toward the pleura, it may be irregular, round or oval.

Infarcts are commonly located at the costophrenic angles, and there they may produce a triangular shadow whose base is directed away from the hilum. Often it presents as a hazy clouding or streaking at one base or as a hump filling the costophrenic angle which may change to a well-defined consolidation. This clouding may be observed within the first 24 hours and may be mistaken for a pleural effusion. When the infarct resolves, it diminishes in size and takes on the appearance of a plate-like atelectasis. The disappearance of the infarct shadow may take from 5 days to 5 weeks. As pointed out above, pleural effusion is not uncommon, and small amounts of fluid may accumulate in one or both pleural cavities. Occasionally pulmonary embolism and infarction may result in a massive hemorrhagic effusion.

Pulmonary hypertension resulting from an embolism causes

dilatation of the main pulmonary arteries and the pulmonary artery trunk. Acute gross dilatation of the right atrium and ventricle is rarely seen radiographically, but an elevated systemic venous pressure may be recognized by dilatation of the superior vena cava and azygos vein. Repeated embolic episodes may lead to marked dilatation of the right ventricle and gross dilatation of the pulmonary artery trunk and hilar arteries, along with diminished vascularity in the lung fields.

FUNCTIONAL MANIFESTATIONS

As a result of occlusion of a branch of the pulmonary artery, alveoli may not be perfused although they may still be ventilated. The air leaving the alveoli has the composition of inspired air and therefore constitutes part of the physiologic dead space. It has been shown that there is bronchoconstriction of the airways supplying the area of lung whose blood supply has been cut off. There is therefore a shift of ventilation away from nonperfused areas, but this is not complete so that there is always some increase in dead-space-like ventilation. Although the mechanism of the bronchoconstriction has not been elucidated, it has been suggested that the regional bronchial constriction results from the low CO_2 concentration in affected segments, loss of surface active material in these segments and release of chemical substances, such as histamine or serotonin, from the thrombus. The increase in airway resistance following a pulmonary embolus can be reduced by intravenous heparin, and the peripheral airway constriction demonstrated after barium sulfate emboli can be reversed by intravenous isoproterenol.

Because the end-tidal gas originates from nonperfused alveoli as well as from well-ventilated and well-perfused alveoli, the mean alveolar carbon dioxide tension is less than that of the arterial blood. This difference in the carbon dioxide tension between the alveolar air and the arterial blood has been recommended by some investigators as a diagnostic test for pulmonary embolism, the extent of the difference largely depending on the size of the artery which has been occluded. However, it must be pointed out that mismatching of ventilation and perfusion for any reason will produce this difference in carbon dioxide tensions.

Hypoxemia, generally of moderate degree, is common following a pulmonary embolus, presumably because of the alteration in ventilation-perfusion ratios, although an increase in physiologic dead space (i.e., high V/Q ratios) per se should not cause a fall in arterial Po_2. Severe hypoxemia is not common, presumably because there is redistribution of blood away from poorly ventilated areas. On the other hand, an abnormally low oxygen tension in many patients suffering from pulmonary emboli, even while breathing 100 per cent oxygen, suggests that true venous admixture may be contributory. Whether this is due to an anatomic right-to-left shunt or perfusion of collapsed, nonventilated alveoli brought about by bronchoconstriction or severe restriction is not known. The oxygen tension falls following acetylcholine infusion, presumably because it causes dilatation of pulmonary vessels which were constricted by local hypoxia so that perfusion of poorly ventilated areas of lung is increased. Rarely, carbon dioxide retention due to alveolar hypoventilation may occur, probably because of either a marked increase in the physiologic dead space or an increased work of breathing.

In patients with multiple pulmonary emboli, the pulmonary vascular bed available for diffusion is reduced. Pathophysiologic correlations have suggested that nearly two-thirds of the pulmonary vascular bed must be obliterated before pulmonary hypertension results, but lesser degrees of mechanical obstruction may be associated with considerable functional pulmonary vasoconstriction so that the pulmonary vascular resistance is usually elevated in patients who have suffered from pulmonary emboli. As a result of the increase in pulmonary vascular resistance, pulmonary hypertension with right ventricular hypertrophy and, eventually, right ventricular failure develop.

PULMONARY ARTERIOVENOUS ANEURYSM

Arteries and veins develop out of a common embryonic capillary plexus so that opportunities are always present for persistent connections, even after birth. There are normally small arteriovenous communications of the vascular systems of most tissues, including the lungs. These communications probably serve as a means of adjustment to changes in the external and the internal environments. For instance, it is believed that such anastomoses in the skin of the fingers and toes play an important part in heat regulation. Their function in the lung is not clear, although it has been suggested that they may act as safety valves to protect the lung capillaries from excessive increases in blood pressure and blood perfusion.

Shunts between large blood vessels and between the chambers of the heart normally only exist during fetal life (see Chapter 6). After birth, the major causes of abnormal vascular shunts are trauma, infection and malignant tumors. In adult life, multiple arteriovenous and other intervascular connections may develop in the lungs in association with chronic infection, such as bronchiectasis.

Normally about 5 to 7 per cent of the total pulmonary blood flow does not become arterialized to the maximum extent and so it acts like venous admixture. In certain pathological conditions, a large volume of blood may be shunted from the pulmonary artery to the pulmonary vein, and considerable hypoxemia results. A pulmonary arteriovenous aneurysm provides an example of true venous admixture. This congenital lesion is a pulmonary manifestation of a generalized systemic vascular disorder, hereditary hemorrhagic telangiectasia, which is characterized by localized dilatations of small vessels forming telangiectases or angiomata that have a tendency to bleed. These tiny ruby lesions are generally seen on the face, the nasopharyngeal and buccal mucous membranes, the lips, the skin of the body and in the nail beds. The gastrointestinal, respiratory or genitourinary tracts and even the brain or spinal cord may be affected.

PATHOGENESIS

Approximately one-half of the patients who have a pulmonary arteriovenous aneurysm have telangiectases of the skin or mucous membranes, and more than one-third of patients with telangiectases have one or more similar lesions in the lungs. About 60 per cent have a family history of cutaneous telangiectasia. The cause of this inherited lesion remains unknown, but it is believed to be transmitted by a single dominant gene. Both sexes are affected and are able to transmit the disease, but females are more frequently involved. Occasionally, a generation may be skipped.

In most cases, the shunt takes place from a pulmonary artery to a pulmonary vein. One or more branches of the artery usually enter a loculated aneurysmal sac which is drained by a greatly enlarged and often tortuous vein. Veins from adjoining lobes may also drain the aneurysm, or it may be drained by completely anomalous veins.

It has been suggested that the vascular dilatation may be a manifestation of a generalized weakening of the ground substance in the vessel wall due to a defect of the normal hyaluronidase-inhibiting mechanism. Another suggestion is that the telangiectasis is produced by 5-hydroxytryptamine, which is normally detoxified in the lungs. According to the latter hypothesis, the 5-hydroxytryptamine escapes detoxification by bypassing the lungs via a pulmonary arteriovenous aneurysm. This postulate suggests, therefore, that the multiple telangiectases develop secondarily as a result of a primary pulmonary arteriovenous aneurysm, rather than vice versa.

CLINICAL MANIFESTATIONS

The pulmonary lesion is usually discovered during the third and fourth decades, although occasionally it has been found in children and even in the newborn. The disease may remain stationary for years, but frequently there is a definite tendency toward progression. There would appear to be two distinct clinical types: the type which is not associated with any clinical signs, and the type associated with the triad of cyanosis, polycythemia and clubbing of the fingers and toes.

If the shunt is small, there may be no noticeable clinical effects. When the shunt is large, the cardinal symptoms are due to the chronic hypoxemia caused by shunting of unoxygenated blood through the aneurysm. The principal symptoms are dyspnea on exertion, which may be slight at first but later progressively increases in severity; weakness; palpitations; and precordial pain. Neurologic complications are not uncommon; these may consist of headaches, vertigo, convulsions, syncope, paresthesias, diplopia, thick speech, and paresis as well as cerebrovascular accidents. The neurologic symptoms have been ascribed to a variety of causes, such as cerebral hypoxia and polycythemia, as well as telangiectasia in the brain with or without associated cerebral thrombosis.

Bleeding is a most important complication, the commonest type being epistaxis from telangiectatic lesions in the nasal mucous membranes. In addition, hemoptysis, hematuria, melena and cerebral hemorrhage may occur because of telangiectatic lesions in the tracheobronchial tree, genitourinary tract, gastrointestinal tract and central nervous system.

Cyanosis, clubbing and occasionally hypertrophic pulmonary osteoarthropathy are present, although cyanosis may be absent.

If the lesion is large, a murmur is often heard on the chest wall over the site. The murmur is limited to a well-circumscribed area on the chest wall which may be quite small and thus easily missed. It is usually continuous, having a systolic accentuation, becoming more intense during deep inspiration and often fading out during expiration. A thrill may also be present. If multiple small aneurysms are present, there may be no abnormal signs at all.

RADIOLOGIC MANIFESTATIONS

The lesions may be so small as to be barely discernible, but a large pulmonary arteriovenous aneurysm is often seen in a routine posteroanterior roentgenogram of the chest. Characteristically, it is a lobulated or spheroid opacity with smooth discrete margins and appears to be connected with the hilus by band-like linear or sinuous opacities, although the afferent and efferent vessels may not be visible. Any segment of either lung may be involved, although there appears to be a predilection for the lower lobes and the right middle lobe. In a few cases, the abnormal shadow may be hidden behind the heart. If multiple tiny lesions are present, no radiologic abnormality may be evident.

Pulsations in the lobulated density, as well as in the hilus, may occasionally be seen on fluoroscopic examination. The vascular nature of the lesion may be demonstrated by certain maneuvers, such as the Valsalva and Mueller tests. Although tomography can often give confirmative evidence, angiography is the most definitive and preferable procedure to establish the diagnosis, for it not only provides information about obvious radiologic lesions but also demonstrates small lesions which may not be seen on a standard roentgenogram.

FUNCTIONAL MANIFESTATIONS

A pulmonary arteriovenous aneurysm produces true venous admixture; some of the blood from the right ventricle returns to the left side of the heart without becoming oxygenated so that hypoxemia develops. Since the lungs themselves are normal and their ventilatory function usually is excellent, the hyperventilation induced by the hypoxemia results in hypocapnia. The presence of true venous admixture is confirmed by the failure of the partial pressure of oxygen in the arterial blood to rise above 500 mm. Hg when the patient inhales 100 per cent oxygen.

The cardiac output is nearly always normal, although it may be increased if the oxygen tension is very low. Erythropoiesis may be stimulated so that both the red blood cell mass and total blood volume are increased. In some cases, the number of erythrocytes may be normal, but anemia, probably due to the chronic or repeated hemorrhages, may be present.

PULMONARY EDEMA

Pulmonary edema is an excessive accumulation of serous or serosanguinous fluid in the alveoli, bronchioles and bronchi. It is remarkable that fluid does not normally accumulate in the lungs, since their structure offers little resistance to the passage of fluid from the capillaries. Ordinarily, in the systemic capillaries the osmotic force of 30 mm. Hg exerted by the proteins is neatly balanced by the intracapillary hydrostatic pressure of about 25 mm. Hg. Even in the most dependent lung capillaries, however, the hydrostatic pressure is only about 10 mm. Hg, so any water or saline introduced into the alveoli is rapidly absorbed. The capillary hydrostatic pressure is even lower in the apices of the lung, indicating a considerable margin of safety for the alveoli.

PATHOGENESIS

Concepts regarding the sequence of events in pulmonary edema have recently undergone considerable change. When capillary hydrostatic pressure is increased by rapid infusion of blood or dextran or when capillary permeability is increased following intravenous injection of Alloxan, fluid first appears in the perivascular interstitial connective tissue and only later appears in the alveolar sacs. Thus, in early pulmonary congestion there may be no fluid in the alveoli, and rales may be absent; later, as fluid enters the alveoli and bronchioles, rales may be apparent. The accumulation of fluid in the terminal respiratory tract leads to increased air-fluid interfaces so that inflation of the lung becomes more difficult. Thus, it has been demonstrated that the pressure required to produce airflow is greatest at the beginning of inspiration in patients suffering from orthopnea.

When edema fluid accumulates in the lungs, the factors responsible are essentially the same as those concerned in the formation of edema fluid elsewhere. These can be any one or a combination of the following: an increase in the capillary hydrostatic pressure, a diminution in the colloid osmotic pressure, an increase in the permeability of the capillary walls, a reduction in the mechanical pressure in the tissues and an interference with the flow of lymph.

INCREASED HYDROSTATIC PRESSURE

When the resistance to the outflow of blood from the lungs is increased, as in mitral stenosis, the level of the capillary hydrostatic pressure may rise above that of the colloid osmotic pressure. A pulmonary venous pressure of 20 mm. Hg is considered to be the upper limit of safety. If the pressure rises above this level, blood pumped into the lung by the right ventricle tends to accumulate behind the obstruction. At high intracapillary pressures, red blood cells are extravasated because of the rupture of capillaries, particularly in the dependent parts of the lungs. When fluid is extravasated at very rapid rates, the ability of the lymphatics to drain the fluid is exceeded, and large amounts of fluid may accumulate in the lung.

The precipitation of pulmonary edema by the intravenous infusion of saline, plasma or blood suggests that pulmonary edema may also be elicited by a sudden increase in the venous return to the lungs, which increases the capillary hydrostatic pressure. Conversely, acute pulmonary edema is often relieved by factors which reduce venous return, such as venesection, intermittent positive pressure or the application of tourniquets to the extremities.

Pulmonary edema may also occur after a traumatic injury to the skull, cerebral hemorrhage or an attack of encephalitis. The pathways are not understood, but it has been proposed that stimulation of the central nervous system induces systemic vasoconstriction through the sympathetic nerves, increasing not only the resistance to the ejection of blood from the left ventricle but also the peripheral venous tone. These act to augment both the pulmonary blood volume and the pulmonary capillary pressure, so that the capillary hydrostatic pressure rises and produces pulmonary edema.

DIMINISHED OSMOTIC PRESSURE

If the osmotic pressure is lowered, pulmonary edema may develop. The extravascular water content of the lung rises when there is a decrease in the colloid osmotic pressure of the plasma. A subacute form of pulmonary edema which is possibly due to reduced colloid osmotic pressure is seen in uremia, acute nephritis and polyarteritis nodosa. It is possible that the rapid infusion of intravenous fluid may also reduce the concentration of the proteins and so cause acute pulmonary edema.

INCREASED CAPILLARY PERMEABILITY

Edema may develop as a result of changes in the permeability of the capillary walls because of chemical, bacterial, thermal or mechanical agents. In addition, it has been shown that capillary dilatation per se favors the outward movement of fluid. As protein escapes into the tissues, the osmotic gradient across the capillary wall is reduced, and further edema is favored. In this situation, the fluid has the characteristics of an exudate, possessing a high protein content.

Hypoxia has been implicated as the most important factor leading to increased capillary permeability in the lungs. Pulmonary edema and pneumonia are frequently found together at postmortem examination. In this case, pulmonary capillary damage is probably produced not only by inflammation but by a local interference with oxygenation as well. It is likely that the pneumonia not only increases the rate of fluid entry into the alveoli but also decreases the rate of fluid resorption by the lymphatics.

The lungs are irritated by acid gases, such as chlorine and sulfur dioxide, and by certain oxides of nitrogen, such as ammonia and phosgene. The inhalation of water and nitric acid fumes or the ingestion of gasoline may also produce pulmonary irritation. The extent

to which such irritants damage the lungs depends upon their solubility in water. A highly soluble gas is readily taken out of the inspired air by the first moist tissue it reaches. The upper respiratory
tract may, therefore, bear the brunt of its action. On the other hand,
a gas with a low solubility is slower in its irritating effect, and the
most important damage usually occurs at the alveolar level. The
effects of gas inhalation may vary, therefore, from slight tracheobronchitis to fatal pulmonary edema.

REDUCED MECHANICAL
PRESSURE

Pulmonary edema may occur in a patient with severe airway
obstruction. During inspiration, the reduced intrapulmonary pressure
may exert a suction effect on the capillaries so that serum exudes into
the alveoli. In addition, the filling of the right side of the heart increases during inspiration, and the flow of blood from the left side
of the heart is hindered. This may result in a progressive accumulation of blood into the lungs and a consequent increase of the hydrostatic pressure in the capillaries. On the other hand, when obstruction
to both expiration and inspiration is present, pulmonary edema does
not develop, presumably because of the positive intra-alveolar pressure during expiration.

INTERFERENCE WITH
LYMPHATIC FLOW

Transuded protein and fluid from the pulmonary capillaries either
can be removed by the numerous lymphatic collecting ducts or
can move into the alveoli and bronchioli and then be expectorated.
Pulmonary edema occurs when the fluid escapes into the lung tissue
faster than it can be removed by the lymphatic system. Any factor
which decreases the resorption of lymph in the lungs or obstructs
the lymphatic channels favors the production of pulmonary edema.
Since the lymphatic vessels empty into systemic veins, an elevated
systemic venous pressure has an adverse effect on the resorption of
transuded lymph from the lungs.

As long as the patient with congestive heart failure is in the
erect position, the high intracapillary pressure in the areas of the
body below the heart protects the lungs, and edema fluid tends to
accumulate in the dependent parts of the body. When he lies down
at night, however, the edema fluid from the peripheral areas enters
the blood stream and increases the venous return to the lungs. As a
result, the pulmonary capillary pressure rises, and pulmonary edema

may develop. Additional factors which may be involved are an increased plasma volume and the increased capillary permeability due to hypoxemia which develops during sleep.

CLINICAL MANIFESTATIONS

By far the commonest form of pulmonary edema encountered clinically is associated with cardiac disease. In patients with hypertensive and arteriosclerotic heart disease or aortic valvular disease, left ventricular failure and paroxysmal attacks of dyspnea frequently occur. The mildest form of dyspneic attack is paroxysmal nocturnal dyspnea, an attack of severe dyspnea and cough which suddenly awakens the patient. Paroxysmal nocturnal dyspnea must be differentiated from the nocturnal attack of dyspnea which may develop in cases of chronic bronchitis. In contrast to the nocturnal dyspnea due to left ventricular failure which improves only after the patient gets up and walks around, the paroxysmal type of nocturnal dyspnea characteristically disappears after the expectoration of a plug of sputum in the patient with bronchitis.

Acute pulmonary edema may begin with terrifying suddenness, or it may develop gradually, starting as a mild form of paroxysmal nocturnal dyspnea with wheezing and then progressing to the full-blown clinical picture, which is characterized by extreme respiratory distress. The breathing is noisy with audible wheezes or gurgling sounds. The patient must sit up to breathe and suffers from a severe cough; the expectoration of frothy, pink-stained sputum may be so profuse that it pours from the nose as well as from the mouth. He may complain of intense precordial oppression or pain, and frequently he becomes panicky as the sense of impending suffocation grows more vivid.

The patient is cyanotic and often is in a cold sweat. Moist bubbling rales may be heard throughout both lungs. The blood pressure is usually elevated unless the patient is in shock, and tachycardia is a constant feature. Mild forms may subside spontaneously after a few minutes, but the attack may last for hours. It may end fatally during the first attack or during a subsequent episode. The chronic form of pulmonary edema may be insidious and often exists with such subtle clinical manifestations that it is easily misdiagnosed by the clinican as asthma or bronchitis.

Recently, pulmonary edema has become an increasing problem in patients with severe respiratory failure, particularly if associated with circulatory shock and acidemia. In many disease disorders, there is damage to the gas exchange membrane, altered alveolar cell function, alveolar collapse, increased capillary permeability and pulmonary edema.

RADIOLOGIC MANIFESTATIONS

Pulmonary edema manifests itself as a dense, fluffy opacity which spreads outward from the hilar areas into the lungs. The peripheral portions of the lungs remain clear so that a butterfly shape is produced. Because the alveoli are filled with fluid, the bronchi which traverse this portion of the edematous lung are revealed as radiotranslucent linear arborizations. The pulmonary vessels are enlarged and hazy in outline and the heart shadow is usually increased in size. The central localization of the edema fluid in the lungs has been attributed both to the relatively greater excursion of the peripheral parts of the lung, so that the removal of lymph and fluid from the periphery is enhanced, and to accessory lymphatic drainage via the pleural lymphatics in these peripheral areas. Another possibility is that the x-rays are penetrating through more tissue centrally than peripherally.

FUNCTIONAL MANIFESTATIONS

Even a very large elevation in mean pulmonary vascular pressure does not greatly affect the distensibility of the lung. When pulmonary edema develops, however, the compliance of the lungs falls considerably and the vital capacity is therefore reduced. As the pulmonary congestion increases, the residual volume falls correspondingly, probably because bubbles of edema fluid at the mouths of the alveoli hinder measurement of the residual volume actually present. When frank pulmonary edema develops, the resistance to airflow increases by approximately three to four times. Edema of the airways and free fluid in the tracheobronchial tree might account for this, although the high resistance found in the early part of inspiration and the late part of expiration suggests that surface tension may also play a part. Because of the increase in nonelastic resistance, the maximal midexpiratory flow rate and the maximal breathing capacity are reduced, and the work of breathing becomes exceptionally great.

In moderate degrees of pulmonary congestion and edema the arterial oxygen tension is usually only slightly lower than normal, but in severe edema it may be very low, presumably because of continued perfusion of areas of lung in which the alveoli are not ventilated because the bronchioles and alveoli are blocked by edema fluid, resulting in venous-admixture-like perfusion. In the "wet lung" syndrome adequate oxygenation may not be achieved even while inhaling 100 per cent oxygen. The arterial carbon dioxide tension is usually lower than normal, presumably because of hyperventilation of well-perfused alveoli which is induced by hypoxemia.

Chapter 16

Pleural Disease

ANATOMY

Normally, the pleural cavity is only a potential space formed by the visceral pleura, which covers the lungs, and the parietal pleura, which invests the inner surface of the thoracic cage. The pleura consists of a serous membrane which is lined on its free surface by a single layer of mesothelium. This layer rests on a subserous, areolar layer which attaches the pleura to the underlying structures. The subserous layer is important, not only because of the considerable elastic tissue which it contains, but also because of its rich network of blood vessels, lymphatics and nerve fibers.

The arterial blood supply of the visceral pleura is derived from the bronchial arteries; the venous return is via the pulmonary venous system. The arterial blood supply of the parietal pleura is derived principally from the intercostal and internal mammary arteries, and its venous return takes place through the corresponding veins. The lymphatics of the pleura are closely connected with those of the lungs and the thoracic cage.

The nerve supply of the visceral pleura is derived from the autonomic pulmonary plexus, but the parietal pleura is supplied by the intercostal nerves. Both contain sympathetic and parasympathetic fibers, and their efferent nerve endings lie near the surface of the pleura. Although the visceral layer is apparently completely devoid of pain fibers, the parietal layer is richly endowed with pain fibers which are derived from the intercostal nerves. Irritation of the parietal pleura produces an exquisitely sharp pain which may be accurately localized to the site of irritation.

Since the outer rim of the parietal layer of the diaphragmatic pleura receives its sensory supply from the lower six thoracic intercostal nerves, irritation of this area results in pain which is referred to the dermatomes of these nerves and is felt in the epigastric region or even in the lower abdomen. The central portion of the diaphragmatic parietal pleura receives its sensory supply from the phrenic nerves, which originate from the third, fourth and fifth cervical nerve roots; therefore, irritation of the central portion of the diaphragm produces pain which is referred to the neck and shoulder along the ridge of the trapezius muscle on the same side.

As has been described in Chapter 1, the pleural pressure is less than atmospheric. The fall in pleural pressure during inspiration produces a sucking effect on the superior and inferior venae cavae, thereby enhancing the venous return to the heart. The inspiratory descent of the diaphragm further assists the return of venous blood from the abdomen by raising the intra-abdominal pressure. Conversely, a rise in pleural pressure, such as occurs normally during a forced expiration or a coughing spell, impedes venous return to the heart. The lymph flow is similarly affected by the pleural pressure during inspiration and is moved from the abdominal cavity into the thoracic portion of the thoracic duct. Because of the valves in the thoracic duct, backward flow is prevented, and the lymph is squeezed into the subclavian vein during expiration.

PLEURAL EFFUSION

In a healthy person the layers of pleura are in close apposition to one another and are separated only by a thin collection of serous fluid, which acts as a lubricant and allows the two layers to slide easily over one another during respiration. The thin layer of lubricating serous fluid represents a balance between transudation from the pleural capillaries and reabsorption by venules and lymphatics in the visceral and parietal layers. An abnormal amount of fluid may accumulate if the venous pressure rises because of cardiac decompensation or pressure on the venae cavae by an intrathoracic tumor. In addition, hypoproteinemia may lead to a pleural effusion because of the low osmotic pressure in the capillary blood. In all of these situations the fluid is a thin, clear transudate with a protein content which is less than 3 per cent and a specific gravity which is less than 1.015. Only a few cells, chiefly lymphocytes, are seen microscopically. It does not clot on standing, and no organisms are grown if the fluid is cultured.

In contrast, a pleural exudate is more viscous, less translucent, and it clots on standing. Its protein content is greater than 3 per cent, and its specific gravity is higher than 1.015. This type of pleural fluid usually collects because the capillary walls are damaged by a disease process, such as pneumonia or tuberculosis, or because there is interference with lymphatic drainage, as with a neoplasm. If it is bacterial in origin, the offending organism can usually be identified. If the effusion is of a recent onset, many polymorphonuclear leukocytes are usually present; whereas, lymphocytes generally predominate if it has been present for some time. If the primary lesion is malignant, tumor cells and red blood cells are frequently demonstrated.

Except for a neoplasm of the pleura itself, a pleural effusion is always secondary to some lesion outside the pleura and may be inflammatory, noninflammatory, hemorrhagic, chylous or chyliform.

INFLAMMATORY PLEURAL EFFUSION

An effusion due to inflammation of the pleura is always secondary to an inflammatory process involving the lung, the mediastinum, the esophagus or the subdiaphragmatic space. In the early stage, there is a "dry" or fibrinous pleurisy (i.e., the inflamed pleural surfaces are covered with fibrin and leukocytes), but there is little increase in pleural fluid. As the lesion progresses, there is an increase in pleural fluid. This fluid is an exudate and possesses the characteristic features which have already been described. In the early stages, the pleural exudate is translucent, has a high fibrinogen content, and is usually described as "serous" or "serofibrinous." In the later stages it may become frankly purulent, more opaque and thicker in consistency as its content of polymorphonuclear cells increases.

EMPYEMA

Empyema, an effusion consisting entirely of pus, constitutes the final stage in the progression of an inflammatory exudate. It should be considered to be an abscess, in that thick, creamy, yellowgreen pus is generally confined by adhesions to a localized area of the pleural cavity. It is important to distinguish a purulent exudate from an empyema. In the former condition, the purulent material is mixed with serous fluid and generally lies free within the pleural space. It is only when the material consists of *pure* pus with no serous fluid that an empyema, or pyothorax, is said to be present. The thick, shaggy, fibrinous exudate which is laid down on both the parietal and visceral pleural surfaces as a result of the suppuration tends to localize the collection of pus.

An empyema is generally situated in the dependent part of the pleural space, usually in the lateral or posterior aspects. It also very frequently tends to localize in one of the fissures between the lobes of the lung.

Aside from an infected traumatic hemothorax or the extremely rare infection of the pleura by a blood-borne septic embolus, all cases of empyema are secondary to a suppurative process in one of the structures adjacent to the pleura, particularly the lungs. Most commonly it develops as a complication of a bacterial pneumonia, chiefly those caused by the pneumococcus *Streptococcus pyogenes* and the *Staphylococcus aureus.* Less frequent causes of empyema are septic infarcts, tuberculosis, a subdiaphragmatic abscess, an amebic abscess of the liver and mycotic infections.

The presence of an empyema should be suspected if a case of pneumonia is not progressing satisfactorily, particularly if fever and constitutional symptoms persist. In general, the clinical picture is one of sepsis associated with a loculated pleural effusion. A small collection of pus may be absorbed gradually, but it usually persists. If a large empyema remains untreated, septicemia frequently develops. Spontaneous evacuation of the pus may occur either by rupture through the lung into a bronchus or by extension through the thoracic wall (empyema necessitans).

A neglected empyema may have disastrous effects on the thoracic cage and its contents. The extensive inflammatory exudate rapidly becomes organized so that thick fibrous adhesions form between the two pleural surfaces. The retracted lung and the displaced mediastinum are anchored, and the overlying thoracic cage is retracted and immobile.

NONINFLAMMATORY PLEURAL EFFUSION

A noninflammatory pleural effusion is a clear, pale, straw-colored serous fluid which does not clot on standing; it is a transudate and is referred to as a "hydrothorax." Always associated with healthy pleurae, it usually develops in diseases in which there is either a diminished osmotic pressure of the blood or retention of sodium. It is, therefore, most commonly found in patients who are suffering from generalized edema secondary to diseases affecting the heart, kidneys or liver. In cardiac decompensation, as well as the nephrotic stage of chronic nephritis, the effusions are usually bilateral. For reasons which are not well understood, the hydrothorax may be unilateral, involving only the right side; even when it is bilateral, it is frequently predominantly right-sided. A unilateral transudate may also result when there is obstruction of the large intrathoracic veins by a neoplasm or enlarged mediastinal lymph nodes.

HEMORRHAGIC PLEURAL EFFUSION

If the fluid in the pleural space consists of frank blood, the condition is referred to as a "hemothorax." It is commonly caused by traumatic penetrating injuries of the chest wall and tearing of the intercostal arteries, but it may also occur spontaneously when a subpleural bleb ruptures or a pleural adhesion is torn. Rarely, it may occur as a result of rupture of an intrathoracic blood vessel, such as an aortic aneurysm. The intrapleural bleeding may be slow, continuing over many hours. The blood usually clots very slowly because of the defibrinating effect of the movements of the lung and the heart. If infection should intervene, however, clotting develops very rapidly.

Pleural fluid which consists of a mixture of serous fluid and blood so that it is pink or red is referred to as "serosanguinous." This type of effusion is most commonly seen following a pulmonary infarction. Other less frequent causes are a neoplasm—either primary (in the pleura) or metastatic (from a primary site elsewhere)—pulmonary tuberculosis, lymphomas and hemorrhagic disorders.

CHYLOUS PLEURAL EFFUSION

The presence of pure chyle in the pleural cavity is known as "chylothorax." This results from obstruction of either the thoracic duct and its tributaries or the left subclavian vein. It is most commonly caused by direct neoplastic invasion of the vessels or by the metastatic involvement of the mediastinal lymph nodes, both of which obstruct the thoracic duct and interfere with the normal flow of chyle. Traumatic rupture of the thoracic duct may result from a penetrating or a nonpenetrating wound of the chest wall. Spontaneous rupture may occur in infants on rare occasions. Although chylothorax occurs more commonly on the left side, it may be bilateral. Since the thoracic duct lies outside the pleural cavity, chyle tends to accumulate in the mediastinum before rupturing into the pleural space.

Chyle consists primarily of emulsified fats and is milky white and opalescent. On standing, a creamy supernatant layer develops. The fat content may be as high as 4 per cent, the fat globules staining easily with Sudan III. Clotting does not usually occur, nor does the fluid putrefy. Its specific gravity is greater than 1.012, and it contains a variable quantity of protein. The cellular content is primarily lymphocytic, and it is sterile on culture.

CHYLIFORM PLEURAL EFFUSION

The type of fluid which is also known as "pseudochyle" has the superficial appearance of chyle. No fat globules can be demonstrated, however, either microscopically or by staining with Sudan III. The milky appearance is due to the fatty degeneration of pus and endothelial cells and occurs in long-standing cases of encysted purulent effusions.

FIBROTHORAX

A fibrothorax is an accumulation of fibrous tissue within the pleural space, usually secondary to a prolonged pleural effusion of any kind, but particularly a hemothorax or an empyema. The fibrosed pleurae inevitably contract and reduce the size of the lung so that the diaphragm becomes elevated and fixed in position. Because of the reduction in lung size, the mediastinum is shifted to the affected side. Movement of the involved side becomes severely limited because of the thickened, fibrosed pleurae. As a result, only a small amount of air enters the underlying lung during breathing, and bronchial drainage is impaired so that chronic infection is a likely complication. Occasionally calcification may be associated with it.

CLINICAL MANIFESTATIONS

The degree of disability produced by a pleural effusion depends not so much on the amount of fluid that is present but on the rapidity of its development. If the fluid accumulates slowly, very little distress may be experienced despite the presence of a very large effusion. On the other hand, a rapidly developing effusion, especially if it is bilateral, may produce extreme respiratory distress.

The degree of breathlessness varies in different patients, but it is a predominant symptom in fibrothorax.

Chest pain can be present if the pleural effusion is associated with or follows a "dry" or fibrinous pleurisy. This pain varies in severity, ranging from a dull, aching discomfort to an excruciatingly severe, sharp, stabbing pain, which tends to restrict the depth of breathing. The characteristic feature of pleural pain is that it is aggravated by a deep inspiration or by coughing. The pain is generally localized to that part of the chest wall overlying the area of pleural inflammation. However, if the lower part of the pleural space or the peripheral area of the diaphragmatic pleura is involved, the pain may be referred to the lumbar region or the abdominal wall. Irritation of the central portion of the diaphragmatic pleura results in pain along the same side of the neck. Since the pain is caused by movement of the inflamed pleural surfaces over each other, it tends to disappear when the two pleural layers are separated by fluid.

Pleural inflammation frequently also causes a dry, nonproductive cough. If a bronchopleural fistula has developed from an empyema, attacks of paroxysmal coughing with the expectoration of considerable amounts of purulent sputum may be noted, particularly with a change in posture.

Depending on the underlying cause, the temperature may be either normal or considerably elevated. If the course of events is favorable, this should subside in a matter of days. The fever associated with an empyema may be continuous, remittent or intermittent and may be accompanied by violent shaking chills as well as slumber sweats. The patient usually feels miserable and has severe anorexia, vague abdominal discomfort, fatigability and progressive weight loss.

Because of its weight, the fluid tends to gravitate to the lowest recesses of the pleural space unless it is hindered by adhesions. The underlying lung is compressed, and its expansion is restricted during inspiration. Since the end-expiratory pressure in the opposite normal pleural space is more negative than that of the affected side, the mediastinum shifts away from the effusion. If the mediastinum is unable to move because of fibrous adhesions, however, the pressure in the affected pleural cavity rises even further, resulting in greater compression of the underlying lung.

The characteristic shift of the mediastinum to the unaffected side when there is a pleural effusion may not be present if there is an underlying atelectasis, such as often occurs with a bronchogenic carcinoma. The mediastinum retains its central position because the elevated pressure produced by the pleural effusion is counterbalanced by the lowered intrapleural pressure induced by the atelectasis.

Depending on the amount of fluid present, vocal fremitus is either diminished or absent, and the percussion note varies from dullness to flatness. When the patient is placed in a lateral decubitus position, free pleural fluid shifts to the most dependent part of the pleural space. No shift occurs if the collection of fluid is confined to a localized area by adhesions.

The breath sounds are usually reduced in intensity or are inaudible, depending on the amount of fluid present. Bronchovesicular breathing is a frequent finding at the upper level of a pleural effusion. Bronchial breath sounds and whispering pectoriloquy may be heard, however, if the layer of fluid is thin and overlies a compressed area of lung in the neighborhood of a patent bronchus.

In a patient with a fibrothorax, the slightly smaller hemithorax, retraction and narrowing of the interspaces and diminished movement are evident. The mediastinum is shifted toward the affected side. Vocal fremitus is diminished or absent, and depending on the degree of fibrothorax present, the percussion note is dull or flat, and breath sounds are distant or absent. Rales or rhonchi may be heard if there is an underlying bronchopulmonary infection.

RADIOLOGIC MANIFESTATIONS

Unless the amount is very small, a pleural effusion is readily distinguishable by the characteristic shadow it produces. This is

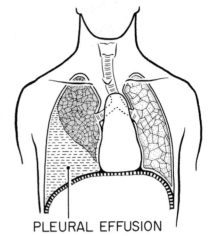

FIGURE 106. Right-sided pleural effusion.

PLEURAL EFFUSION

illustrated in Figure 106. The fluid casts a shadow which has the
same density as the heart. It appears as a dense homogeneous mass
occupying the lowest area of the chest, its upper border being hazy
and gradually blending into the lung above it. The costophrenic
angle is the first area to be obliterated. The upper border has a concave downward curve with the highest level in the axillary region.
The presence of air above the fluid can be implied if the upper level
of the fluid is straight and horizontal. If the air has not been introduced accidentally during an attempted aspiration, this finding indicates the presence of a bronchopleural fistula.

A shift of the mediastinum toward the normal side is usually
evident, and the degree of the shift depends on the amount of fluid
present. If no shift is demonstrable, it is likely that the mediastinum
has become fixed by adhesions or that an underlying atelectatic lobe
is present in association with the fluid. If the pleural effusion is
massive, the ribs may be widely separated and may have a more
horizontal configuration than they have normally.

If the quantity of fluid is small, it tends to collect in the costophrenic space and produces a shadow which is often difficult to distinguish from adhesions between the diaphragmatic and parietal
pleurae. Fluid occasionally accumulates between the lung and the
diaphragm, where it is called an infrapulmonary effusion, and this
may be overlooked. This difficulty can be overcome if an x-ray is
taken in the lateral decubitus position.

In a fibrothorax the opacity produced by the thickened pleura
may be as dense as that of a pleural effusion, and occasionally there
may be areas of calcification. It is distinguished from a pleural effu-

sion, however, in that the interspaces between the ribs are narrower, the mediastinal structures are shifted to the affected side, and the diaphragm is considerably elevated and fixed.

FUNCTIONAL MANIFESTATIONS

The degree of functional impairment depends on the size of the pleural effusion. As the fluid accumulates and the underlying lung becomes more compressed, the elastic resistance to distention increases. This is reflected by a reduction in the vital capacity. Unless secretions accumulate in the tracheobronchial tree or kinking of the bronchi occurs, the nonelastic resistance is frequently unimpaired, and the $FEV_{1.0}$ and MMF may be normal. The maximal breathing capacity is usually slightly reduced but not to the same extent as the vital capacity.

Because of lung compression, there may be local variations in the distensibility of the lung so that the distribution of inspired air is impaired. Venous-admixture-like perfusion may occur if the compressed lung continues to be perfused; hypoxemia may result, but there will be no carbon dioxide retention if the remainder of the alveoli are hyperventilated.

In patients with fibrothorax the vital capacity may be markedly reduced, but there is little increase in the resistance to airflow. Since ventilation is reduced in the affected lung, the ventilation-perfusion ratios are considerably altered, and hypoxemia and possibly some hypercapnia may develop.

ABSORPTION OF A PLEURAL EFFUSION

The absorption of a pleural effusion depends on the character and amount of fluid present as well as on the state of the pleurae. If the pleurae are healthy, as they usually are when a transudate is present, absorption is rapid once the initial cause of the effusion has been removed. Water, electrolytes and other diffusible substances are absorbed into the capillaries of the subserous areolar layer of the pleurae; protein and other particulate matter are carried away by the lymphatic channels.

Absorption becomes more complicated when an exudate is present, for it is considerably hindered by thickening and fibrosis of the pleurae. The fibrin in the fluid must first become liquefied and the obstructed lymphatics must again become patent before the fluid can be absorbed. If an empyema is present, no absorption whatsoever may take place.

PNEUMOTHORAX

The presence of gas in the pleural space is referred to as pneumothorax; for practical purposes, this gas is always the atmosphere. Air can enter the pleural space through a bronchopleural fistula, through an opening in the thoracic wall due to a traumatic injury, or it may be deliberately introduced through a needle for therapeutic or diagnostic reasons. Rarely, anaerobic organisms may produce gas within the pleural space when a putrefactive pulmonary abscess ruptures through the visceral pleura.

OPEN PNEUMOTHORAX

In this type of pneumothorax, there is a persistent communication between the pleural space and the atmosphere so that air can pass freely in and out of the pleural cavity. The most common cause is a traumatic injury of the chest wall which results in an external communication. A bronchopleural fistula, which is an internal communication between the pleural space and the tracheobronchial tree, also causes an open pneumothorax. Such a fistula may be produced by any condition which causes destruction of alveolar walls and visceral pleura. It can therefore occur in inflammatory disease of the lung, such as tuberculosis; malignant disease, such as bronchogenic carcinoma; vascular disease, such as a pulmonary infarction; loss of lung elasticity, as in emphysema; or rupture of a bronchial stump following operative removal of a lung or a portion of a lung.

An open pneumothorax, particularly if it is caused by a traumatic injury to the chest wall, presents a serious problem. Because of the free communication between the pleural cavity and the atmosphere, the pleural pressure on the affected side is equal to that of the atmosphere. Since the elastic forces of both the chest wall and the lung are now unopposed, the chest cage enlarges while the affected lung collapses. If the mediastinum is mobile and is not bound by fibrous adhesions, it will move to the unaffected side where the pressure is lower and thus will produce varying degrees of compression of the opposite lung. During inspiration, contraction of the respiratory muscles lowers the pleural pressure on the unaffected side. The pressure on the affected side may also fall slightly and some air may enter through the opening in the chest wall and cause a further shift of the mediastinum toward the unaffected side. During inspiration, the pressure in the pleural space on the affected side usually rises above that of the atmosphere, and air escapes from the pleural space. The mediastinum may then move back toward its original position. This is illustrated in Figure 107, which also shows that

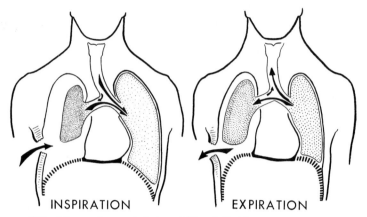

INSPIRATION   EXPIRATION

FIGURE 107.   The mediastinal shift and "Pendelluft" in an open pneumothorax.

some of the air expired from the normal lung may enter the collapsed lung, causing it to expand slightly. During the next inspiration, this "rebreathed air" may again be inspired into the normal lung. This paradoxical movement of air, or "Pendelluft," and the recurrent swing of the mediastinum, or "flutter," can be a serious menace to the patient's life.

CLOSED PNEUMOTHORAX

A closed pneumothorax implies that the air in the pleural cavity is not in communication with the atmosphere. This condition occurs after the rupture of a subpleural bleb, the tear in the visceral pleura having been sealed off, or after the induction of an artificial pneumothorax. Once a pneumothorax becomes established, the gas is usually uniformly distributed, and the pleural pressure is then essentially the same throughout the pleural cavity. If the pleura is diseased, however, adhesions may prevent the uniform distribution of the gas so that it remains localized in one or several areas.

A closed pneumothorax may be spontaneous, traumatic, therapeutic or diagnostic.

SPONTANEOUS PNEUMOTHORAX

A pneumothorax which develops suddenly in a person, with or without obvious underlying pulmonary disease, is usually referred to as a "spontaneous pneumothorax." The patient may have been free of respiratory symptoms and may have had no apparent clinical or radiologic evidence of an underlying pulmonary lesion. A spontaneous pneumothorax occurs predominantly in young people, particularly males, who are between 15 and 35 years of age. Although the right lung is most commonly affected, it is not unusual for recurrent attacks to affect either one or both lungs.

Since the healthy pleura is impervious to air, it is obvious that these apparently idiopathic cases of pneumothorax can only be secondary to a rent in the pleura and that this must be produced by some pathological process. Rupture of a subpleural bleb or bulla is the cause of spontaneous pneumothorax in approximately 85 per cent of the cases. The remaining 15 per cent are produced by rupture of a tuberculous or pyogenic subpleural abscess, a tear in the esophagus during esophagoscopy, or erosion of the esophageal wall by a malignant process.

Subpleural blebs may be congenital, but more frequently they are found in association with scar formation which is due to some inflammatory disease, such as tuberculosis. In such cases, no symptoms are evident until the rupture of the bleb takes place. Subpleural blebs may also be found in association with other pulmonary diseases, such as asthma, bronchiectasis, emphysema and the pneumoconioses. Under these circumstances, the symptoms preceding the event are those of the particular disease.

It has been suggested that a bleb may rupture because of a sudden increase in the intrathoracic pressure, such as may occur during an unusual exertion, coughing or sneezing. It is more likely that the rupture results from the repeated deep inspirations which precede these acts, particularly if, as is usually the case, the bleb has been caused by a check-valve obstruction.

Alveoli may rupture if they become greatly overdistended as a result of a check-valve obstruction. The air escaping from the ruptured alveoli then tracks along the sheaths of the perivascular structures, the bubbles of air traveling either peripherally (toward the pleural surface) or medially (toward the mediastinum). In either case a pneumothorax may result because of the rupture of either the visceral or mediastinal pleura. This may explain the occasional delay between the time of the actual exertion and the development of pneumothorax.

TRAUMATIC PNEUMOTHORAX

Mention has already been made of the type of pneumothorax associated with an open, sucking wound of the chest wall. Pneumothorax may also be associated with a nonpenetrating injury of the chest wall. The sharp edges of fractured ribs may lacerate the parietal and visceral pleura and the underlying lung parenchyma, thereby allowing air to escape into the pleural space. Such injuries frequently cause a hemothorax as well.

THERAPEUTIC PNEUMOTHORAX

Prior to the introduction of antituberculous chemotherapeutic agents, the deliberate introduction of air into the pleural space was one of the most effective methods of treatment of pulmonary tuberculosis. It was surmised, without definite confirmatory evidence, that reducing the size of the lung and restricting its excursions resulted in a reduction in the flow of blood and lymph so that hematogenous spread of the disease was prevented, and growth of the tubercle bacilli was inhibited by the decreased supply of oxygen. In addition, the retardation of lymphatic flow was considered to favor the development of fibrous tissue.

DIAGNOSTIC PNEUMOTHORAX

When there is radiologic evidence of a peripheral intrathoracic opacity and its anatomic site is difficult to determine, an artificial pneumothorax may be induced for purely diagnostic purposes. If the lesion is intrapulmonary, an x-ray taken after the induction of the pneumothorax will show the opacity in the collapsed lung. If the lesion is attached to a rib or the parietal pleura, the opacity will project into the pneumothorax. Tumors arising from the diaphragm or the intercostal nerves can also be distinguished by this procedure.

VALVULAR PNEUMOTHORAX

A tear in the visceral pleura may behave like a check-valve, and air from the tracheobronchial tree may enter the pleural space during inspiration but be unable to leave during expiration. Large quantities of air may therefore accumulate in the pleural cavity within a short time, rapidly increasing the pleural pressure, which may reach or surpass that of the atmosphere. A pneumothorax in which the pressure is greater than atmospheric is known as a "tension pneumothorax." This condition is dangerous, since in addition to complete collapse of the affected lung, there is also a decided shift of the mediastinum to the opposite side. This, in turn, compresses the opposite lung and can kink and obstruct the great veins. As a result, the venous return to the heart may be retarded so that the cardiac output falls.

CLINICAL MANIFESTATIONS

The severity of the symptoms produced by a pneumothorax depends on the amount of air that has collected in the pleural space and the degree of collapse of the underlying lung. A small pneumothorax may often be asymptomatic and may produce no abnormal physical findings.

The onset of spontaneous pneumothorax is usually abrupt and dramatic. The picture of a young man in apparently good physical health who, for no obvious reason, is suddenly overwhelmed by exquisite chest pain and respiratory distress is very striking. The pain, which is generally confined to the affected side of the chest, is presumed to be caused by the sudden abrupt increase in pleural pressure and tension on any adhesions that may be present. It is usually sharp and stabbing in character and is aggravated by breathing and coughing. On occasion, however, it may be only a dull, aching discomfort. If the pain is very severe, it may be associated with symptoms of shock, apprehension and a feeling of chilliness. An irritative cough, which is due to stimulation of nerve endings in the pleural space or in the walls of the collapsed bronchi, may also be present.

A patient with a large pneumothorax is frequently in great respiratory distress, is breathing rapidly and shallowly, and may be cyanosed. If shock is present, the skin is cold and clammy, the pulse rapid and thready, and the blood pressure is low. Under these circumstances, the possibility of associated bleeding into the pleural space should be considered as well.

The affected hemithorax moves poorly or not at all and may be larger than the normal side because of the unopposed elastic recoil of the chest wall. Movement of the costal margin is also impaired because the rise in pleural pressure restricts the expiratory ascent of the diaphragm and flattens its contour. If the case is traumatic in origin and there are numerous rib fractures, there may be paradoxical movement of the chest cage, the affected side collapsing during inspiration and enlarging during expiration (see Chapter 17). The mediastinum is deviated toward the normal side of the chest. Because of the increased ratio of air to solid tissue the percussion note is hyperresonant, vocal fremitus is diminished or absent and the breath sounds are usually faint or inaudible over the affected side. When a right-sided tension pneumothorax develops, downward displacement of the liver may be demonstrated by percussion of the upper limit of its dullness. If a bronchopleural fistula is present, the breath sounds may have a bronchial quality.

If a significant collection of fluid is present in conjunction with the pneumothorax, this settles to the bottom of the pleural cavity, and the percussion note over it will be dull or flat. In this situation, the upper limit of the flat note is horizontal so that the change from resonance to dullness is abrupt. Since both air and fluid are present, a "succussion splash" may be heard with a stethoscope when the patient is given an abrupt shake.

RADIOLOGIC MANIFESTATIONS

A pneumothorax, unless it is very small, presents a characteristic and easily recognizable radiologic picture in the upright postero-anterior view. If the collection of air is small, it may not be demonstrable when the x-ray is taken at full inspiration, but it often becomes visible if the exposure is made at the end of a maximal expiration because the translucency of the air in the pleural space is more apparent when contrasted with the density of the deflated lung.

The underlying deflated lung appears somewhat denser than the opposite normal lung, and its periphery is recognized as a thin, fine line running parallel to the lateral margin of the chest cage. The pneumothorax space has a uniform translucency which is characterized by the complete absence of lung markings, although linear strands caused by adhesions may occasionally be seen running from the periphery of the lung to the costal margins. The collection of air is usually predominant in the upper part of the pleural cavity if the film has been taken while the patient is in the upright position but may be localized by adhesions and confined to a portion of the pleural space. If it is complicated by an effusion, the fluid occupies the lowest part of the space, the upper border being straight and horizontal.

During fluoroscopy of a closed pneumothorax, it may be noted that, unlike the opposite normal lung, the partially deflated lung may only enlarge slightly during inspiration so that the mediastinum moves toward the pneumothorax side. This paradoxical movement of the mediastinum is presumably caused by the considerably larger change in the size of the normal lung during inspiration. This is in contrast to the mediastinal movement, which takes place in an open pneumothorax, in which it moves toward the normal side during inspiration.

FUNCTIONAL MANIFESTATIONS

The degree of functional impairment resulting from a pneumothorax depends upon its size. As the pressure in the pleural space rises toward that of the atmosphere, the lung collapses and the chest cage expands because of its elastic properties. The vital capacity decreases proportionally with the amount of air introduced into the pleural space.

If perfusion of the collapsed lung persists, venous admixture and consequent hypoxemia are present. It has been shown that this state persists for only a few hours, after which the arterial oxygen tension rises. Apparently blood is diverted from the collapsed lung to the opposite functioning lung, and only well-oxygenated blood reaches the left side of the heart. If there is a paradoxical movement of the chest, air may be shunted back and forth between the normal and the collapsed lung. Air which has already taken part in gas exchange is rebreathed, so that there is an increase in physiologic dead space, and alveolar hypoventilation with hypoxemia and hypercapnia may result.

ABSORPTION OF A PNEUMOTHORAX

The air of a pneumothorax is usually absorbed gradually, provided there is no communication between the pleural cavity and the atmosphere. Absorption of the air takes place through the subpleural venous channels, and the speed of absorption depends primarily on the state of health of the pleural surfaces. It is most rapid when the pleurae are healthy and is retarded if they are thickened and fibrosed as a result of disease. If the pleurae are calcified, no absorption may occur at all.

The process of absorption of air from a pneumothorax is similar to that which takes place in atelectasis. The pleural surfaces act as wet membranes, allowing oxygen, carbon dioxide and nitrogen to diffuse through them. Since the partial pressures of the gases in the pneumothorax approximate those of the atmosphere and those in the venous blood are substantially lower, the gases in the pleural space diffuse into the venous blood until the pneumothorax becomes completely absorbed. As the pneumothorax diminishes in size, the lung gradually expands and the chest cage becomes smaller, and the total pressure within the space is maintained. Expansion of the lung can be prevented, however, if it has become fibrosed or if the visceral pleura has become thickened through the deposition of fibrin. As with atelectasis, absorption of gas can be accelerated if the air is replaced by oxygen.

Chapter 17

Diseases of the Chest Wall and Diaphragm

Any disease which interferes with the function of the respiratory muscles or increases the resistance to distention of the chest cage may lead to interference with gas exchange and respiratory insufficiency even though there is no underlying bronchopulmonary disease.

In the early stages, mismatching of the distribution of blood and gas may be only moderate so that although hypoxemia is present, it is not associated with carbon dioxide retention. However, the development of even a minor respiratory infection may precipitate acute respiratory failure with severe hypoxemia and hypercapnia because the patient is unable to maintain an alveolar ventilation sufficient to cope with the increased carbon dioxide production. In the later stages of many of these diseases, alveolar hypoventilation is common, although the mechanisms producing it may be different in individual cases. If the alveolar hypoventilation persists for a length of time, it may lead to retention of bicarbonate and secondary polycythemia; ultimately, pulmonary hypertension and right-sided heart failure may develop.

THE SKIN AND SUBCUTANEOUS TISSUES

When scleroderma involves the respiratory system, it is usually because of pulmonary fibrosis which results in marked mismatching of ventilation and perfusion. The pulmonary insufficiency which develops in this disease may occasionally be complicated by involvement of the extrapulmonary structures. In scleroderma the skin of the chest wall has a waxy sheen, is taut and cannot be lifted from the underlying structures; it occasionally becomes so thickened, fibrosed and stiff that respiratory excursion of the chest wall may be limited.

When this is severe, the tidal volume will be low, and alveolar hypoventilation, hypoxemia and hypercapnia may develop.

408

OBESITY

An excess deposition of fat over the chest wall and abdomen may also limit the respiratory excursion of the thorax, and even when there is no obvious pulmonary or cardiac disease, pulmonary function may be altered to such an extent that respiratory and cardiac failure occurs. The increased body mass in obesity leads to an increased oxygen consumption and carbon dioxide production and a resulting stress on the gas transport mechanisms, even at rest. During exercise the increments in oxygen consumption, ventilation, cardiac output and work of the heart for any level of activity are greater in the obese person than in one who is not obese. The increased need of obese persons for oxygen at rest, and particularly during exercise, must be met in the face of an elevated work of breathing, an increased blood volume, a high pulmonary vascular resistance, and with an inefficient gas exchange in the lung.

The cardiac transverse diameter is increased in proportion to the body weight, but the precise mechanisms underlying the development of the cardiac enlargement have not been defined completely. Since hypoxemia results in pulmonary vasoconstriction, it might be expected that the increased pulmonary vascular resistance plays a role in the etiology of the cardiomegaly. However, although pulmonary hypertension is frequently present at rest or during exercise in the majority of obese persons, there is no correlation between the level of the pulmonary artery pressure and the arterial oxygen tension. In fact, exercise in these persons is often associated with a rise in arterial Po_2, despite the rise in pulmonary artery pressure. Many of the patients with pulmonary hypertension also have systemic hypertension, and the rise in pulmonary artery pressure during exercise is almost regularly accompanied by a rise in pulmonary wedge pressure of the same magnitude, suggesting a change in the left ventricular filling pressure. However, the increase in heart size in obese persons bears no relationship to the presence or absence of systemic hypertension either.

In severe obesity a syndrome which consists of cyanosis, twitching, a tendency toward excessive lethargy and drowsiness, and periodic breathing has been observed. In a fashion analogous to myxedema, these features usually develop insidiously and may be present for a long time before the patient or his relatives realize their significance. Functional assessment of such patients has revealed that the total lung capacity and its subdivisions are frequently reduced. In addition, there may be alveolar hypoventilation with hypoxemia and hypercapnia. It has been demonstrated that two-thirds of "normal" obese persons are hypoxemic and that one-third have associated hypercapnia. The low functional residual capacity and shallow respirations result in marked mismatching of ventilation and perfusion with considerable areas of the lungs being underventilated but still perfused so that hypoxemia results. Often the arterial PO_2 may not rise to expected values during oxygen breathing. If the hypoxemia has been present for some time, secondary polycythemia may become a complication. The pulmonary vascular resistance is often increased, presumably because of the vasoconstrictive effect of hypoxemia and acidemia. There may be marked pulmonary hypertension so that the work of the right ventricle of the heart increases, and in some cases, right ventricular hypertrophy develops. In the more advanced stages, congestive heart failure may occur.

Although excessive obesity is considered to be the prime factor in the development of this condition, the exact mechanism by which excessive weight can lead to respiratory failure has not been adequately elucidated. The compliance of the lung-thorax system is considerably reduced in the obese subject entirely because of an increase in elastic resistance of the extrapulmonary structures. This elastic resistance increases even further when the patient assumes the supine position, a finding which may possibly explain why obese patients are nursed more easily in the sitting position and why their condition tends to deteriorate if they are kept supine.

It has been generally accepted that the basic physiologic defect in the cardiopulmonary syndrome of obesity is the gross mismatching of ventilation and perfusion and the alveolar hypoventilation. The work of breathing probably plays an extremely important role in the development of alveolar hypoventilation in excessive obesity. As described in Chapter 1, an increased work of breathing has far-reaching effects on the control of breathing and the ability to maintain a normal arterial PCO_2. The respirations are usually rapid and shallow in obesity; this is to be expected in view of the high elastic resistance. This change in respiratory pattern results in alveolar hypoventilation. Thus, the rapid respiratory pattern is, in part, responsible for the development of hypoxemia and hypercapnia in obesity. Furthermore, it has been demonstrated that the oxygen cost of breathing is approximately three times as great in obese persons as it is in healthy persons. This is illustrated in Figure 108, where it can be seen that a slight increase in ventilation raises the oxygen consumption considerably in obesity and that this rise becomes precipitous when the ventilation is increased still further. This high cost of breathing is probably due to the increased mechanical work of breathing, although it has also been suggested that the efficiency of the respiratory apparatus is lower than normal. A similar reduction in efficiency is seen in normal subjects who are made to breathe at lower lung volumes by applying pressure around the chest. It has been estimated

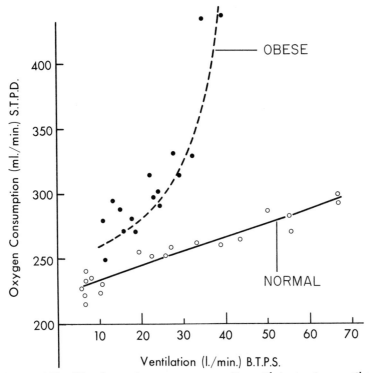

FIGURE 108. The change in oxygen consumption with increasing ventilation in a normal subject and in an obese subject. (From Cherniack, R. M.: Respiratory effects of obesity. Canad. Med. Ass. J. *80*:613, 1959. By permission.)

that the full-blown cardiopulmonary syndrome occurs in about 10 per cent of those with uncomplicated gross obesity, but the type of obese patient who is prone to develop it has yet to be established. The favorable effect of weight loss supports the theory that excessive obesity is the prime factor in its development. Many of the manifestations of the cardiopulmonary syndrome appear to accompany the uncomplicated obese state, and the full-blown syndrome may merely be an accentuation of these manifestations by one or more additional factors. Drowsiness and periodic breathing may be pronounced in obese patients without CO_2 retention or heart failure. However, pronounced CO_2 retention, which is known to be accompanied by drowsiness, may aggravate the previously existing tendency. Similarly, heart failure, which in itself may result in Cheyne-Stokes respirations, may accentuate the periodic breathing seen in the obese state. The congestive heart failure which develops in extremely obese patients, even in the absence of an elevated systemic pressure, is usually characterized by a high cardiac output and "failure" of both ventricles. Venous thrombosis and pulmonary embolism occur frequently in obese patients, and this may account for the clinical picture of chronic cor pulmonale in some patients. The exact mechanism leading to alveolar hypoventilation has not been adequately evaluated. Some believe that alveolar hypoventilation never occurs in uncomplicated obesity and that it is always associated with myxedema or a lung disease such as asthma, emphysema or a pulmonary infarction.

It would appear that when the obese state, with its increased work of breathing, is complicated by mild, and perhaps even clinically insignificant, disturbances in respiratory function due to lung disease, malfunction of the muscles of respiration, or a central nervous system lesion, cardiorespiratory failure and its consequences develops. The converse is also true, for the superimposition of obesity on pre-existing lung disease may increase the work of breathing sufficiently to lead to alveolar hypoventilation.

DEFORMITIES OF THE BONY THORAX

Any condition which increases the resistance of the ribs to movement is liable to produce respiratory insufficiency. Examples of these conditions are chronic diseases of the thoracic spine, such as kyphoscoliosis and rheumatoid spondylitis, and acute conditions such as traumatic chest injuries. If the disorder leads to a considerable reduction of the chest movement and an increased work of breathing, alveolar hypoventilation becomes a prominent feature, and severe hypoxemia, hypercapnia and cardiac failure may develop.

Although there is a wide variation in the general contour of the rib cage, its bony structure is normally symmetrical, largely because of the thoracic spine, which is also normally straight. An abnormality of the thoracic vertebrae will result in distortion of the chest configuration. Thus, bizarre distortions of the thoracic cage may result following paralysis of the back muscles due to poliomyelitis, tuberculous osteomyelitis of the vertebrae or a traumatic injury of the spine. All grades of spinal deformities can occur, and lesser forms may easily be overlooked unless the thoracic spine is examined routinely, both by inspection and by the palpation of its spinous processes.

Several types of spinal deformity may be encountered, the important ones being scoliosis, kyphosis and kyphoscoliosis.

SCOLIOSIS

The commonest deformity of the thoracic spine is scoliosis, a gradual lateral curvature of the thoracic spine which is usually associated with some degree of rotation or torsion of the vertebrae in their longitudinal axes. This type of deformity most frequently results from improper postural habits. If a person constantly shifts his body weight to one leg while standing, the body tends to be bent laterally, and one shoulder assumes a higher position than the other. This causes unequal tension on the muscles attached to the thoracic vertebrae and results in a lateral curvature of the thoracic spine. At the same time, the asymmetrical pull on the transverse spinous processes of the thoracic vertebrae also causes a rotation of the vertebral bodies in the direction of the convexity of the lateral curvature. For reasons which are not fully understood, approximately 75 to 80 per cent of the cases of scoliosis have a convexity to the right. This deformity can initially be corrected by voluntarily straightening the spine, but if the faulty posture is maintained for long periods of time, a permanent deformity may result.

With the more severe forms of scoliosis of the thoracic spine, the rib cage becomes distorted in a characteristic fashion. On the convex side of the scoliotic spine the ribs are widely separated as a result of the lateral deviation of the thoracic vertebrae, and the rotation of the vertebrae produces an angulation of the ribs on their posterior aspect. The altered position and the shape of the ribs result in a bulging of the posterior aspect of the rib cage on the convex side while its anterior aspect is flattened. In contrast, the ribs are crowded together on the concave side of the spine, and their insertions into the vertebrae are rotated so that the anterior aspect of the hemithorax on that side bulges while its posterior aspect is flattened.

KYPHOSIS

Kyphosis is a curvature of the thoracic spine; the convexity is directed posteriorly. Kyphosis frequently develops in elderly persons because of degenerative osteoarthritis of the thoracic spine. This type of curvature is also present in the "barrel-chest" deformity of chronic obstructive pulmonary disease.

An angular kyphosis, which is less common, is due to a destructive lesion of one or more vertebral bodies which follows tuberculous osteomyelitis. This produces a characteristic angulated hump which is made up solely by the spine and is known as a "gibbus." This causes chest cage deformity by crowding the ribs so that the anterior portion of the chest and sternum bulge forward in a pigeon-breast type of deformity.

KYPHOSCOLIOSIS

As the name implies, this deformity of the thoracic spine is caused by a combination of both kyphosis and scoliosis. Approximately 1 per cent of the population is affected by some degree of kyphoscoliosis, although the deformity is usually so mild that no medical attention is required. In most cases the cause of kyphoscoliosis is unknown, although postural abnormalities have been implicated, and there is apparently a hereditary tendency in about 25 per cent of cases. Poliomyelitis often leads to kyphoscoliosis because of the involvement and weakening of the spinal muscles.

In a severe form of kyphoscoliosis, one side of the chest may be so retracted that there is extensive compression of the underlying lung, and protrusion of the opposite side of the chest may cause marked overdistention of the lung on that side (Fig. 109).

Minor forms of kyphosis and scoliosis do not appear to produce significant alterations in pulmonary function. Severe cardiorespiratory disability develops only in patients who have advanced spinal deformities (a kyphosis with an angle of curvature greater than 20 degrees or a scoliosis with a curvature greater than 100 degrees). On the other hand, when there is a combination of these two deformities—i.e., kyphoscoliosis—the effects on the circulation and the respiration appear to be additive. In a kyphoscoliosis in which each of these components is present in only a moderate degree the alteration of pulmonary function may be equivalent to that produced by a severe form of either kyphosis or scoliosis alone.

When kyphoscoliosis is present there is an increased elastic resistance to distention of both the lungs and the chest wall, and the vital capacity and the total lung capacity are reduced. The nonelastic resistance is only moderately increased so that the $FEV_{1.0}$ and MMF are usually within normal limits. Both the mechanical work of breathing and the oxygen cost of breathing are high because of the raised elastic resistance. The minute ventilation is often increased, and the breathing pattern is typically rapid and shallow.

Although the distribution of inspired air is only moderately im-

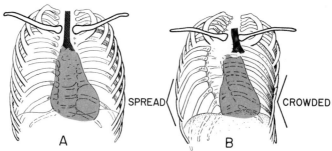

FIGURE 109. The normal contour of the chest cage (A) and that seen in kyphoscoliosis (B).

paired, the compression of the lung causes uneven perfusion so that there is gross mismatching of the distribution of ventilation and perfusion and a resultant hypoxemia. The size of the physiologic dead space is usually unaltered, but because of the breathing pattern and the increased work of breathing, alveolar hypoventilation often occurs so that hypoxemia and hypercapnia develop.

In the early stages of kyphoscoliosis the pulmonary arterial pressure is usually normal at rest, but the requirement of an increased blood flow (i.e., during exercise) may be associated with a considerable rise in the mean pulmonary artery pressure. In the later stages of this condition, pulmonary hypertension may be present even at rest. The increased pulmonary vascular resistance is probably due to mechanical compression of the pulmonary vessels as well as hypoxemia and acidosis. The work of the right ventricle is increased because of the elevated pulmonary vascular resistance, and hypertrophy of the right ventricle and eventually right-sided heart failure frequently develop.

CONGENITAL DEFORMITIES

Certain deformities of the anterior aspect of the thoracic cage have been almost conclusively shown to be hereditary in nature, for the same type of chest deformity may appear in a family over several generations. These deformities arise because of the impaired development of the septum transversum in the embryo which later forms the anterior portion of the diaphragm. Two factors seem to be involved in the production of these deformities—an abnormal pull of the diaphragm on the anterior chest wall, along with a disproportionate elongation of the ribs. The type of deformity which develops will depend on which factor is predominant.

FUNNEL CHEST OR "PECTUS EXCAVATUM"

In the infant, the cartilages and bony structures of the chest cage are softer and more mobile than those of the adult. Consequently, a congenitally shortened anterior portion of the diaphragm usually causes a retraction of the lower anterior chest wall during inspiration. The apex of the inspiratory depression is situated at the xiphisternal junction. As the child develops, its thoracic bony structure becomes more rigid and the sternal depression becomes fixed. In a fully developed funnel-chest deformity the body of the sternum is curved backward, forming a deep depression on the anterior chest wall around the xiphisternal junction and resulting in a reduced anteroposterior diameter of the chest cage.

A funnel-chest deformity, even of moderate severity, is generally asymptomatic, even though there may be some compression of the heart so that it appears enlarged radiologically. In some persons, the body of the sternum may be so depressed that it is in actual contact with the vertebral column. In such cases, the heart is distorted and displaced into the left hemithorax, causing the left lung to become compressed. The distortion of the bronchi may impair drainage, rendering the patient more susceptible to respiratory infections. In severe deformities there may be symptoms resulting from compression of the heart or lungs, such as dyspnea, palpitation and cough, and compression of the esophagus may cause dysphagia and other digestive disturbances.

PIGEON BREAST OR "PECTUS CARINATUM"

Protruding deformities of the anterior chest wall occur considerably less frequently than do the funnel-chest deformities. In this deformity, both the sternum and the costal cartilages are projected anteriorly and both sides of the chest are depressed so that it resembles the breast of a pigeon. The transverse diameter of the thoracic cage is narrowed, and the costal cartilages, which are attached to the sternum, extend forward obliquely.

CHEST TRAUMA

Approximately 25 per cent of deaths caused by traffic accidents result from chest injuries. Most such injuries are nonpenetrating, crushing or compression injuries, although occasionally a closed penetrating wound and, very rarely, an open penetrating wound may occur.

NONPENETRATING INJURIES

Crush injuries of the chest are usually nonpenetrating. These may consist of a single rib fracture, multiple rib fractures, multiple fractures involving a single or several ribs, or a fracture of the sternum. These chest injuries may result from direct crushing or compression beneath a heavy object, such as an automobile, a direct blow to the chest, or a deceleration type of compression injury caused by a head-on collision so that the person is forcefully thrown against the steering wheel, a seat or panel.

Even though there is no fracture of either the ribs or the cartilages, the chest cage may be compressed in an anteroposterior direction to such an extent that the sternum is practically in contact with the vertebrae. Fracture of the ribs is most likely to occur in the mid-axillary region. If the compressive force is applied in an oblique direction, the rib fractures may be situated posteriorly on one side and anteriorly on the other. Compression of the chest cage, particularly in an elderly person, may result in bilateral fractures of the anterior ends of the ribs, which may or may not be associated with separation of the costochondral or chondrosternal junctions or even with a fracture of the cartilages.

A "flail" chest results from fractures of multiple ribs or the disruption of several costosternal cartilages. Figure 110 demonstrates that this kind of injury usually causes paradoxical movement of the chest wall at the site of the fractures so that the affected area is drawn in during inspiration and is pushed out during expiration. Because the fractured ribs are abnormally mobile, the flail area is pushed inward by the atmospheric pressure surrounding the chest when the pleural pressure becomes more negative during inspiration. During expiration the intrathoracic pressure becomes greater than atmospheric and causes the flail area to bulge outward. Because of the paradoxical movement of the affected lung, air may be shunted backward and forward from one lung to another during respiration so that the patient actually inspires a portion of his expired air. This shunting, called "Pendelluft," is equivalent to rebreathing from a dead space. In addition, although the flail lung is poorly ventilated, it continues to be perfused, and gross hypoxemia may develop. The patient often increases the respiratory rate with a resultant increase in CO_2 elimination, but this has little effect on the arterial P_{O_2} because most of the inspired air enters the lung on the intact side. Thus, it is not uncommon to find considerable hypoxemia and a low P_{CO_2} in the patient

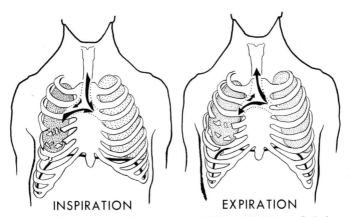

INSPIRATION   EXPIRATION

FIGURE 110.   Paradoxical movement and "Pendelluft" in a flail chest.

who is suffering from a flail chest injury. If there are bronchial secretions or the patient fatigues, the alveolar ventilation may be inadequate to cope with the carbon dioxide production, and severe hypoxemia and hypercapnia may develop.

In severe cases, the paradoxical movement of the chest cage may also cause the mediastinum to swing to and fro during respiration and interfere with the venous return to the heart. Because the flow of blood into the great veins of the thorax depends to a certain extent on the inspiratory sucking action of the negative pleural pressure, the cardiac output may fall, bringing on peripheral vascular collapse.

PENETRATING INJURIES

When there is a free communication between the outside air and the pleural cavity through a wound in the thoracic wall, an "open" pneumothorax exists. Air may enter the pleural cavity during inspiration and leave during expiration, causing the mediastinum to shift toward the affected side during expiration (see Fig. 107). The distensibility of the two lungs will be grossly unequal, and the pendulum movement of the mediastinum may cause air to be shunted backward and forward from one lung to the other. As a result, there will be a marked alteration of ventilation-perfusion ratios within the lung; the arterial oxygen tension will be low, and in some cases, the arterial carbon dioxide tension may rise. If this communication should become sealed off, the air in the pleural space constitutes a "closed" pneumothorax.

If the wound is small and acts as a check-valve, air may enter the pleural cavity during inspiration but may be prevented from escaping during expiration. Consequently, the pleural pressure rises, producing what is called a "tension" pneumothorax. Because of the elevated pleural pressure on the affected side, the mediastinum is displaced to the opposite side, and the normal lung is compressed. In addition, the raised pleural pressure and the deviated mediastinum may impede the venous return to the right side of the heart and result in a serious reduction in cardiac output and hypotension.

COMPLICATIONS OF
THORACIC INJURY

In addition to the severe physiologic imbalances created by mismatching of ventilation and perfusion and the drop in alveolar ventilation, other complications may develop which can further aggravate the already disturbed gas exchange. If the injury has caused a hemothorax or a pneumothorax, the alteration in pulmonary function is greatly aggravated, particularly if the air in the pleural space is under tension. In addition pulmonary edema may occur within a few hours after a serious accident. The mechanism of the development of pulmonary edema under such circumstances is not clearly understood.

The cough reflex may be affected because of "splinting" of the injured side so that it is difficult to expel bronchial secretions. The accumulation of blood or edema fluid in the smaller air passages may completely obstruct the small bronchi with resultant atelectasis of lobules, segments or even lobes of the lung. These atelectatic areas are liable to become infected, especially if there already is sepsis in the tracheobronchial tree.

The presence of air in the muscle planes and the subcutaneous tissues is a common accompaniment of nearly all chest injuries. The air may track through the subcutaneous tissues over long distances and may even involve the scalp or the lower extremities. Mediastinal air results from the rupture of air vesicles within the lung, the escaped air dissecting its way along the pulmonary vessels into the mediastinum and the neck. It may also be produced by rupture of the trachea or an intramediastinal portion of a bronchus. If mediastinal air is present in large quantities, it may compress the great veins, thereby causing serious impairment of the venous return to the heart, and a fall in cardiac output. This is usually associated with evident respiratory embarrassment, severe substernal pain and occasionally a "crowing" type of respiration due to compression of the trachea. A crunching sound which is synchronous with the heart beat may be detected by auscultation over the sternum.

Extravasation of blood into the pericardial sac as a result of rupture or a wound affecting either a heart chamber or one of the great vessels in the pericardium may also compress the heart and reduce the cardiac output. The blood pressure falls, the pulse pressure becomes smaller, and the cardiac sounds may have a distant quality. The jugular venous pressure may rise during inspiration and fall during expiration, presumably because the right atrium cannot enlarge sufficiently to accommodate the increased venous return during inspiration. In severe cases the patient may lose consciousness as a result of the cerebral ischemia and hypoxia which develop and are secondary to the reduced cardiac output.

THE RESPIRATORY MUSCLES

Any disease process which interferes with the normal function of the respiratory muscles may lead to a serious alteration in pulmonary function and the development of respiratory insufficiency. The disturbances in function may vary from a mild ventilation-perfusion abnormality due to the unequal expansion of areas of lung tissue to severe alveolar hypoventilation.

In patients suffering from dermatomyositis, myasthenia gravis or muscular dystrophy the thoracic muscles may contract asymmetrically because of the varying strength of the intercostal muscles. Different areas of the lung are therefore unequally or asymmetrically inflated, and the inspired gas is distributed abnormally. There is mismatching of ventilation and perfusion ratios throughout the lung, and hypoxemia develops. Occasionally, polycythemia and cor pulmonale may be the presenting clinical features. Carbon dioxide retention does not occur as long as there is hyperventilation of a sufficient number of perfused alveoli. On the other hand, if excessive muscular weakness should develop, or if an acute respiratory infection should supervene in the above-mentioned conditions, provision of an adequate alveolar ventilation may become impossible; consequently, severe hypoxemia and carbon dioxide retention occur.

Provision of an adequate alveolar ventilation may become impossible because of paralysis of the respiratory muscles in patients suffering from poliomyelitis, polyneuritis, spinal injuries or while muscle relaxants are being administered. As a consequence, unless artificial respiration is instituted, severe hypoxemia and hypercapnia may develop. If hypoxemia, either alone or together with hypercapnia, is present for a prolonged period of time, it may lead to the development of secondary polycythemia and in severe cases pulmonary hypertension and cor pulmonale.

THE DIAPHRAGM

The diaphragm, which occupies the floor of the thoracic cavity and acts as a partition between the contents of the thoracic cage and those of the abdominal cavity, is formed by two thin, dome-shaped sheets of striated muscles, each of which arises from the inner surface of the xiphoid process, the ipsilateral costal margin and the bodies of the upper lumbar vertebrae. It is the principal muscle of respiration. Although its primary function is to enlarge the chest cage vertically during inspiration, it also plays a part in its transverse enlargement by elevating the lower ribs and the costal margin. Both leaves of the diaphragm move approximately equally, going through a range of about 2 cm. during quiet breathing. At the end of a normal expiration, the upper limit of the dome of the right hemidiaphragm is at the level of the fifth rib, and that of the left hemidiaphragm is at the level of the fifth interspace. The ascent of the diaphragm during expiration is a purely passive phenomenon, being produced by the elastic recoil of the inflated lungs and the tone of the abdominal muscles. In a healthy person, a change from the erect to the supine position may result in as much as a 6 cm. rise of the resting level of the diaphragm. When the lateral decubitus position is assumed, the lower hemidiaphragm rises further, particularly if the subject lies on his right side.

A disease process involving the diaphragm may result in either its elevation or its depression. Both conditions are associated with a decrease in its mobility.

PARALYSIS OF THE DIAPHRAGM

Interruption of a phrenic nerve results in paralysis of the ipsilateral hemidiaphragm, and provided there are no adhesions, it rises from 3 to 10 cm. higher than the hemidiaphragm on the nonparalyzed side. This paralysis is permanent if the nerve is cut or avulsed and results in muscle atrophy and gradual replacement by fibrous tissue.

The phrenic nerves may become paralyzed by disease processes affecting the anterior horn cells, such as meningitis or tuberculous caries of the spine; the nerves directly, such as in diphtheria, lead poisoning, alcoholic neuritis or beriberi; or by direct extension of a malignant intrathoracic tumor. Before the advent of chemotherapy and excisional surgery, crushing of the phrenic nerve was one of the methods used to induce relaxation of the lung in the treatment of pulmonary tuberculosis. Motor activity usually returns within a period of approximately six months following a phrenic nerve crush.

EVENTRATION OF THE DIAPHRAGM

The term "eventration" is actually a misnomer, for there is no protrusion of abdominal viscera through an opening in the diaphragm, as the name would imply. In this condition, the diaphragm is a thin, atrophic sheet of fibrous tissue with no muscle fibers. It assumes an abnormally elevated position but still arches smoothly from its costal attachments. The acquired form of eventration is commonly seen as the end result of paralysis of the phrenic nerve. In an infant it may develop as a result of a birth injury affecting the brachial plexus. Because of its occurrence in the newborn, a congenital origin has been postulated for a small percentage of the cases. The congenital hypothesis is enhanced by the occasional association of hypoplasia and other congenital abnormalities of the corresponding lung, as well as congenital abnormalities elsewhere.

INFLAMMATION OF THE DIAPHRAGM

Although primary myositis of the diaphragm probably occurs, it is rare in comparison with secondary inflammation. The difference in incidence is easily understood if one considers the intimate relationship between the diaphragm and the pleural, pericardial and peritoneal membranes. The exceedingly rich plexus of the lymphatics which traverse the diaphragm forms communications between the pleural and peritoneal spaces and thus permits the spread of infection from one space to the other. The diaphragm can become secondarily involved by even the smallest collection of inflammatory exudate in the pleural space. This is not true of inflammatory exudate in the peritoneal cavity, which tends to gravitate toward the pelvis.

Subdiaphragmatic Abscess. Although involvement of the subdiaphragmatic space is exceedingly rare in pleural or pulmonary suppuration, a subdiaphragmatic abscess very commonly extends into the thorax and may lead to a serous pleural effusion, empyema, pyopneumothorax and pulmonary suppuration. Although thoracic extension is usually due to lymphatic spread, it may also follow perforation of a necrotic portion of the diaphragm.

A localized collection of purulent exudate or pus in the subdiaphragmatic space may follow any form of intra-abdominal suppuration and most commonly occurs as a result of peritonitis following perforation of a portion of the gastrointestinal tract. The right subdiaphragmatic space is involved five times more frequently than the left. The most common causal organisms are the *Bacillus coli,* the staphylococcus and occasionally gas-forming bacilli. The gas produced by the latter organisms collects within the abscess cavity under the diaphragm and produces a characteristic radiologic appearance which is suggestive of a pneumoperitoneum.

An elevated hemidiaphragm is easily recognized on the x-ray. If a diaphragmatic hernia is present, the contour of the affected diaphragm appears abnormal. The space-occupying abdominal viscus in the lower thorax may be solid or air-containing, and the mediastinum is usually displaced away from the side of the hernia (Fig. 111). It appears low and flattened and the costophrenic angles are widened.

One leaf of the diaphragm may be depressed by a pleural effusion, a pneumothorax or unilateral overdistention due to a check-valve bronchial obstruction. Both hemidiaphragms are usually depressed in emphysema or during a severe exacerbation of asthma.

Diaphragmatic movement during respiration can be assessed by fluoroscopic examination. The elevated hemidiaphragm associated with an atelectasis, a pulmonary infarction or a subdiaphragmatic

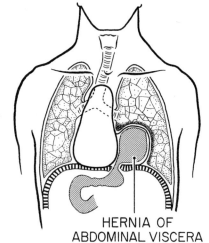

FIGURE 111. Diaphragmatic hernia.

HERNIA OF
ABDOMINAL VISCERA

abscess has restricted movement but in a normal direction. When a hemidiaphragm is paralyzed, it is practically motionless during quiet breathing and may even move paradoxically upward when a deep inspiration or a sniff is carried out. This "paradoxical movement" of the paralyzed diaphragm is produced by several factors. Inspiratory elevation of the ribs lowers the pressure, and this has a sucking effect on the paralyzed diaphragm. In addition, the inspiratory descent of the normal diaphragm increases the intra-abdominal pressure, which is transmitted through the abdominal viscera to the undersurface of the paralyzed diaphragm.

Even bilateral paralysis of the phrenic nerves may produce minimal impairment in respiratory function if there is little or no paradoxical movement. When there is considerable paradoxical movement, however, the vital capacity and the maximal breathing capacity are decreased and the residual volume is increased. There may be gross maldistribution of inspired air and altered ventilation-perfusion ratios so that hypoxemia is present. In severe cases, hypercapnia may be associated with the hypoxemia.

RESPIRATORY FAILURE AND ITS MANAGEMENT

RESPIRATORY FAILURE

MANAGEMENT OF CHRONIC
RESPIRATORY FAILURE

MANAGEMENT OF ACUTE
RESPIRATORY FAILURE

Chapter 18

Respiratory Failure

Respiratory disease imposes an increased load on the respiratory system. By increasing the amount of work done by the respiratory muscles or the heart, patients can often compensate for the increased load and maintain normal levels of arterial oxygenation and carbon dioxide elimination. When the respiratory system is unable to compensate adequately for the increased load, it fails to maintain normal arterial blood gas tensions. This situation is termed respiratory failure. The earliest manifestation of respiratory failure is often a defect in oxygen transfer; an associated defect in carbon dioxide elimination usually develops later. Severe respiratory failure frequently induces cardiac abnormalities, and conversely, primary cardiac disease may lead to respiratory failure.

Although hypoxemia which is not associated with hypercapnia is often not considered to be respiratory failure, a partial pressure of oxygen below 50 mm. Hg in the arterial blood, particularly when the hypoxemia is progressing, should also be considered as evidence of a severe gas exchange abnormality which is life-threatening. Severe progressively increasing hypoxemia occurs in a variety of acute pulmonary conditions, which have been termed "wet-lung syndrome" and "shock lung," in which there is damage to the gas exchange membrane, resulting in alveolar edema and collapse.

PATHOPHYSIOLOGY OF RESPIRATORY FAILURE

INADEQUATE OXYGENATION

Inadequate oxygenation of tissues may be a consequence of the low arterial oxygen tension and oxygen content occurring in patients suffering from severe pulmonary disease. This may result from diffusion defects, venous-to-arterial shunts, unequal ventilation-perfusion ratios, alveolar hypoventilation or any combination of these abnormalities.

A pure diffusion defect is probably rare, but it may develop when the quality of the membrane is markedly altered, as in pul-

427

monary fibrosis or congestion, or when there is a reduced capillary bed available for diffusion, as in pulmonary emboli, following pneu-monectomy or as a result of the degenerative processes in emphy-sema. In most instances, a low diffusing capacity is due to mismatch-ing of the distribution of blood and gas rather than a diffusion defect. Carbon dioxide retention does not develop in a diffusion defect because this gas diffuses across the alveolocapillary membrane 20 times more readily than oxygen. In fact, the arterial carbon dioxide tension is usually low when there is a diffusion defect because the hypoxic stimulus induces hyperventilation. Consequently, the total carbon dioxide content is low, and the pH tends to be high. The inhalation of 100 per cent oxygen completely relieves hypoxemia due to this type of disturbance.

True venous admixture occurs in congenital or acquired venous-to-arterial shunts within either the heart or the lungs. The hypoxemia which results may induce hyperventilation, and since the lungs are usually healthy, the arterial carbon dioxide tension is often low and the pH is high, but the increased ventilation is not sufficient to cor-rect the hypoxemia. Hypoxemia due to this type of disturbance is not completely corrected by the inhalation of 100 per cent oxygen.

Ventilation-perfusion ratios may vary because of uneven ventila-tion, uneven perfusion or both. When areas of lung are adequately ventilated but poorly perfused (dead-space-like ventilation), hypoxe-mia does not result, unless the ventilation of the remainder of the lung is inadequate to cope with the increased perfusion. Many patients compensate for increased dead-space-like ventilation by hyper-ventilation so that the arterial carbon dioxide tension and carbon dioxide content are frequently low and the pH is high. When areas of lung are poorly ventilated but relatively well perfused, venous-admixture-like perfusion is present, the P_{O_2} in the blood leaving these areas is low and the P_{CO_2} is elevated. However, the carbon dioxide tension in the mixed arterial blood may still be normal or even low if a sufficient number of adequately perfused alveoli are hyper-ventilated. Such "compensatory" hyperventilation of certain regions is not, however, effective in correcting the hypoxemia resulting from hypoventilation of other regions.

DEFECTS IN BOTH OXYGENATION AND CARBON DIOXIDE ELIMINATION

As has been pointed out previously in Chapter 3, the amount of carbon dioxide eliminated from the lungs in a minute ($\dot{V}_{CO_2}$) can be calculated from knowledge of the alveolar ventilation ($\dot{V}_A$) and the fractional concentration of carbon dioxide in the alveoli ($F_{A_{CO_2}}$). The partial pressure of carbon dioxide (P_{CO_2}) depends upon two factors. These are the alveolar ventilation and the metabolic production of carbon dioxide or oxygen consumption.

$$\text{PCO}_2 = \frac{\dot{V}_{CO_2}}{\dot{V}_A} \times 0.863 = \frac{\dot{V}_{O_2} \times R}{\dot{V}_A} \times 0.863$$

Thus, retention of carbon dioxide, or hypercapnia, develops whenever the alveolar ventilation is inadequate in relation to the level of metabolic CO_2 production. The hypercapnia is always accompanied by hypoxemia unless the patient is inhaling an oxygen-enriched mixture. The term *alveolar hypoventilation* is used to denote a situation in which the alveolar ventilation is inadequate to cope with the level of metabolism. Insufficiency of both oxygen exchange and carbon dioxide elimination or alveolar hypoventilation develops whenever the alveolar ventilation diminishes without a proportionate fall in metabolism or if there is a rise in oxygen consumption and carbon dioxide production without a proportionate increase in alveolar ventilation.

The minute volume is composed of both a dead space component, which does not take part in gas exchange, and an alveolar component, which supplies oxygen to and takes up carbon dioxide from the pulmonary capillary blood. Table 14 indicates the effect on the alveolar ventilation of an increase in physiologic dead space (tidal volume and respiratory rate remaining constant), a decrease in minute ventilation or a change in respiratory pattern (minute ventilation remaining constant).

The three situations depicted in Table 14 are often encountered

TABLE 14

EFFECT ON ALVEOLAR VENTILATION OF CHANGE IN (A) DEAD SPACE, (B) MINUTE VENTILATION AND (C) RESPIRATORY PATTERN

$\dot{V}_E$ (l./min.)	V_T (l.)	f (No./min.)	V_D (l.)	$\dot{V}_A$ (l./min.)
a. 8.0	0.50	16	.15	5.6
8.0	0.50	16	.25	4.0
8.0	0.50	16	.35	2.4
b. 8.0	0.50	16	.15	5.6
6.4	0.40	16	.15	4.0
4.8	0.30	16	.15	2.4
c. 8.0	0.80	10	.15	6.5
8.0	0.50	16	.15	5.6
8.0	0.25	32	.15	3.2

in patients with respiratory insufficiency. The physiologic dead space is frequently abnormally increased in patients suffering from a variety of bronchopulmonary diseases. Rapid shallow breathing is a common finding in patients suffering from bronchopulmonary disease or diseases affecting the chest wall and thoracic cage, particularly if the work of breathing is increased. The minute ventilation falls when the central response to carbon dioxide is depressed, as in patients suffering from a cerebral injury or vascular accident (particularly if the cerebrospinal fluid pressure is elevated), an overdose of depressant drugs, or chronic hypoxemia and hypercapnia.

The work of breathing is particularly important in the genesis of alveolar hypoventilation. As was demonstrated in Figure 28, the cost of an increase in minute ventilation in a healthy subject is only about 1 to 2 ml. per liter of ventilation, and this constitutes only about 2 to 8 per cent of the total oxygen consumption. The cost of an increase in ventilation in patients with increased mechanical resistances to breathing is often much higher, and in some patients the oxygen consumption of the respiratory muscles may amount to as much as 50 per cent of the total oxygen consumption when ventilation is increased.

If the relationship between ventilation and oxygen consumption is considered in the light of the relationship between alveolar ventilation and carbon dioxide production, it becomes clear that, in patients suffering from cardiopulmonary insufficiency, the increased work of breathing may contribute to hypoxemia and hypercapnia by increasing CO_2 production and oxygen consumption.

When alveolar hypoventilation develops, arterial acidemia results as predicted by the Henderson-Hasselbalch equation (see Chapter 3).

In acute respiratory failure, the carbon dioxide content is normal and the pH is low. The acidosis may be severe, particularly if there is marked tissue hypoxia which leads to the accumulation of lactic acid. In chronic respiratory failure, the effect of the elevated CO_2 is compensated for by increased retention of bicarbonate by the kidneys. If the renal compensatory mechanisms are normal, the retention of bicarbonate is sufficient to bring the pH to a low normal value.

CARDIAC INSUFFICIENCY

Heart failure is a frequent manifestation of severe respiratory insufficiency. Although right ventricular failure is the earliest and most frequent event, left ventricular failure may also develop in the

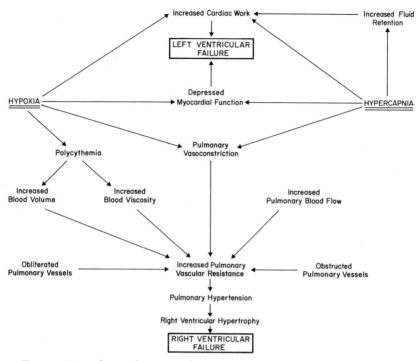

FIGURE 112.   The mechanism of development of right heart failure in respiratory disease and possible factors which may lead to left heart failure.

later stages of respiratory insufficiency. The mechanisms by which these conditions may be brought about are illustrated in Figure 112.

RIGHT VENTRICULAR FAILURE

Right ventricular failure, a frequent consequence of respiratory insufficiency, develops because of a high pulmonary vascular resistance. Although the pathogenetic mechanisms by which pulmonary vascular resistance is increased may vary from patient to patient, it is believed that hypoxemia and acidemia, which can lead to pulmonary vasoconstriction, are important factors. In addition, pulmonary vascular resistance may be elevated by the increased blood volume and viscosity due to secondary polycythemia; by obliteration of pulmonary capillaries, as in kyphoscoliosis, pulmonary fibrosis and emphysema; or by obstruction of the pulmonary vessels, as in pulmonary embolism. It may be further aggravated by anastomoses between the bronchial and pulmonary circulation, as in bronchiectasis.

The high pulmonary vascular resistance leads to pulmonary

hypertension, right ventricular hypertrophy and eventually right heart failure, the manifestations of which include jugular venous distention, hepatic enlargement and peripheral edema. It has been suggested by some that edema rarely develops unless the arterial carbon dioxide tension is elevated, and it has been postulated that the compensatory retention of bicarbonate and sodium leads to expansion of the extracellular space and tissue edema. This may explain why edema is most frequently encountered in patients who have hypoxemia and hypercapnia and is rarely seen in those who maintain nearly normal blood gas tensions.

LEFT VENTRICULAR FAILURE

Although there is no concrete evidence regarding the frequency of development of left ventricular failure in cases of respiratory disease, it is not uncommon to find small areas of fibrosis in the myocardium of the left ventricle in patients with respiratory disease. These may be the result of chronic hypoxemia and hypercapnia. When cardiovascular disease is present, it is possible that left ventricular function is depressed by any associated hypoxemia and acidemia. The resultant pulmonary congestion in turn further increases the work of breathing and aggravates the hypoxemia so that gross right and left heart failure may be present.

MANIFESTATIONS OF RESPIRATORY FAILURE

As mentioned earlier, there is frequently an initial stage of compensation for any abnormal blood and gas distribution by an increase in ventilation and cardiac work. Patients with obstructive pulmonary disease in this phase are often termed "pink puffers." Later, because of the marked increase in the resistances to breathing, there is alveolar hypoventilation with hypoxemia and carbon dioxide retention. (Patients with obstructive pulmonary disease in whom alveolar hypoventilation is associated with right-sided heart failure have been termed "blue bloaters"). The tempo of progression from the first to second stage is highly variable, and indeed, the order in which they appear may vary.

There is no correlation between the degree of compensation and the severity of the patient's symptoms. In fact, many patients who are maintaining relatively normal blood gas tensions but at the cost of a marked increase in respiratory work (i.e., pink puffers) are much more disabled than others with hypoxemia and hypercapnia who tolerate these marked alterations in blood gas tensions rather than work harder to improve them (blue bloaters). Nevertheless, progressive decompensation is almost invariably associated with an increasing severity of symptoms and is attended by secondary effects of hypoxemia and acidosis and, in some instances, hypercapnia, all of which further compromise respiratory and cardiac function.

The physical signs elicited in respiratory insufficiency are related to the underlying disease process; precipitating factors, such as infection, embolism or pneumothorax; and those related to the hypoxemia, hypercapnia and acidosis.

Though acute respiratory insufficiency is frequently precipitated by an acute infection, constitutional signs of infection are usually minimal or absent, the temperature being subnormal in many cases and the white blood count being low, normal or only slightly elevated.

The manifestations of altered blood gas tensions vary considerably and depend largely on its severity and duration. The central nervous system is particularly vulnerable to hypoxia and hypercapnia, and neurologic signs usually predominate; headache, lassitude, slurred speech, incoordination, restlessness, irritability, tremors and mood fluctuations varying between anxiety, depression and euphoria may be present. Hyperpnea, dyspnea, tachycardia and cyanosis may also be dominant features in some patients.

Asterexis and papilledema may also occasionally develop. The headache, the papilledema and some of the mental changes may be related to the increase in cerebral blood flow and the elevated cerebrospinal fluid pressure which occurs when the arterial carbon dioxide tension rises. The cause of the mental changes is uncertain, although both hypoxia and the narcotic effect of carbon dioxide probably play a role.

Catecholamine release results in tachycardia and systolic hypertension. Acute hypoxemia and acidosis increase the pulmonary vascular resistance and may precipitate acute right ventricular heart failure. In severely ill patients, in whom the P_{CO_2} is markedly elevated, generalized cardiovascular collapse with hypotension, profuse sweating and cyanosis produce a picture resembling other forms of shock.

RECOGNITION OF RESPIRATORY FAILURE

Respiratory failure may develop in a wide variety of patients who are suffering from a multitude of conditions (Table 15). As is illustrated in Figure 113, these conditions may be divided into three major groups, and although the respiratory failure may be produced by different mechanisms, the end result is always hypoxemia, either alone or in association with hypercapnia.

TABLE 15

DISEASES ASSOCIATED WITH RESPIRATORY FAILURE

I. DISEASES WITH PREDOMINANT DIFFUSE OBSTRUCTIVE DISORDER
  a. Chronic bronchitis
  b. Emphysema
  c. Asthma
  d. Bronchiectasis
  e. Cystic fibrosis
II. DISEASES WITH PREDOMINANT DIFFUSE PULMONARY RESTRICTIVE DISORDER
  a. Due to acute alveolocapillary dysfunction
    1. Pulmonary edema
    2. Shock lung
    3. Fat embolism
    4. Gram-negative septicemia
    5. Hyaline membrane disease
  b. Due to "interstitial disease"
    1. Sarcoidosis
    2. Fibrosing alveolitis
    3. Extrinsic allergic alveolitis
    4. Pneumoconiosis
    5. Lupus, rheumatoid arthritis
    6. Histiocytosis "X"
    7. Radiation fibrosis
    8. Idiopathic pulmonary hemosiderosis, etc.
  c. Due to "vascular disease"
    1. Multiple pulmonary emboli
    2. Polyarteritis
    3. Mitral stenosis and other cardiac diseases
  d. Due to pleural disease
    1. Pleural effusion
    2. Pneumothorax
III. DISEASES PRIMARILY AFFECTING THE CHEST WALL
  a. Kyphoscoliosis
  b. Thoracoplasty
  c. Obesity
  d. Chest trauma
IV. DISEASES AFFECTING THE NEUROMUSCULAR SYSTEM
  a. Muscular disorders
    1. Muscular dystrophy
  b. Neuronal disorders
    1. Poliomyelitis
    2. Polyneuritis
  c. Respiratory center dysfunction
    1. Sedation, narcotics, anesthesia
    2. Cerebral injury, hemorrhage, tumor
    3. Encephalitis
    4. Chronic hypoxia and hypercapnia

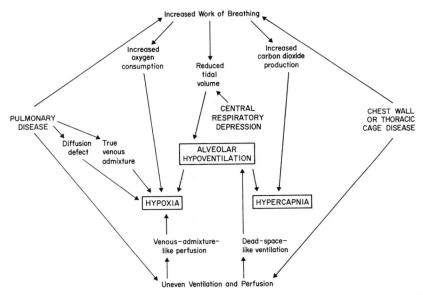

FIGURE 113. The mechanism of development of inadequate oxygenation and defects in both oxygenation and CO_2 elimination.

BRONCHOPULMONARY DISEASE

Respiratory insufficiency is commonest in patients with airway obstruction. In parenchymal or pleural diseases mismatching of blood and gas distribution results in hypoxemia, but the alveolar ventilation is usually sufficient to provide an adequate elimination of carbon dioxide at rest. However, the added ventilatory demands of heavy exercise or a superimposed bronchial obstruction, infection or pulmonary congestion may precipitate acute respiratory failure with severe hypoxemia and carbon dioxide retention. Respiratory failure is especially ominous in patients with asthma.

CHEST WALL OR THORACIC CAGE DISEASES

Diseases affecting the spinal cord, motor nerves, neuromuscular junction and respiratory muscles, such as poliomyelitis, polyneuritis, myasthenia gravis or the muscular dystrophies, and conditions affecting the thoracic cage, such as kyphoscoliosis, severe obesity or traumatic chest injuries, may lead to gross alterations in the distribution of ventilation and perfusion and also may result in alveolar hypoventilation.

CENTRAL RESPIRATORY DEPRESSION

Excessive administration of barbiturates, narcotics, opiates, tranquilizers or anesthesia, all of which depress the sensitivity of the respiratory center, will cause a fall in minute ventilation and alveolar hypoventilation. A similar situation may occur in patients suffering from a CNS infection or increased cerebrospinal fluid pressure as a result of an intracranial tumor, vascular accident or a head injury. In addition, as has been pointed out earlier, the respiratory system may lose its ability to respond to excessive levels of carbon dioxide in patients with chronic hypoxemia. and carbon dioxide retention.

DIAGNOSIS OF RESPIRATORY FAILURE

Early identification of respiratory failure is extremely important and is facilitated by being aware of the conditions that cause it. Unless hypoventilation is extremely severe, clinical assessment of the adequacy of the alveolar ventilation is virtually impossible. The presence of slow gasping respirations and cyanosis may make the diagnosis of acute respiratory failure easy but, in the majority of cases, it may not be recognized unless there is a high index of suspicion on the part of the attending physician. Visual assessment of the apparent adequacy of chest movement or lung aeration is not to be relied upon. The presence or absence of cyanosis may also be misleading because its recognition is notoriously difficult; as pointed out earlier, it may not develop until hypoxemia is severe, and severe hypoxemia may be present without cyanosis, particularly in the presence of anemia.

Acute respiratory failure should be suspected in any patient who is suffering from bronchopulmonary, chest wall, thoracic cage or central nervous system disease if an acute respiratory infection, asthma or acute heart failure has developed. Chronic respiratory failure frequently develops insidiously, but it should be suspected when chronic right-sided heart failure and polycythemia are present, since they are frequently associated with chronic hypoxemia and carbon dioxide retention.

The definitive diagnosis of respiratory failure depends heavily on the demonstration of hypoxemia with or without CO_2 retention by analysis of the arterial blood. The arterial oxygen and carbon dioxide tensions and the pH can be determined readily with electrodes. If blood gas electrodes are not available, the arterial carbon dioxide tension can also be determined indirectly by measurement of the arterial pH and the total carbon dioxide content, or it can be estimated from the mixed venous P_{CO_2} by the rebreathing technique.

The findings in the arterial blood in acute and chronic alveolar hypoventilation are presented in Table 16. In acute alveolar hypo-

TABLE 16

ARTERIAL BLOOD FINDINGS IN ACUTE AND CHRONIC ALVEOLAR HYPOVENTILATION

ARTERIAL BLOOD	ACUTE	CHRONIC
PO_2	↓↓*	↓↓*
PCO_2	↑↑	↑↑
HCO_3^-	⟷	↑↑
CO_2 content	⟷	↑↑
pH	↓↓	⟷

*Unless on oxygen therapy.

ventilation, there is hypoxemia (unless oxygen is being administered), and the arterial PCO_2 is elevated. The plasma bicarbonate and carbon dioxide content are normal, and the pH is low (acute respiratory acidosis). In chronic alveolar hypoventilation, hypoxemia (unless oxygen is being administered) and hypercapnia will be present. In this situation, however, there has been compensation for the elevated partial pressure of carbon dioxide by elimination of chloride and retention of base and bicarbonate. As a result, the bicarbonate and the carbon dioxide content are elevated, the serum chloride is low, and the pH is restored to low normal values.

SUMMARY

Respiratory failure implies that the respiratory system is unable to provide adequate arterial oxygenation, with or without an inadequate elimination of carbon dioxide. These situations can occur in patients with bronchopulmonary disease, chest wall or thoracic cage disease, or central respiratory depression. The manifestations of respiratory failure are nonspecific and definitive recognition of this condition requires analysis of the arterial blood gas tensions and pH. The management of respiratory failure is based upon knowledge of the disturbances present and is directed at improving pulmonary function.

Although there are specific adjuncts to the therapy of any of the conditions which may be associated with abnormal gas exchange, the management of respiratory failure can be discussed in general terms. The principles of therapy are equally applicable to acute and chronic failure, but for the sake of clarity, management of the two conditions will be dealt with separately in the following two chapters.

Chapter 19

Management of Chronic Respiratory Failure

The management of chronic respiratory failure is discussed before that of acute respiratory failure because it presents a far greater therapeutic challenge to the physician. Although the challenge of acute respiratory failure, with its requirement for sophisticated equipment and personnel, has resulted in the development of "intensive care" units in many hospitals, it is not as well recognized that the patient with chronic respiratory disease also requires intensive care and the attention of a sophisticated health team.

The results may not be as dramatic as in acute respiratory failure, but the application of intensive therapy directed at improving altered respiratory function can result in considerable improvement both in function and in well-being of the patient with chronic respiratory failure. It must be emphasized that the patient with chronic respiratory failure, like one with diabetes or heart failure, is suffering from a chronic condition. Although the disease may not be curable, its progression can be slowed considerably by appropriate management.

To achieve even a modicum of success in the management of chronic respiratory failure, it is imperative that the patient and his family understand as much as possible about the condition, the alterations in function present, and the therapeutic measures which are necessary to prevent acute exacerbations. Often a patient receives excellent attention and care while in hospital because of an acute exacerbation but is then discharged from the hospital without proper advice about the need for continuing attention to details of treatment. It is relatively common for many patients to be readmitted to hospital in an acute exacerbation and report that, since they had felt so well, they stopped taking medications.

The management of respiratory failure is an on-going affair, and although its intensity may be reduced under optimal conditions, it should never be stopped. The therapeutic approach to respiratory failure is based on the nature of the derangement in respiratory function and the effects of the altered blood gas tensions and acid-base state on other organ systems in the body. Often maximal improvement in respiratory function only occurs when effective treatment of the secondary phenomena is instituted. The measures utilized are directed at a reduction of the work of breathing, an increase in alveolar ventilation, improvement in exercise tolerance and the prevention of acute exacerbations.

MEASURES DESIGNED TO REDUCE WORK OF BREATHING

In the majority of patients with chronic respiratory failure, the work of breathing is increased. A reduction of the work of breathing will result in a lowering of the oxygen uptake and carbon dioxide production of the respiratory apparatus. The measures utilized depend on whether the increased work of breathing is due to an increased resistance to airflow in the airways or to an increased resistance to distention of the lungs or the chest cage.

RELIEF OF AIRWAY OBSTRUCTION

The measures used to relieve airway obstruction depend on the site of the obstruction and its cause. If excessive secretions, whether allergic, irritative or infective in nature, are obstructing airways, the measures utilized are directed at reducing secretions by diminishing their production and increasing their elimination. If bronchoconstriction is present, pharmacological agents which will lead to bronchodilation should be administered.

REDUCTION OF SECRETIONS

Removal of Irritants or Allergens. The removal of all possible bronchial irritants or allergens is essential. Avoidance of dusty working conditions or environmental pollution is important, and a change in residence away from a dusty or smoggy area may be necessary. Cessation of smoking, particularly of cigarettes (even a single cigarette may cause a measurable increase in airway resistance), is imperative and particularly effective in lessening symptoms. Similarly, removal of any incriminating allergens, such as household pets, may result in virtually complete recovery from symptoms.

It is almost impossible to treat lower airway obstruction effectively without concomitant therapy directed at the upper respiratory tract, for both are frequently affected by irritants or allergens. The persistent drainage of secretions from the upper respiratory tract into the tracheobronchial tree (postnasal discharge) is frequently responsible for irritative cough, sputum and wheezing attacks. Under these circumstances nasal saline douches in the morning and at night and, if necessary, the instillation of vasoconstrictive agents should be carried out whenever a postnasal discharge is present, even though x-rays of the sinuses may demonstrate no abnormality.

Control of Infection. Pulmonary infections with thick viscid secretions, which may be difficult to expectorate, and inflammatory swelling of the bronchial mucosa result in airway obstruction and predispose to the development of severe hypoxia and hypercapnia. Each episode of infection may leave behind it a residuum of incompletely resolved infection and some permanent structural damage. Even a minor cold should be regarded seriously in patients with chronic respiratory failure. Upper respiratory infection, particularly involving the sinuses, may progress to pneumonia or to a life-threatening bronchitis and bronchiolitis. It is therefore important not only to search for evidence of infection and to treat it effectively but also to prevent infections. Mild chronic respiratory infection is fairly common in patients with chronic bronchitis and even though the sputum appears clear and mucoid during the day, it is often yellow or green in the mornings after the inhalation of a bronchodilator permits the expectoration of retained secretions.

Whenever the sputum is yellow or green, a sample should be examined by Gram stain, the sensitivity of the organisms to antibiotics determined by culture techniques, and the infection treated. The choice of antibiotic administered is dictated by proper identification of the organisms concerned. Antibiotic therapy should be continued for at least a week after the sputum shows sustained reduction of pus cells and bacteria and the patient is clinically improved.

Chronic prophylactic antibiotic therapy has been advocated because, although acute infections are not prevented, their severity is reduced. However, if proper attention is paid to "bronchial toilet" and retention of secretions is prevented, most acute exacerbations can be prevented, and treatment with antibiotics is recommended only when the sputum is infected.

Thinning of Secretions. Hydration of the patient with a fluid intake of 30 to 40 ml. per kg. of body weight daily can prevent the formation of thick, viscid and crusted secretions. Warming and saturation of the inspired air with water vapor also helps to liquefy secretions and makes them easier to expectorate, especially if bronchodilators are also administered. Oral expectorants, such as potassium iodide, ammonium chloride or guaiacol, may also thin secretions, but in most instances these agents are not necessary if adequate hydration and humidity are provided. The inhalation of detergent aerosols or mucolytic agents has been recommended, but they must be administered over most of the day to produce benefit and have not been proved to be more effective than aerosols of water or saline solution. Furthermore, such agents must be used with caution in asthma, since they can induce bronchoconstriction.

Postural Drainage. Postural drainage at frequent intervals often helps eliminate secretions, particularly if the disease involves a localized area of lung. When postural drainage is being carried out, elimination of secretions can be facilitated by chest pummeling with rapid repetitive strokes and vibration of the chest, following which the patient is encouraged to cough and expectorate secretions. The predominant posture to be adopted for drainage will depend upon the area of lung involved. The upper lobe bronchus is drained best in the upright position. Drainage of the bronchi of the right middle lobe or the lingular segment of the left upper lobe, which run horizontally and anteriorly, is best in the supine position with the involved lung uppermost and the body tilted at an angle of 45 degrees with the head lowermost. The prone position is best for drainage of the superior segments of both lower lobes, since they run horizontally and posteriorly. Drainage of the remaining segments of the lower lobes is best while prone in the Trendelenburg position.

RELIEF OF BRONCHOCONSTRICTION

Contraction of the smooth muscle in small and medium-sized airways increases the work of breathing and should be vigorously treated. In most instances a combination of agents which result in maximum bronchodilation with minimal side effects is desirable.

Bronchodilators. By far the greatest relief of airway obstruction due to bronchoconstriction is obtained when a bronchodilator is inhaled into the tracheobronchial tree. Prompt relief often follows the proper administration of racemic epinephrine, epinephrine, isoproterenol, orciprenaline or solbutamol by means of a nebulizer which delivers sufficiently small droplets.

The effectiveness of nebulized bronchodilator is directly dependent upon the mode of administration. Following a maximal expiration, the nebulizer is placed in the open mouth, and the bulb squeezed repeatedly while the patient makes a slow maximal inspiration, as though he were "sipping" hot soup. The breath is held at full inspiration for a few seconds, and then expiration is carried out slowly through pursed lips. After each inhalation of bronchodilator the patient should attempt to cough up secretions so that the fine droplets delivered by the ensuing nebulization can exert their effect in the smaller bronchi and bronchioli.

If the patient is unable to coordinate the squeezing of the nebulizer bulb with a slow maximum inhalation, the bronchodilator aerosol should be nebulized with a compressed air or oxygen source. In this case occlusion of a **Y** tube, which is placed between the pressure source and the nebulizer, allows the patient to control the nebulization. If a patient is not able to take a big breath, the nebulized bronchodilator can be administered by a positive-pressure breathing machine. Once again, slow deep inspirations should be encouraged.

The nebulization of bronchodilator should be repeated until the patient feels subjective relief in the lower lateral thoracic areas or until he notes tachycardia or shakiness. The number of inhalations necessary will depend upon the severity of the obstruction and, thus, will vary from patient to patient and, in a given patient, from day to day. Even in the chronic patient who appears to be relatively free of difficulty, administration of aerosol bronchodilator should be continued at least twice daily—every morning on arising and before retiring. In addition, the bronchodilator should be inhaled when the patient has episodes of cough or breathlessness or before he undertakes any activity which is known to precipitate symptoms.

Oral bronchodilating agents such as ephedrine sulfate, theophylline or a combination of these are exceedingly useful once an acute exacerbation has subsided. They are irregularly absorbed in an acutely ill patient, and even after the acute episode, they are best taken on an empty stomach (i.e., ½ to 1 hour before meals and at bedtime) because the absorption of aminophylline is slowed in an alkaline medium. For the patient who has considerable difficulty during the night, the sustained action oral bronchodilators, rectal aminophylline suppositories or aminophylline dissolved in water are often of great benefit.

REDUCTION OF ELASTIC RESISTANCE

Reduction of an increased work of breathing resulting from a high elastic resistance of the lungs is not achieved often except in some patients with diffuse pulmonary infiltration due to sarcoidosis or allergic alveolitis. In these conditions, the administration of steroids and, if possible, removal of a responsible allergen may diminish the infiltrations and the work of breathing, thereby leading to a reduction in dyspnea and an improvement in gas exchange.

REDUCTION OF PULMONARY CONGESTION

Right ventricular failure and fluid retention are important consequences of respiratory failure and the hypoxemia and hypercapnia resulting from it. However, the fluid retention and pulmonary congestion increase the respiratory work further and thus aggravate respiratory failure. Treatment with diuretics and a restricted salt intake is often sufficient to overcome the fluid retention and heart failure associated with respiratory failure. If improvement does not occur after the administration of a diuretic and serum electrolyte concentrations are normal, digitalis should be given. The reduction in pulmonary congestion brought about by this therapy lowers the work required to overcome the resistance to lung distention and leads to improved blood and gas distribution and, consequently, an improvement of arterial blood gas tensions. Clearly then, a dual approach to therapy of respiratory failure is required; treatment of the basic disturbances in pulmonary function decreases the tendency to heart failure, and treatment of heart failure improves pulmonary function.

WEIGHT LOSS

Obesity is associated with an increased work of breathing due to a reduced distensibility of the thorax. This increased work of breathing may predispose to marked abnormalities in gas exchange. Not only can obesity, per se, lead to respiratory failure, but it can aggravate respiratory failure due to other causes. In persons with chronic lung disease and an increased work of breathing, the superimposition of obesity leads to a marked increase in the work of breathing and contributes to the development of alveolar hypoventilation with consequent hypoxemia and hypercapnia. The therapy of such situations consists of intensive efforts to bring about weight reduction. Loss of weight diminishes the work of breathing, leads to a change in respiratory pattern so that alveolar ventilation is increased, and improves the matching of ventilation and perfusion so that arterial blood gas tensions improve. It is therefore extremely important to bring about weight reduction in any patient who is obese.

MEASURES DESIGNED TO INCREASE ALVEOLAR VENTILATION

Along with reduction in oxygen uptake and carbon dioxide production, measures must be instituted to increase the alveolar ventilation in relation to the CO_2 production when hypoxemia and hypercapnia are present. In order to achieve this it is essential to ensure a patent tracheobronchial tree. Thus, the therapy directed at the reduction of airway obstruction, which has been outlined, is an integral component of the measures directed at provision of an adequate alveolar ventilation.

ASSISTED VENTILATION

As pointed out earlier, intermittent positive pressure breathing may be necessary to deliver bronchodilator to the tracheobronchial tree in some patients. It is debatable whether the routine use of IPPB is of any benefit in the usual case of chronic respiratory failure. There is considerable evidence that the proper administration of bronchodilating agents with a nebulizer is just as beneficial as a bronchodilator delivered with a positive pressure apparatus. The beneficial results can, for the most part, be attributed to the bronchodilators which are used in conjunction with the apparatus. Nevertheless, in the severely disabled or uncoordinated patient, the use of IPPB to deliver a nebulized bronchodilator can be of marked benefit.

BREATHING RETRAINING

In patients suffering from obstructive lung disease, the lungs are frequently hyperinflated, the diaphragms are low and scarcely move, and the accessory respiratory muscles are active during breathing. Physical relaxation and "breathing retraining" are an integral part of the therapy. The patient should go through a series of exercises to relax the accessory muscles and should carry out "diaphragmatic breathing" exercises simultaneously.

Breathing retraining is difficult, and the benefit derived varies directly with the amount of time actually spent by the physician and physiotherapist in teaching the patient. In order to develop more effective diaphragmatic activity during breathing, the diaphragm must be restored to a more expiratory position. This is initially achieved most easily in the Trendelenburg position at an angle of approximately 20 degrees at which the weight of the abdominal viscera raises the diaphragm. Inspiration should be carried out by sniffing, and expiration should take place through pursed lips in association with contraction of the abdominal muscles. Pursing the lips during expiration increases the resistance to airflow, thereby maintaining a slightly elevated pressure in the airway so that the tendency of the airways to collapse is reduced. These breathing maneuvers result in a considerable slowing of breathing. The reduction in respiratory rate lessens the work of breathing and often results in an improvement in ventilation and perfusion distribution and therefore improves gas exchange. The patient should be supervised during his "breathing exercises" at frequent intervals first while lying, then while sitting, and finally while walking until he has mastered the technique. Even when mastered, the patient should practice whenever he thinks of it and for 30 to 40 minutes at least three times each day.

RESPIRATORY STIMULANTS

There have been enthusiastic reports about the use of "respiratory stimulants" to increase alveolar ventilation in patients with respiratory failure. Such stimulants may be appropriate if the hypoventilation is the result of a diminished respiratory drive in a patient whose respiratory capacity is adequate. However, respiratory stimulants may actually be harmful in patients with gross ventilatory abnormalities because stimulation of nonrespiratory as well as respiratory muscles results in a marked increase in carbon dioxide production, which the respiratory apparatus may be incapable of eliminating. As a result, respiratory acidosis may be aggravated rather than improved when stimulants are administered.

SEDATION

The administration of sedation to patients suffering from acute or chronic respiratory failure will aggravate the respiratory disturbances, for ventilation will be further reduced. Central nervous system depressants (i.e., sedatives, narcotics, tranquilizers, excessive alcohol and even antihistamines) not only induce alveolar hypoventilation but also suppress the cough reflex and may lead to retention of secretions and further deterioration. If a night sedative is required, an ounce or two of whiskey or wine can usually be tolerated.

MEASURES DESIGNED TO INCREASE EXERCISE TOLERANCE

Although excessive physical activity should be avoided during an acute illness, it is very important that invalidism be discouraged. General physical activity is of great importance in maintaining muscular strength and normal vasoregulation. Inactivity leads to atrophy of the voluntary muscles and vasoregulatory disorders.

In patients with respiratory failure, a graded exercise program should be instituted to improve general physical fitness. The program must be suited to the age and general condition of the patient, and excessive physical exertion should be avoided.

Recovery from an episode of acute respiratory failure will be accelerated if the patient exercises on a bicycle ergometer or "walks on the spot" at the bedside, even if he is being ventilated mechanically. In chronic respiratory failure, the graded exercises should begin with the patient walking on the level and should progress through increasing intensities of work using a cycle ergometer, a treadmill or stair climbing.

It has been demonstrated that exercise tolerance improves if oxygen is breathed during exertion, and this is very useful when the patient first undertakes the program of graded activity. Portable oxygen units have also been recommended for home use in patients with chronic respiratory failure, but in most cases, they are not necessary on a long-term basis.

The marked improvement in exercise tolerance which can be achieved in patients with chronic cardiorespiratory failure cannot be correlated with improvement in pulmonary function. The increased exercise tolerance is apparently due to the more efficient use of available oxygen by the exercising muscles. Whatever the explanation, the patient's ability to perform his daily tasks is increased considerably, and his mental outlook is greatly improved.

MEASURES DESIGNED TO PREVENT ACUTE EXACERBATIONS

The course of chronic respiratory disease is punctuated with acute episodes requiring repeated hospital admissions. Intensive care of the patient with chronic respiratory failure will prevent most acute exacerbations of respiratory insufficiency so that admission of many patients with chronic respiratory failure to "intensive care" units can be avoided.

Further acute respiratory insults can be prevented by continued and aggressive therapy directed at ensuring patent airways and at the prevention and treatment of infection. The patient should be instructed regarding the importance of removal of all antigens and irritants, particularly cigarettes, the administration of oral and nebulized bronchodilators on a regular basis and adequate hydration as well as improvement in exercise tolerance. In addition, they should be taught how to recognize signs of deterioration early and to institute corrective measures immediately.

HOME CARE

Repeated hospital admissions or permanent hospitalization because of the necessity of frequent medical supervision or mechanical aids to respiration can be prevented if both the patient and his attending physician are meticulous in their attention to details. Unfortunately, such "intensive care" for the nonhospitalized patient may be difficult to provide by even the most highly motivated physician. The management of chronic respiratory failure is time-consuming and fraught with frustration; the patient often becomes a

TABLE 17

RESPIRATORY HOME CARE TEAM

Inhalation therapist
Physiotherapist
Respiratory medical resident
Private physician
Nurse
Social worker
Occupational therapist
Family

burden, and the attending physician tends to "slough" him off. However, regular supervision and guidance for the patient suffering from severe respiratory failure can be provided primarily by allied health professionals who ensure that the patient is continuing all modes of therapy (Table 17). Through frequent visits and counseling by specially trained nurses, physiotherapists and, when necessary, inhalation therapists, early recognition of deterioration is facilitated, and proper therapy is immediately instituted or intensified. Air compressors, positive pressure machines, mist tents, and occasionally home humidifiers should be provided when they are indicated. In some cases a homemaker can assist the family with the housekeeping.

The benefits of intensive home care programs have been well demonstrated in the management of patients with cystic fibrosis. Such programs have changed the prognosis of such patients markedly. This disease which was frequently fatal in early childhood can now be controlled even through adulthood. The experience with adult patients suffering from severe respiratory failure due to chronic obstructive pulmonary disease has been more disappointing. The morbidity and mortality rates of patients with chronic bronchitis or emphysema have been rising precipitously over the past decade. The life expectancy of patients with these diseases does not appear to have been altered by home care programs. Nevertheless, it is clear that intensive home therapy and the prevention of acute exacerbations has reduced the requirement for frequent hospital admissions and has allowed the patient to lead a more useful existence. It is possible that the early institution of such continuous and intensive therapy in patients who have only minimal disability would reduce morbidity considerably and ultimately reduce the mortality rate.

Chapter 20

Management of Acute Respiratory Failure

The development of acute respiratory failure with hypoxemia and hypercapnia represents a medical emergency which clearly requires immediate therapy. Although only the development of hypercapnia is considered by many to constitute respiratory failure, it must be emphasized that acute hypoxemia even without carbon dioxide retention, particularly if it is progressive, can also be life-threatening and requires immediate action.

The management of acute respiratory failure, like that of chronic respiratory failure, is designed to reverse the physiologic disturbances that are present. The aim of therapy should be to restore the patient to health, not merely to achieve "normal gases." Improvement of blood gas tensions and treatment of the underlying respiratory disorder should go hand in hand. The therapy that is instituted consists primarily of measures to improve oxygenation and the elimination of carbon dioxide through reduction of the work of breathing and through the provision of an adequate alveolar ventilation.

OXYGENATION

Hypoxemia is the single most lethal consequence of acute respiratory failure and should be dealt with as an emergency. When the cause of hypoxemia is simply the result of a reduction in alveolar ventilation, provision of an adequate ventilation will restore the arterial PO_2 to normal levels. However, in most instances, oxygen enrichment of the inspired air is required in order to correct the hypoxemia because of the mismatching of ventilation and perfusion distribution resulting from respiratory disease.

The primary aim of oxygen therapy is to increase the amount of oxygen carried in the blood to normal or nearly normal levels by increasing the concentration of oxygen in the alveolar gas. In patients who are suffering from hypoxic hypoxia, alveolar oxygen concentrations which raise the arterial oxygen tension to normal levels will suffice. In cases of circulatory or anemic hypoxia, an adequate arterial oxygen supply may require alveolar oxygen concentrations which raise the arterial PO_2 above normal values.

The concentration of oxygen necessary to raise the arterial oxygen tension to normal levels differs from patient to patient, depending on the type of physiologic disturbance present and the severity of the hypoxemia. In most cases a concentration of 30 to 40 per cent oxygen is more than adequate to return the arterial oxygen tension to normal levels.

There are numerous methods of administering oxygen, and no single method has gained universal favor. The level of oxygenation desired, the reliability and simplicity of the method and the patient's comfort dictate the optimal method. No matter which mode of administration is chosen, adequate humidification, preferably with jet humidifiers, is essential.

OXYGEN IN LOW CONCENTRATIONS

In some patients with chronic hypoxemia and hypercapnia, oxygen administration results in depression of ventilation and a further rise in arterial PCO_2. Many physicians restrict administration of oxygen to such patients because they fear that the increased oxygen level will eliminate the hypoxic stimulus to breathing and will result in a fatal depression of ventilation. This hazard of oxygen administration has been overemphasized. The judicious administration of oxygen to patients with chronic hypoxemia and hypercapnia with venturi masks, which deliver preset low concentrations of oxygen, or oxygen delivered at flow rates of 1 to 2 liters per minute via relatively simple devices, such as a nasal catheter or cannula, generally corrects severe hypoxemia without unduly depressing ventilation. Even if it does, a slight rise in arterial PCO_2 during adequate oxygenation is not associated with significant deleterious effects and is in no way comparable to the potential danger of severe hypoxemia. A rise in PCO_2 while oxygen is being administered is not an indication for cessation of oxygen therapy but rather for intensification of concomitant therapy directed at reducing the work of breathing and increasing the alveolar ventilation. If increasing mental stupor or confusion, a decrease in ventilation, or an increase in arterial carbon dioxide tension develop during oxygen therapy, intensive measures directed at clearing the airways and reducing the work of breathing are indicated. A reduction in the work of breathing will lower the carbon dioxide production at any given ventilation and counteract the tendency toward further carbon dioxide retention which may be brought about by oxygen administration.

It is important that oxygen be delivered continuously to patients with acute respiratory failure, for intermittent oxygen therapy may have deleterious effects. Sudden cessation of oxygen breathing, particularly if the arterial P_{CO_2} has been lowered acutely by assisted ventilation (e.g., by IPPB), may be followed by a precipitous fall in arterial oxygen tension. The P_{O_2} may fall to dangerously low levels because the oxygen stores in the body, represented almost entirely by oxygen in the lungs and arterial blood, are relatively small. On the other hand, the arterial P_{CO_2} rises relatively slowly when ventilation is depressed because the carbon dioxide stores in the body fluids are large.

OXYGEN IN HIGH CONCENTRATIONS

When a higher oxygen concentration is necessary to correct hypoxemia, the open top, clear plastic face hoods, head tents or high humidity oxygen tents can be utilized, although these devices rarely achieve oxygen concentrations above 50 per cent. The oxygen tent is an appropriate means of administering oxygen to infants, but it is important that the concentration of oxygen delivered be monitored carefully. Retrolental fibroplasia may develop if newborn infants are exposed to high concentrations of oxygen continuously for several days, but this will not occur if the arterial oxygen tension is kept below 100 mm. Hg. As long as the arterial P_{O_2} is below 100 mm. Hg, one should not be deterred from using high concentrations of oxygen in inspired air in situations, such as hyaline membrane disease, in which there is considerable venous admixture.

Even high concentrations of oxygen may fail to restore the oxygen tension to normal in both the adult pulmonary hypoperfusion syndrome (shocked lung, adult respiratory distress syndrome) and the respiratory distress syndrome of infants because of the gross right-to-left shunting. If a concentration of oxygen approaching 100 per cent is necessary, the oxygen must be delivered from a non-rebreathing system through a well-fitted oronasal mask or mouthpiece or from an intermittent positive-pressure breathing device (IPPB). In some cases, it may have to be administered along with controlled ventilation.

HYPERBARIC OXYGEN

Until recently there was considerable enthusiasm for the use of oxygen under greater than atmospheric pressure (hyperbaric oxygen) in the treatment of many conditions. The rationale of this form of oxygen therapy is to raise the partial pressure of oxygen in the arterial blood so that the oxygen needs of the tissues can be supplied almost entirely from the oxygen in physical solution in the plasma. For instance, when oxygen is breathed at a pressure of 3 atmospheres about 6 ml. of additional oxygen are present in physical solution in the plasma.

The therapeutic usefulness of hyperbaric oxygen therapy appears to be limited to the treatment of the bends, carbon monoxide poisoning, gas gangrene and in association with tumor irradiation. However, the possible harm to both patient and operator with this form of therapy must be appreciated, for the theoretical advantage of improved tissue oxygenation is counterbalanced by the problems of oxygen toxicity.

COMPLICATIONS OF OXYGEN THERAPY

In all patients receiving oxygen therapy, the lowest inspired oxygen concentration which will result in an arterial PO_2 between 80 and 100 mm. Hg should be administered. As has been pointed out by many, the administration of oxygen may result in cellular toxicity if given in too high a concentration for more than 48 to 72 hours. In addition to the retrolental fibroplasia which may be precipitated by high oxygen concentrations in the newborn infant, lung congestion, consolidation, atelectasis and alveolar exudates have been described following administration of high concentrations of oxygen to adult patients suffering from respiratory failure. In addition, the inhalation of oxygen-enriched air, particularly in high concentrations, leads to a washout of nitrogen from the lungs. If airway obstruction develops in this situation, gas is rapidly absorbed from the distal alveoli. A fall in the arterial PO_2 despite the continued inhalation of a constant concentration of oxygen may signal the development of focal areas of atelectasis which may still be perfused.

REDUCTION OF WORK OF BREATHING

As indicated in the management of chronic respiratory failure, the oxygen uptake and carbon dioxide production of the respiratory apparatus should be lowered by measures directed at reducing the mechanical resistances to breathing. This is achieved through relief of airway obstruction and pulmonary congestion if they are present.

RELIEF OF AIRWAY OBSTRUCTION

Airway obstruction is usually increased because of accumulation of secretions or bronchoconstriction. Thus, therapy must be directed at reducing the production and increasing the elimination of secretions as well as alleviating bronchoconstriction.

REDUCED PRODUCTION OF SECRETIONS

To reduce the production of secretions requires elimination of all irritants and eradication of infection. In many cases severe hypoxemia and hypercapnia is precipitated by infection with increased airway resistance due to thick purulent secretions and inflammatory swelling of the bronchial mucosa. It is essential to identify the offending organisms by smear and culture of the secretions and to assess their sensitivity to antibiotics so that the appropriate antibiotic can be administered. Since most of the gram-positive organisms are sensitive to penicillin, this is usually the antibiotic of choice. If gram-negative bacilli predominate, a broad-spectrum antibiotic is indicated.

INCREASED ELIMINATION OF SECRETIONS

Improved elimination of bronchial secretions is facilitated by efforts to reduce their viscosity and by physiotherapy. If this is not successful, the secretions should be aspirated.

Thinning of Secretions. Thinning of bronchial secretions and prevention of crusting are integral requirements for improving elimination of secretions. The most important measure in this regard is provision of adequate hydration. An intake of 3 liters of fluids per day should be provided to ensure adequate hydration. In some cases, warm humdification of the inspired air will also help liquefy secretions so that they are easier to expectorate. As pointed out earlier, nebulized liquefying agents, enzymes or detergents or the administration of oral liquefying agents such as potassium iodide have not been shown to be more effective than water or saline mists or good hydration.

Physiotherapy. The role of physiotherapy in the management of acute respiratory failure cannot be overemphasized. When airway obstruction is associated with the accumulation of secretions postural drainage is particularly useful in order to expedite elimination of secretions. The foot of the bed should be elevated about 12 inches, and the patient is turned from side to side every half hour to facilitate drainage of secretions. Postural drainage should be carried out at frequent regular intervals during the acute situation. While this is being carried out, the chest should be pummeled with rapid repetitive strokes and vibrated. During these procedures, the patient should be encouraged frequently to cough and expectorate secretions.

Endotracheal Suction. If the patient's cough mechanism is adequate, but secretions are particularly difficult to evacuate, percutaneous insertion of a small plastic catheter into the trachea either through the cricothyroid or between the first tracheal interspace is a useful maneuver. This also will permit periodic instillation of warm isotonic saline solution to promote thinning and easier evacuation of thick tenacious secretions.

In the patient who has an ineffective cough, nasotracheal suction and, in some cases, bronchoscopy may be necessary in order to clear accumulated secretions. To accomplish nasotracheal suctioning a catheter is inserted into the nose as far as the larynx (usually the distance from the tip of the nose to the ear pinna) with the neck extended and then is advanced into the trachea during an inspiration. Bronchoscopy, which is the most effective means of removing accumulated secretions from the main-stem bronchi, is best performed while the patient is awake, using a local anesthetic. If bronchial obstruction is severe, the use of a general anesthetic, such as halothane or ether, during the bronchoscopy may relieve any associated bronchoconstriction. Whenever nasotracheal suction or bronchoscopy is carried out adequate oxygenation of the patient must be ensured.

RELIEF OF BRONCHOCONSTRICTION

When bronchospasm is present, the administration of bronchodilating agents will result in a marked reduction in airflow resistance. As pointed out earlier, aerosol bronchodilators should be administered effectively by means of a nebulizer which delivers small droplets. IPPB may be necessary to deliver the nebulized bronchodilator if the patient is unable to take a big breath or if he cannot coordinate his breathing to allow the inhalation of bronchodilator agents which are delivered by nebulizer with either a handbulb or a pressure source. In acute situations the aerosol bronchodilator should be administered every 30 to 60 minutes. After improvement occurs, the frequency of administration can be reduced.

If severe persistent bronchospasm is present and the patient is not in a state of peripheral vascular collapse, it is appropriate to administer intravenous aminophyllin directly. In most instances 500 mg. of aminophyllin in intravenous fluid can be infused slowly every 6 to 8 hours. In patients with severe bronchial obstruction, particularly those in status asthmaticus, it may be necessary to administer high doses of corticosteroids, such as hydrocortisone or prednisone, intravenously in order to reduce the markedly increased airflow resistance.

The administration of aerosol or intravenous bronchodilator agents can sometimes result in an initial worsening of hypoxemia, presumably because of a redistribution of ventilation. However, the transient decrease in arterial PO_2 is usually not great, and bronchodilators should not be withheld on this account. Clearly, the administration of oxygen together with the bronchodilators is essential in patients suffering from acute respiratory failure.

RELIEF OF PULMONARY CONGESTION

As has been pointed out, right ventricular failure is a major complication of chronic respiratory failure. It may also develop acutely in severe respiratory failure. This is frequently accompanied by fluid retention and pulmonary congestion, particularly in elderly patients who are also suffering from arteriosclerotic cardiovascular disease. The pulmonary congestion further increases the work of breathing and aggravates the disturbances of gas exchange. The administration of diuretics, digitalis and a salt-free diet in such circumstances frequently results in improvement in ventilatory function and arterial blood gas tensions, presumably because of a reduction in pulmonary congestion.

PROVISION OF ADEQUATE ALVEOLAR VENTILATION

In order to ensure an adequate alveolar ventilation, it is essential that a patent airway be maintained.

THE AIRWAY

Insertion of an endotracheal tube is frequently life-saving in patients with laryngeal or tracheal obstruction; in the seriously ill patient with generalized airway obstruction who is comatose an artificial airway is also indicated when it is obvious that a safe and effectively patent airway will be difficult to maintain otherwise. This allows oxygenation and provision of assisted or controlled ventilation if it is required and facilitates the aspiration of secretions. The introduction of a bronchoscope also provides an airway, facilitates aspiration of secretions and, in addition, permits examination of the tracheobronchial tree and the application of adrenalin directly to edematous mucous membranes.

ENDOTRACHEAL INTUBATION

The nasotracheal tube is more comfortable than the orotracheal tube, but the latter is technically easier to insert. In addition, the orotracheal tube can be shorter and wider so that it offers less flow resistance and permits better tracheobronchial toilet. Intubation of the right main bronchus, which will lead to collapse of the left lung, should be avoided. The position of the tube should be determined immediately after insertion by auscultation over the lateral aspects of both lower lobes and palpation of the upper trachea while the tube is slowly withdrawn and the cuff is simultaneously inflated and deflated. When the endotracheal tube has been properly positioned, its upper end should be taped securely to the skin and the position then confirmed by a chest x-ray.

It is possible to leave an endotracheal tube in the airway for a number of days, but the risk of laryngeal edema increases if it remains in place for longer than 48 to 72 hours. The decision as to how long a tube should be left in place depends on many factors, including the underlying condition, the likely duration of the acute problem, and the difficulty of coping with accumulating secretions. Generally, if frequent tracheal suctioning or prolonged ventilatory assistance is required, a tracheostomy should be performed as soon as the patient is stable.

TRACHEOSTOMY

When it has been decided that the acute situation will be prolonged or that despite intensive attention to the tracheobronchial tree, with repeated nasotracheal suction and physiotherapy, the accumulation of secretions continues to present a problem in management, a tracheostomy is indicated. However, it must be stressed that intensive physician and nursing care directed at the tracheobronchial tree with repeated nasotracheal suction and physiotherapy may frequently obviate the necessity for tracheostomy.

In addition, it is important to point out that a tracheostomy is not without complications and should not be carried out in haste or without proper precautions. Complications of tracheostomy occur most frequently in cases in which the procedure is done hastily in poor surroundings. A tracheostomy, per se, is not an emergency; rather it is the need for a patent airway that is the true emergency; as has been pointed out, this emergency can be corrected by the installation of an endotracheal tube Tracheostomy should always be performed over a cuffed endotracheal tube or a bronchoscope and should be carried out under sterile conditions in an operating room with the advantage of good assistance, lighting and position of the patient.

The largest possible endotracheal or tracheostomy tube which fits easily into the trachea should be used. In addition, the tube should be fitted with a large, easily distensible cuff which will make contact over a large area of the tracheal wall, so that mucosal compression is minimized. A large tube facilitates aspiration of secretions and prolongs the life of the cuff. In addition to effectively preventing aspiration of oropharyngeal or gastric secretions the cuffed tube makes it possible to assist or control the ventilation. Metal tracheostomy tubes are largely being replaced by plastic, nylon and rubber tubes, for these usually have a cuff built into their wall. These tubes are preferable to the metal tube because the possibility of life-threatening airway obstruction due to a cuff which has slipped off the end of the tube no longer exists. Their stiff cuffs may be made more pliable by overinflation with water while the tube is in hot water.

CARE OF THE AIRWAY

By far the majority of complications of an endotracheal or tracheostomy tube result from improper care and lack of attention to details. It is important to provide adequate humidity and to prevent infection and traumatic damage to the tracheobronchial tree.

Provision of Humidity. As was pointed out in Chapter 8, when dry gas is inhaled there is approximately 650 ml. of water per day added to the inspired gas by the upper respiratory tract, particularly the nasal mucosa. When an endotracheal or tracheostomy tube is in place, the inspired air bypasses the upper respiratory tract, and unless evaporation of water from the tracheobronchial tree is prevented, bronchial secretions will become viscid and thick, and crusting may develop. By increasing the moisture content of the inspired air and ensuring adequate hydration of the patient, complications of an artificial airway will be minimized.

If the patient is breathing spontaneously, humidification of the inspired air is best achieved by a heated nebulizer containing water or saline and powered by oxygen or compressed air. The nebulizer can be connected to the tracheostomy or endotracheal tube through wide-bore tubing connected to a "T" connector or a perforated plastic chamber which is placed over the tracheostomy opening. Another apparatus which fits into the tracheostomy or endotracheal tube traps warm water vapor from each expiration so that the ensuing inspiration is humidified and warmed. If the patient is being ventilated artificially, the gas should be delivered through a heated bypass humidifier of the cascade type.

Prevention of Infection. In addition to bypassing the humidifying properties of the upper respiratory tract an artificial airway eliminates many of the defenses of the respiratory tract to contamination and infection. The ability to eliminate secretions is reduced when an artificial airway is in place, and suctioning of the tracheobronchial tree is often necessary. As a result, pathogenic bacteria may be introduced into the tracheobronchial tree. Clearly then, it is essential to use aseptic technique during tracheobronchial suctioning. The donning of sterile gloves whenever suctioning is carried out, although ideal, is usually impractical. Nevertheless, frequent hand washing is essential, and if possible, a gown and mask should be worn by those in contact with the patient and his bed.

A separate sterile catheter should be used each time the patient requires suctioning. A trap attached to the catheter will allow collection of secretions for bacteriologic examination, which should be performed every other day during the acute situation or whenever there is a change in the character of the secretions. In addition, it must be pointed out that all inhalation therapy equipment, particularly humidifiers and nebulizers, may become contaminated with organisms, such as *Pseudomonas aeruginosa,* and may result in pulmonary infections. This can be avoided by daily sterilization of all tubing and humidifiers or nebulization of weak acetic acid through the humidifiers and nebulizers.

On the basis of a gram-stained smear and culture, as well as antibiotic sensitivity tests, the appropriate antibiotic should be administered. However, it must be emphasized that antibiotic treatment should be given only when the secretions are purulent and are associated with clinical and radiologic evidence of infection. "Chasing" the culture reports with broad-spectrum antibiotics frequently hastens the appearance of resistant strains of bacteria and their associated infections.

Prevention of Trauma. Endotracheal suctioning can cause considerable trauma to the trachea and bronchi. It should not be performed at predetermined intervals, since it may often be unnecessary. Instead, it should be performed when accumulation of secretions is detected by auscultation. A rise in the respirator pressure necessary to derive a given tidal volume in patients being artificially ventilated should also lead one to suspect the presence of accumulated secretions.

The suction catheter should be directed as far down the tracheobronchial tree as possible and into the appropriate bronchus. It can be directed into either the left or right main bronchus at will by suitable positioning of the head and tracheostomy tube. A curved catheter should be used, since it passes easily into the left main bronchus. The tube should have only a single opening at its tip because the tracheal mucosa may be sucked into side openings and be torn when the catheter moves, especially if a mucous plug blocks the distal opening. A **Y** tube at the proximal end of the catheter will ensure that the negative pressure is not exerted during insertion of the catheter. The suction catheter should not be left in the tracheobronchial tree for longer than 5 to 10 seconds, particularly in severely hypoxemic patients, and suction is applied only while the catheter is withdrawn smoothly in a twisting motion.

The mode of inflation of the cuff on the tube is also extremely important in preventing trauma. The cuff should be inflated while a positive-pressure breathing machine is attached to the tracheostomy tube, and the smallest volume of air which will allow minimal air leakage during the inspiratory phase should be introduced into the cuff. The state of inflation of the cuff should be checked hourly. With proper precautions, pressure necrosis can be avoided, and patients can be ventilated indefinitely without tracheal complications. Fortunately, tracheal stenosis is not a common occurrence. However, it is so serious that all patients who have had a tracheostomy or endotracheal intubation should be examined for tracheal stenosis by x-ray at intervals following decanulation.

MECHANICAL VENTILATION

A ventilator may be necessary to manage the patient with acute respiratory failure under the following conditions: persistent marked alveolar hypoventilation despite intensive therapy directed at reducing the work of breathing; excessive fatigue on the part of the patient; severe progressive hypoxemia which is refractory to conservative therapy and liable to cause the death of the patient; or internal fixation of a "flail chest."

Ventilators vary in their capabilities, complexities and costs, and a knowledge of their characteristics is essential in order to obtain optimal results. Ventilators can be used as assistors, controllers, or assistor-controllers. When used as an assistor, the ventilator inflates the lungs in response to an inspiratory effort by the patient and is usually triggered by the inspiratory reduction in airway pressure. When used as a controller, the ventilator cycles automatically at a preset pattern and is not affected by inspiratory efforts by the patient. When used as an assistor-controller, the ventilator not only controls the respiratory pattern but also assists inspiration when an inspiratory effort is made out of phase with the ventilator. In effect, this type of ventilator acts as an assistor as long as the patient's breathing efforts are at a higher rate than the preset respirator rate and as a controller if the respiratory rate drops below the preset value.

Most ventilators are either pressure-limited (i.e., the delivery pressure is preset) or volume-limited (i.e., the volume of air delivered with each breath is preset).

Pressure-limited ventilators provide a constant inspiratory flow rate until a preset cutoff pressure is reached. The resultant tidal volume will diminish in the face of increased resistance to inflation. Most ventilators of this type are oxygen powered and can function as an assistor, or an assistor-controller.

Volume-limited ventilators, with a few exceptions, are electrically powered and deliver a preset volume of gas at a variable pressure depending on the resistance to inflation. The simplest volume-limited ventilators are strictly controllers. Newer volume-limited ventilators can assist or control and offer variable inspiratory flow and inspired oxygen concentrations, an inspiratory hold, programmed large inflations, and an end-expired pressure plateau, all of which are useful in the management of severely ill patients.

ASSISTED VENTILATION

In most instances it is preferable to allow the patient to trigger the ventilator, provided that a respiratory rate between 10 and 20 breaths per minute can be maintained. The patient-triggered, intermittent positive-pressure breathing apparatus (IPPB) is purely an assistor, but it provides a convenient and effective means of administering nebulized bronchodilators and humidity and is an exceedingly useful adjunct to the management of the patient with respiratory failure. However, it is important to recognize that the patient who is extremely fatigued, or whose respiratory muscles are weak or paralyzed, may be unable to activate the machine, and it is then preferable to use a ventilator which operates as an assistor-controller in such patients. The assistor-controller type of respirator should be set at a rate which is a little below that of the patient so that if breathing slows or stops, the ventilator will take over.

CONTROLLED VENTILATION

A ventilator which can control ventilation is necessary to restore the alveolar ventilation to normal levels if the patient is apneic, excessively fatigued, performing excessive respiratory work or unable to achieve an adequate alveolar ventilation with assisted respiration.

USE OF THE VENTILATOR

The majority of patients suffering from acute respiratory failure can be managed without resorting to the use of a ventilator. If a ventilator is necessary, the ventilatory requirements (i.e., tidal volume and respiratory rate) of the patient may be estimated initially from a Radford nomogram, remembering that respiratory disease generally increases the dead space—tidal volume ratio. The effectiveness of ventilator therapy and the adjustment of the ventilator should be based upon blood gas analysis.

If a conscious patient resists the ventilator, reassurance and adjustment of tidal volume and flow should be attempted. When large tidal volumes are necessary in order to maintain adequate oxygenation, the use of an artificial external dead space will prevent undue lowering of the arterial P_{CO_2}. If these measures fail, control of ventilation can usually be achieved after sedation with small intravenous doses of morphine or diazepam, which can be repeated as necessary. In patients with a high respiratory drive in whom all other measures have failed, curare (administered intravenously when necessary) will paralyze the patient so that ventilation may be controlled. For obvious reasons patients who are being ventilated, particularly those receiving curare, should never be left unattended.

MONITORING OF THE PATIENT WITH ACUTE RESPIRATORY FAILURE

The therapy of acute respiratory failure is directed at the immediate provision of oxygenation and gradual reduction of the arterial PCO_2. The effect of the therapy is assessed by monitoring of arterial blood gas tensions and pH as well as other parameters at regular intervals.

In patients with hypercapnia the arterial PCO_2 should be lowered slowly enough to maintain the pH between 7.35 and 7.50. If the PCO_2 is reduced rapidly to normal levels by artificial ventilation, particularly in patients with compensated chronic hypercapnia and an elevated plasma bicarbonate, severe alkalemia may result, and the patient may develop convulsions or coma. In such patients, the intravenous administration of a carbonic anhydrase inhibitor such as acetazolamide can hasten the renal excretion of bicarbonate and prevent the development of severe alkalemia. Since excessive haste in the reduction of arterial carbon dioxide tension may produce dire consequences, it is clear that the management of respiratory failure should be directed not at the arterial PCO_2 but rather at the arterial PO_2 and any associated hydrogen ion disturbance.

MONITORING ARTERIAL PCO_2

Analysis of the arterial PCO_2 at frequent intervals will indicate the adequacy of the alveolar ventilation in relation to the CO_2 production. If ventilation is being controlled, the ventilator should be adjusted to provide an alveolar ventilation which will maintain the PCO_2 at normal levels. Once the patient becomes stable, the interval between arterial PCO_2 determinations can be lengthened.

MONITORING ARTERIAL PO_2

As long as the oxygen concentration of the gas being inspired is constant, the arterial PO_2 is a sensitive indicator of minute pathologic change in the lung. In patients with severe respiratory failure, particularly if they are being ventilated at a constant tidal volume, small areas of focal atelectasis may develop, and perfusion of the atelectatic areas often persists (i.e., venous-admixture-like perfusion increases) and the arterial oxygen tension falls. This may precede clinical or radiologic signs of atelectasis by several days.

When this situation develops, two measures are required. Sufficient oxygen must be added to the inspired air in order to restore the arterial PO_2 to safe levels, and vigorous efforts must be made to expand the lungs in order to inflate small areas of atelectasis. Frequent large inflations of the lungs may prevent or reverse, at least in part, the focal pulmonary collapse. In addition, as is shown in Figure 114, continuous positive pressure breathing (i.e., the application of pressure during expiration) which does not allow the pressure in the chest to fall below 5 to 10 cm. H_2O has been shown to be particularly effective in preventing airway closure and allowing a lower inspired oxygen concentration to be delivered. Similarly, the application of a positive end-expiratory pressure is of value in the management of hyaline membrane disease of the newborn and has resulted in a marked reduction in the mortality of that condition.

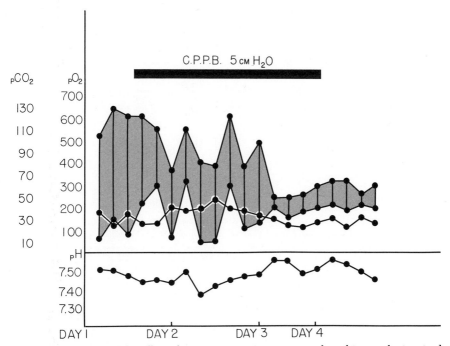

FIGURE 114. The effect of continuous positive pressure breathing on the inspired-to-arterial partial pressure of oxygen gradient (shaded area) in "shock lung." Note that a high inspiratory concentration of O_2 was necessary to maintain a normal level of arterial oxygen tension. The administration of CPPB permitted reduction of inspired oxygen concentrations and led to improvement in gas exchange.

MONITORING HYDROGEN ION CONCENTRATION

Alterations in acid-base balance exert important effects on the cardiorespiratory system, and these may influence the therapeutic regimen adopted. The presence of acidosis is particularly significant, for an increased hydrogen ion concentration, particularly when hypoxemia is present, can cause pulmonary vasoconstriction and may precipitate cardiac failure and arrhythmias. In addition, it has been shown that an increase in hydrogen ion concentration reduces the efficiency of bronchodilator agents. Acidosis may be present even when carbon dioxide retention is not marked, since severe hypoxemia may lead to increased glycolysis and lactic acid production by the tissues.

MONITORING THE VENTILATOR

If a patient is being ventilated artificially, the airway pressure, tidal volume and respiratory rate should be monitored at frequent intervals once an adequate alveolar ventilation is ensured. This will allow recognition of alterations in mechanical resistance in the respiratory system.

An increase in ventilatory resistance will affect different parameters, depending on whether a volume-limited or a pressure-limited

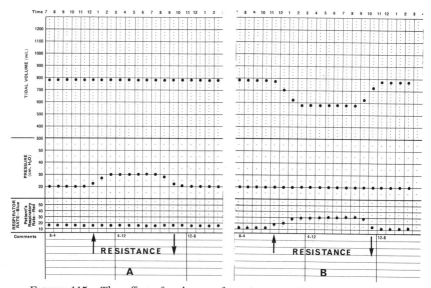

FIGURE 115. The effect of a change of respiratory resistance on respirator pressure, tidal volume and respiratory rate when a volume-limited ventilator (A), and a pressure-limited ventilator (B) are being utilized. Note that when a volume-limited ventilator is in use, an increase in resistance results in a rise in pressure; when a pressure-limited ventilator is in use, an increase in resistance results in a fall in tidal volume and a rise in respiratory rate. (From Cherniack, R. M.: The management of acute respiratory failure. Chest 58:427, 1970. By permission.)

ventilator is being used. Since the force generated by the ventilator during inspiration is, to a large extent, expended against the elastic and nonelastic resistances of the lung and chest wall, the force necessary to provide the same tidal volume will change if any of these resistances change.

As long as there is no change in resistance to inflation or a leak in the airway, both the pressure-limited and volume-limited ventilators will deliver a constant tidal volume. If the resistance of the lung rises, the volume-limited ventilator will continue to deliver the preset tidal volume to the patient by generating a higher pressure in order to overcome the increased resistance to inflation. The pressure-limited ventilator will be unable to deliver the same tidal volume under these circumstances because the pressure cutoff has been preset so that the amount of gas delivered will fall reciprocally. Thus, an increased resistance to inflation or a leak in the airway is reflected by a rise or fall in airway or monitoring pressure when a volume-limited ventilator is being utilized and by a fall in tidal volume and a rise in respiratory rate when a pressure-limited ventilator is being used (Fig. 115).

CARDIAC MONITORING

Monitoring of the electrocardiogram and heart rate is essential when acute respiratory failure is being treated because the incidence of arrhythmias is high when severe hypoxemia, acidemia, alkalemia, or hypokalemia is present.

FLUID AND ELECTROLYTE MONITORING

Improvement in alveolar ventilation with relief of hypoxemia and hypercapnia usually results in a diuresis. Occasionally the use of ventilators and intravenous fluid administration may negate the effect of improved alveolar ventilation, and fluid retention may persist or become worse. The need to ensure good hydration in the management of respiratory failure, while avoiding fluid overload, requires adjustment of fluid intake on the basis of an accurate daily record of the gain and loss of fluids and body weight.

As pointed out earlier, there may be considerable loss of chloride and depletion of the potassium stores in patients with respiratory failure so that the serum electrolyte concentrations should also be monitored daily.

MONITORING WHILE WEANING FROM A VENTILATOR

Successful treatment of the underlying pathology and the factors which precipitated respiratory failure will allow a patient to be weaned from a ventilator if this has been necessary to maintain adequate oxygenation and elimination of carbon dioxide. Patient fatigue is common, particularly in the early stages of weaning, and it is therefore best to employ short intervals off the ventilator at increasingly frequent intervals rather than long periods off the ventilator at infrequent intervals.

Weaning from a ventilator should be undertaken cautiously, and adequate oxygenation and humidity should be ensured. Blood gases should be monitored repeatedly during the weaning period, and if possible, tidal volume and vital capacity are assessed at intervals. Short periods of spontaneous ventilation can usually be tolerated if the patient has an adequate tidal volume and vital capacity of about 1000 ml. (in the adult).

THE INTENSIVE CARE UNIT

From the previous section, it is clear that the management of acute respiratory failure consists of measures directed at improvement of disturbances of function and requires close attention to minute details with continuous monitoring of vital parameters. The continuous availability of personnel who are sufficiently trained to understand basic mechanisms of disturbed function and the sophisticated equipment used to treat or monitor the critically ill patient is virtually impossible on a general medical or surgical ward of a hospital. A coordinated effort and continuity of care particularly is difficult on such wards because of the frequent staff changes. The members of the staff have divided responsibilities in that they are responsible for care of other patients on the ward and therefore cannot devote sufficient attention to the minute details which are so important in the management of acute respiratory failure. For these reasons, it is now recognized that these critically ill patients should be cared for in a special area staffed by highly trained personnel.

As has been pointed out previously, respiratory failure may complicate diseases of other systems, and disorders of other systems may complicate respiratory failure. Thus, the attending staff in a special unit must be able to recognize and manage not only acute respiratory failure, but also acute circulatory, acid-base, fluid and electrolyte disturbances. From the foregoing it is clear that there is little to recommend a special unit which is dedicated solely to the management of acute respiratory failure. By the same token, disturbances in function are similar in critically ill medical and surgical patients and many management requirements are common so that the establishment of separate medical and surgical units involves unnecessary duplication of equipment and trained personnel. It is therefore preferable to establish a single intensive care unit for the management of all critically ill patients.

FACILITIES

This single intensive care unit has certain requirements which differ from those of the general wards. The area should be air-conditioned, with frequent air changes, and temperature and humidity should be easily controlled. There must be ample outlets for oxygen, compressed air, suction and electricity at each bed station. Since ventilators and monitoring equipment may be necessary during the course of management, there must be sufficient space around each bed to permit easy utilization of such equipment. A portable x-ray unit is essential, and if it is feasible, equipment for electroencephalography, radioisotope lung scans and cardiac output should be available. Facilities for electronic monitoring of essential parameters must be present at each bed station to help the nurse manage the patient. The use of monitoring equipment to assist the nurse must be emphasized, for under no circumstances should one consider that electronic monitors serve as a replacement for the nurse at the bedside.

A laboratory with facilities for measurement of blood gas tensions and pH, blood volume, serum electrolytes and osmolality, as well as for examination of blood smears, sputum or urine, is an integral component of the unit. There should also be a conference room, living quarters for residents or physicians, a waiting room for relatives, an electronic work shop, and storage space for bulky equipment such as respirators, cooling apparatus, circo-electric beds and pacemakers.

ORGANIZATION

The details of the organization of a unit designed to care for critically ill patients is necessarily different in various centers, but there are certain general principles that are applicable in most units.

The duties of the personnel in the unit are, in some respects, different from those in a general ward. The staff members are under constant pressure and are continually directing and continually assessing the patient or undertaking measures aimed at maintaining or improving respiratory, cardiovascular, renal and cerebral function as well as acid-base, fluid, electrolyte and nutritional status. Continuous attention to minute details is necessary, changes in patient status must be recognized immediately, and emergencies handled quickly and effectively. In many cases, completely new directions in therapy must be undertaken. Clearly, this kind of attention and care must be provided throughout the day and night and cannot be a part-time occupation on the part of the attending personnel, particularly the nurse or the physician. Although it seems to be recognized that a full-time trained nursing staff is necessary to provide the technical competence required for the care of the very ill patient, this concept is much less readily accepted for residents and medical staff.

It is important to point out that, like the nurse, a doctor who is not constantly involved in such care cannot maintain the technical competence and expertise necessary. The busy practicing physician or surgeon and his residents also have divided responsibilities, and these may keep them occupied with patients in the office, the general wards, and, in the case of the surgeon, the operating room. As a result, they are not always immediately available when they are needed. Consequently, their suggestions or direction for treatment often come after the crisis situation has been dealt with, and therapy has already been instituted. Thus, the responsibility for care of the critically ill patient should be turned over to a full-time attending staff.

To ensure continuous advances and innovations in the investigation and care of the critically ill patient, repeated evaluation of procedures and clinical research are necessary, and this can only proceed effectively if those involved in the evaluation and research are in control of the management of the patients. In addition, the full-time personnel in the unit, under a director, are best equipped to evaluate potential admissions and discharges and to initiate a discharge if necessary. If control of admissions and discharges is not exercised by the staff of the unit, inappropriate deployment of resources may result.

In order to ensure that the resources of the entire health team are readily available to each critically ill patient, an experienced nurse must be at the bedside to coordinate the care of the patient, and an experienced physician or resident must be immediately available. There are very few physicians who have expertise in the pathophysiology of all systems, pharmacology and electronics and who are capable of applying new techniques of assessment and treatment. Thus, the full-time resident or, if residents are not available, the full-time physician whose efforts are wholly devoted to the unit, along with the nurse at the bedside, should form the core of a team which includes specialists in various fields as well as the referring doctor. This team, acting through the full-time resident or physician, should be responsible for investigation and total care of all patients admitted to the unit. Only one person should have the responsibility for coordinating suggestions and writing orders in the chart so that conflict or duplication is avoided and so that the nurses and other staff members have a coherent treatment and investigation plan to follow.

The number of trained bedside personnel required will vary,

depending on the particular type of patient being managed. Since the care of critically ill patients is on a moment-to-moment basis, there should be at least one nurse for every two patients if they are in cubicles or a large ward and one nurse for every patient in an isolation room. The nurse at each bedside should be responsible for applying the therapeutic measures decided upon by the attending team and should coordinate the activities of physiotherapists, inhalation therapists, occupational therapists and social workers, who play a vital role in both the management and rehabilitation of the patients. The inhalation therapy technicians on the unit, who maintain and quality control ventilators and other inhalation equipment, are often also trained to perform laboratory techniques, such as arterial blood gases. Since the electronic engineer and technician maintain and quality control all electronic equipment, they must also be members of the care "team." In order to modify or develop new techniques of monitoring, it is essential that they understand the disturbances being treated and the problems encountered by the nurse. Finally, it is clear that an adequate number of nurses' assistants, such as aides and orderlies, as well as clerical workers are necessary to ensure optimum care and record keeping.

Organization of an "intensive care" unit in the manner described, with a full-time staff, facilitates virtually continuous teaching at the bedside. Through orderly rounds all personnel can gain an insight into the capabilities and limitations of equipment or monitoring apparatus. Patients can be discussed by all members of the health team, and procedures and their rationale, as well as the therapeutic plan, can be explained to the health team. In this way, a true "esprit de corps" is developed, and all feel that they are truly taking an active role in the planning process and in the management of the critically ill patients.

SUGGESTED ADDITIONAL READING

SECTION 1. Basic Considerations

Acid Base Terminology. Report by ad-hoc committee of the New York Academy of Sciences Conference. Lancet 2:1010–1012, 1965.

Adams, W., and Veith, I.: Pulmonary Circulation. New York, Grune & Stratton, 1959.

Anthonisen, N. R., Danson, J., Robertson, P. C., and Ross, W. R. D.: Airway closure as a function of age. Resp. Physiol. 8:58–65, 1969.

Anthonisen, N. R., and Milic-Emili, J.: Distribution of pulmonary perfusion in erect man. J. Appl. Physiol. 21:760–766, 1966.

Astrand, P. O., and Rodahl, K.: Textbook of Work Physiology. New York, McGraw-Hill, 1970, p. 669.

Astrup, P., Jorgensen, K., Andersen, O. S., and Engel, K.: Acid-base metabolism. A new approach. Lancet 1:1035, 1960.

Avery, M. E.: The Lung and Its Disorders in the Newborn Infant. 2nd ed. Philadelphia, W. B. Saunders Co., 1968.

Aviado, D. M.: The Lung Circulation. (2 vols.) New York, Pergamon Press, 1965.

Bates, D. V., Macklem, P. T., and Christie, R. V.: Respiratory Function in Disease. 2nd ed. Philadelphia, W. B. Saunders, 1971.

Briscoe, W. A., and DuBois, A. B.: The relationship between airway resistance, airway conductance and lung volume in subjects of different age and body size. J. Clin. Invest. 37:1279, 1958.

Brockett, N. C., Jr., Cohen, J. J., and Schwartz, W. B.: Carbon dioxide titration curve of normal man. New Eng. J. Med. 272:6–12, 1965.

Brodovsky, D. M., Macdonell, J. A., and Cherniack, R. M.: The respiratory response to carbon dioxide in health and emphysema. J. Clin. Invest. 39:724, 1960.

Bryan, A. C., Bentivoglio, L. G., Beerel, F., MacLeish, H., Zidulka, A., and Bates, D. V.: Factors affecting regional distribution of ventilation and perfusion in the lung. J. Appl. Physiol. 19:395, 1964.

Campbell, E. J. M., Westlake, E. K., and Cherniack, R. M.: Simple methods of estimating the oxygen consumption and efficiency of the breathing muscles. J. Appl. Physiol. 11:303, 1957.

Campbell, E. J. M., Westlake, E. K., and Cherniack, R. M.: The oxygen consumption and efficiency of the respiratory muscles of young male subjects. Clin. Sci. 18: 55, 1959.

Campbell, E. J. M., Agostoni, E., and Davis, J. N.: The Respiratory Muscles: Mechanics and Neural Control. Philadelphia, W. B. Saunders Co., 1970, p. 348.

Cander, L., and Moyer, J. (Eds.): Aging of the Lung, Perspectives. The Tenth Hahnemann Symposium. New York, Grune and Stratton, 1964.

Caro, C. G. (Ed.): Advances in Respiratory Physiology. London, Edward Arnold Publishers, 1966.

Cherniack, R. M.: Ventilatory function in normal children. C.M.A.J. 87:80, 1962.

Cherniack, R. M.: The oxygen consumption and efficiency of the respiratory muscles in health and emphysema. J. Clin. Invest. 38:494, 1959.

Cherniack, R. M.: The physical properties of the lung in chronic obstructive pulmonary emphysema. J. Clin. Invest. 35:394, 1956.

Cherniack, R. M., Farhi, L. E., Armstrong, B. W., and Proctor, D. F.: A comparison of esophageal and intrapleural pressure in man. J. Appl. Physiol. 8:203, 1955.

468

Cherniack, R. M., and Snidal, D. P.: The effect of obstruction to breathing on the ventilatory response to CO_2. J. Clin. Invest. 35:1286, 1956.

Clements, J. A.: Surface phenomena in relation to pulmonary function. Physiologist 5: 11–28, 1962.

Comroe, J. H., Jr., Forster, R. E., II, DuBois, A. B., Briscoe, W. A., and Carlsen, E.: The Lung: Clinical Physiology and Pulmonary Function Tests. 2nd ed. Chicago, Year Book Medical Publishers, 1962.

Conference on Ciliary Function. Amer. Rev. Resp. Dis. 93:No. 3, Part 2, 1966.

Cotes, J. E.: Lung Function: Assessment and Application in Medicine. 2nd ed. Oxford, Blackwell Scientific Publications, 1968.

Cumming, G.: Gas mixing efficiency in the human lung. Resp. Physiol. 2:213–224, 1967.

Cumming, G., and Hunt, L. B. (Eds.): Form and Function in the Human Lung. Baltimore, Williams and Wilkins Company, 1968, p. 259.

Cunningham, D. J. C., and Lloyd, B. B. (Eds.): The Regulation of Human Respiration: Proceedings of the J. S. Haldane Centenary Symposium, Oxford, 1961. Oxford, Blackwell Scientific Publications, 1963.

Davenport, H. W.: The A B C of Acid-Base Chemistry. 4th ed. Chicago, University of Chicago Press, 1958.

DeReuck, A. V. S., and O'Connor, M. (Eds.): Ciba Foundation Symposium on Pulmonary Structure and Function. London, J. & A. Churchill Ltd., 1962.

DeReuck, A. V. S., and Porter, K. (Eds.): Ciba Foundation Symposium. Development of the Lung. London, J. & A. Churchill Ltd., 1967.

Dill, D. B.: Physiological adjustments to altitude changes. J.A.M.A. 205:123, 1968.

Donald, K. W., Renzetti, A., Riley, R. L., and Cournand, A.: Analysis of factors affecting concentrations of oxygen and carbon dioxide in gas and blood of lungs: results. J. Appl. Physiol. 4:497, 1952.

DuBois, A. B.: New concepts in cardio-pulmonary physiology, developed by the use of the body plethysmograph (Third Bowditch Lecture). Physiologist 2:8, 1959.

Effects of Altitude on Physical Performance. International Symposium, The Athletic Institute, Albuquerque, New Mexico, 1967.

Fenn, W. O.: Mechanics of respiration. Amer. J. Med. 10:77, 1951.

Ferris, B. G., Mead, J., and Opie, L. H.: Partitioning of respiratory flow resistance in man. J. Appl. Physiol. 19:653–658, 1964.

Filley, G. F., Bower, G. C., and Mitchell, R. S.: Report on the Second Aspen Conference on Research in Emphysema. The morphologic basis of pulmonary mechanics. Amer. Rev. Resp. Dis. 81:734, 1960.

Finley, T. N., Swenson, E. W., and Comroe, J. H., Jr.: The cause of arterial hypoxemia at rest in patients with "alveolar-capillary block syndrome." J. Clin. Invest. 41: 618–622, 1962.

Finley, T. N., Tooley, W. H., Swenson, E. W., Gardner, R. E., and Clements, J. A.: Pulmonary surface tension in experimental atelectasis. Amer. Rev. Resp. Dis. 89:372, 1964.

Fishman, A. P., Turino, G. M., and Bergofsky, E. H.: The syndrome of alveolar hypoventilation. Amer. J. Med. 23:33, 1957.

Flenley, D. C., and Millar, J. S.: The effects of carbon dioxide inhalation on the inspiratory work of breathing in chronic ventilatory failure. Clin. Sci. 34:385–395, 1968.

Forster, R. E., II: Exchange of gases between the alveolar air and pulmonary capillary blood: pulmonary diffusing capacity. Physiol. Rev. 37:391, 1957.

Fowler, W. S.: Intrapulmonary distribution of inspired gas. Physiol. Rev. 32:1, 1952.

Gaensler, E. A., and Wright, G. W.: Evaluation of respiratory impairment. Arch. Environ. Health 12:146–189, 1966.

Gray, J. S.: Pulmonary Ventilation and its Physiological Regulation. Springfield, Ill., Charles C Thomas, 1950.

Gray, J. S.: The multiple factor theory of the control of respiratory ventilation. Science *103*:739, 1946.

Hackney, J. D., Sears, C. H., and Collier, C. R.: Estimation of arterial CO_2 tension by rebreathing technique. J. Appl. Physiol. *12*:425, 1958.

Handbook of Physiology. (Section 3, Vols. I and II.) Respiration Section. Washington, D. C., American Physiological Society, 1964.

Harris, P., and Heath, D.: The Human Pulmonary Circulation; Its Form and Function in Health and Disease. Edinburgh, E. and S. Livingstone, 1962.

Hatcher, J. D., and Jennings, D. B. (Eds.): Proceedings of the International Symposium on the Cardiovascular and Respiratory Effects of Hypoxia. New York, S. Karger, 1966.

Hickam, J. B., and Ross, J. C.: Respiratory acidosis in chronic pulmonary heart disease: pathogenesis, clinical features and management. Progr. Cardiovasc. Dis. *1*:309, 1959.

Hultgren, H. N., and Grover, R. F.: Circulatory adaptation to high altitude. Ann. Rev. Med. *19*:119–152, 1968.

Hyatt, R. E.: The interrelationships of pressure, flow, and volume during various respiratory maneuvers in normal and emphysematous subjects. Amer. Rev. Resp. Dis. *83*:676, 1961.

Hyatt, R. E., and Flath, R. E.: Relationship of airflow to pressure during maximal respiratory effort in man. J. Appl. Physiol. *21*:477–482, 1966.

Jones, N. L.: Exercise testing. Brit. J. Dis. Chest *61*:169–189, 1967.

Jones, N. L., Campbell, E. J. M., McHardy, G. J. R., Higgs, B. E., and Clode, M.: The estimation of carbon dioxide pressure of mixed venous blood during exercise. Clin. Sci. *32*:311–327, 1967.

Lenfant, C.: Measurement of ventilation/perfusion with alveolar-arterial differences. J. Appl. Physiol. *18*:1090–1094, 1963.

Lindskog, G. E.: Collateral respiration in the normal and diseased lung. Yale J. Biol. & Med. *23*:311, 1951.

Lilienthal, J. L., Jr., and Riley, R. L.: Circulation through the lung and diffusion of gases. Ann. Rev. Med. *5*:237, 1954.

Macklem, P. T.: Airway obstruction and collateral ventilation. Physiol. Rev. *51*:(No. 2) 368–436, 1971.

Macklem, P. T., Woolcock, A. J., Hogg, J. C., Nadel, J. A., and Wilson, N. J.: Partitioning of pulmonary resistance in the dog. J. Appl. Physiol. *26*:798–805, 1969.

Marshall, R.: The physical properties of the lungs in relation to the subdivisions of lung volume. Clin. Sci. *16*:507, 1957.

Mead, J.: Mechanical properties of lungs. Physiol. Rev. *41*:281, 1961.

Mead, J., and Whittenberger, J. L.: Physical properties of human lungs measured during spontaneous respiration. J. Appl. Physiol. *5*:779, 1953.

Michel, C. C., Lloyd, B. B., and Cunningham, D. J. C.: The in vivo carbon dioxide dissociation curve of the plasma. Resp. Physiol. *1*:121–137, 1966.

Milic-Emili, J., Henderson, J. A. M., Dolovich, M. B., Trop, D., and Kaneko, K.: Regional distribution of inspired gas in the lung. J. Appl. Physiol. *21*:749–759, 1966.

Milic-Emili, J., and Tyler, J. M.: Relation between work output of the respiratory muscles and end-tidal CO_2 tension. J. Appl. Physiol. *18*:497–504, 1963.

Naimark, A., and Cherniack, R. M.: Compliance of the respiratory system and its components in health and obesity. J. Appl. Physiol. *15*:377, 1960.

Negus, V.: Protection of the respiratory tract. Brit. Med. J. *2*:723, 1961.

Otis, A. B.: The work of breathing. Physiol. Rev. *34*:449, 1954.

Otis, A. B., McKerrow, C. B., Bartlett, R. A., Mead, J., McIlroy, M. B., Selverstone, N. J., and Radford, E. P., Jr.: Mechanical factors in distribution of pulmonary ventilation. J. Appl. Physiol. *8*:427, 1956.

Pattle, R. E.: The lining layer of the lung alveoli. Brit. Med. Bull. *19*:41, 1963.

Permutt, S., and Riley, R. L.: Hemodynamics of collapsible vessels with tone: The vascular waterfall. J. Appl. Physiol. *18*:924, 1963.

Peterson, D. I., Lonergan, L. H., and Hardinge, M. G.: Smoking and pulmonary function. Arch. Environ. Health *16*:215–218, 1968.

Petty, T. L., Ryan, S. F., and Mitchell, R. S.: Cigarette smoking and the lungs. Arch. Environ. Health *14*:172–177, 1967.

Porter, R. (Ed.): Hering-Breuer Centenary Symposium. Ciba Foundation Symposium. London, J & A Churchill, 1970, p. 402.

Pride, N. B., Permutt, S., Riley, R. L., and Bomberger-Barnea, B.: Determinants of maximal expiratory flow from the lungs. J. Appl. Physiol. *23*:646–662, 1967.

Riley, R. L.: The work of breathing and its relation to respiratory acidosis. Ann. Int. Med. *41*:172, 1954.

Roughton, F. J. W.: Respiratory functions of blood. *In* Handbook of Respiratory Physiology. Randolph Air Force Base, Texas, U. S. School of Aviation Medicine, 1954.

Rudolph, A. M., and Yuan, S.: Response of the pulmonary vasculature to hypoxemia and H^+ ion concentration changes. J. Clin. Invest. *45*:399–411, 1966.

Scarpelli, E. M.: The Surfactant System of the Lung. Philadelphia, Lea and Febiger, 1968, p. 269.

Severinghaus, J. W.: Electrodes for blood and gas pCO_2, pO_2 and blood pH. Acta Anaesthesiol. Scand. (Suppl.) *11*:207, 1962.

Severinghaus, J. W., Bainton, C. R., and Carcelen, A.: Respiratory sensitivity to hypoxia in chronically hypoxic man. Resp. Physiol. *1*:308–334, 1966.

Sinclair, M. J., Hart, R. A., Pope, H. M., and Campbell, E. J. M.: The use of the Henderson-Hasselbalch equation in routine medical practice. Clin. Chim. Acta *19*:63–69, 1968.

Stein, M., Tanabe. G., Rege, V., and Khan, M.: Evaluation of spirometric methods used to assess abnormalities in airway resistance. Amer. Rev. Resp. Dis. *93*:257–263, 1966.

Weibel, E. R.: Morphometry of the Human Lung. New York, Academic Press, 1963.

West, J. B.: Ventilation/Blood Flow and Gas Exchange. Oxford, Blackwell Scientific Publications, 1965.

West, J. B., Dollery, C. T., and Naimark, A.: Distribution of blood flow in isolated lung; relation to vascular and alveolar pressures. J. Appl. Physiol. *19*:713–724, 1964.

Woolcock, A. J., Vincent, N. J., and Macklem, P. T.: Frequency dependence of compliance as a test for obstruction in small airways. J. Clin. Invest. *48*:1097–1107, 1969.

Woolmer, R.: Symposium on pH and Blood Gas Measurement. London, J. & A. Churchill, 1959.

SECTION 2. The Manifestations of Respiratory Disease

Bates, D. V., Macklem, P. T., and Christie, R. V.: Respiratory Function in Disease, 2nd ed. Philadelphia, W. B. Saunders Co., 1971.

Campbell, E. J. M., and Howell, J. B. L.: The sensation of breathlessness. Brit. Med. Bull. *19*:36, 1963.

Cherniack, L.: Chest movements in respiratory diseases. C.M.A.J. *62*:266, 1950.

Cherniack, R. M., Cuddy, T. E., and Armstrong, J. B.: The significance of pulmonary elastic and viscous resistance in orthopnea. Circulation *15*:859, 1957.

Christie, R. V.: Dyspnea: a review. Quart. J. Med. *7*:421, 1938.

Comroe, J. H., Jr.: Dyspnea. Mod. Concepts Cardiovasc. Dis. *25*:347, 1956.

Conn, H. O.: Asterekis: Its occurrence in chronic pulmonary disease, with a commentary on its general mechanism. New Eng. J. Med. *259*:564–569, 1958.

Coope, R.: Diseases of the Chest. 2nd ed. Edinburgh, E. S. Livingston, 1951.

Coury, C.: Hippocratic fingers and hypertrophic osteoarthropathy: A study of 350 cases. Brit. J. Dis. Chest 54:202–209, 1960.

Crofton, J., and Douglas, A.: Respiratory Diseases. Oxford, Blackwell Scientific Publications, 1969.

Delp, M. H., and Manning, R. T.: Major's Physical Diagnosis. 7th ed. Philadelphia, W. B. Saunders Co., 1968.

Forgacs, P.: Crackles and wheezes. Lancet 2:203–205, 1967.

Fraser, R. G., and Paré, J. A. P.: Diagnosis of Diseases of the Chest. (2 vols.) Philadelphia, W. B. Saunders Co., 1970, p. 1388.

Fritts, H. W.: Clinical implications of cyanosis. Bull. N.Y. Acad. Med. 37:291, 1961.

Godfrey, S., Edwards, R. H. T., Campbell, E. J. M., Armitage, P., and Oppenheimer, E. A.: Repeatability of physical signs in airways obstruction. Thorax 24:409, 1969.

Huckstep, R. L., and Bodkin, P. E.: Vagotomy in hypertrophic pulmonary osteoarthropathy associated with bronchial carcinoma. Lancet 2:343–345, 1958.

Hurtado, A., Velasquez, T., Reynafarje, C., Lozano, R., Chavez, R., Salazar, H. A., Reynafarje, B., Sanchez, C., and Muñoz, J.: Mechanisms of natural acclimatization; studies on the native resident of Morococha, Peru, at an altitude of 14,900 feet. Randolph Air Force Base, Texas, School of Aviation Medicine. Report No. 56–1, 1956, pp. 1–62.

Husson, G. S., and Otis, A. B.: Physiological Adaptation to Chronic Hypoxia. Randolph Air Force Base, Texas, School of Aviation Medicine, 1956.

Jackson, C., and Jackson, C. L.: Diseases of the Nose, Throat and Ear. Philadelphia, W. B. Saunders Co., 1958.

Langlands, J.: The dynamics of cough in health and in chronic bronchitis. Thorax 22: 88–96, 1967.

Leopold, S. S.: The Principles and Methods of Physical Diagnosis. Philadelphia, W. B. Saunders Co., 1957.

MacBryde, C. M.: Signs and Symptoms. Philadelphia, J. B. Lippincott Co., 1957.

McIlroy, M. B.: Dyspnea and the work of breathing in diseases of the heart and lung. Progr. Cardiovasc. Dis. 1:284, 1959.

Porter, R. (Ed.): Hering-Breuer Centenary Symposium. Ciba Foundation Symposium. London, J & A Churchill, 1970, p. 402.

Prior, J. A., and Silberstein, J. S.: Physical Diagnosis. St. Louis, C. V. Mosby Co., 1959.

Schneider, I. C., and Anderson, A. E., Jr.: Correlation of clinical signs with ventilatory function in obstructive lung disease. Ann. Int. Med. 62:477–485, 1965.

Selzer, A.: Chronic cyanosis. Am. J. Med. 10:334, 1951.

Smyllie, H. C., Blendis, L. M., and Armitage, P.: Observer disagreement in physical signs of the respiratory system. Lancet 2:412–413, 1965.

Vogl, A., and Goldfischer, S.: Pachydermoperiostosis: primary or idiopathic hypertrophic osteoarthropathy. Amer. J. Med. 33:166–187, 1962.

SECTION 3.   The Assessment of Respiratory Disease

Abrams, L. D.: A pleural-biopsy punch. Lancet 1:30–31, 1958.

Andersen, H. A., Fontana, R. S., and Harrison, E. G., Jr.: Transbronchoscopic lung biopsy in diffuse pulmonary disease. Dis. Chest 48:187–192, 1965.

Baldwin, E. deF., Cournand, A., and Richards, D. W., Jr.: Pulmonary insufficiency. II. A study of 39 cases of pulmonary fibrosis. Medicine 28:1, 1949.

Bronnestam, R., and Hallberg, T.: Precipitins against an antigen extract of aspergillus fumigatus in patients with aspergillosis or other pulmonary disease. Acta Med. Scand. 177:385–392, 1965.

Carlens, E.: Mediastinoscopy: a method for inspection and tissue biopsy in the superior mediastinum. Dis. Chest 36:343–352, 1959.

Carr, D. T., Karlson, A. G., and Stilwell, G. G.: A comparison of cultures of induced sputum and gastric washings in the diagnosis of tuberculosis. Mayo Clin. Proc. 42:23–25, 1967.

Cherniack, L.: Chest movements in respiratory diseases. C.M.A.J. 62:266, 1950.

Comroe, J. H., Jr., Forster, R. E., II, Dubois, A. B., Briscoe, W. A., and Carlson, E.: The Lung. Clinical Physiology and Pulmonary Function Tests. 2nd ed. Chicago, Year Book Medical Publishers, 1962.

Cooley, R. N.: Pulmonary thromboembolism—the case for the pulmonary angiogram (editorial). Amer. J. Roentgen. 92:693–698, 1964.

Coope, R.: Diseases of the Chest. Edinburgh, E. S. Livingston, 1951.

Cope, C.: New pleural biopsy needle; preliminary study. J.A.M.A. 167:1107–1108, 1958.

Cope, C., and Bernhardt, H.: Hook-needle biopsy of pleura, pericardium, peritoneum and synovium. Amer. J. Med. 35:189–195, 1963.

Delarue, N. C., and Strangway, D. W.: Open lung biopsy. C.M.A.J. 91:271–281, 1964.

Delp, M. H., and Manning, R. T.: Major's Physical Diagnosis. 7th ed. Philadelphia, W. B. Saunders Co., 1968.

Donohoe, R. F., Katz, S., and Matthews, M. J.: Aspiration biopsy of the parietal pleura: results in 45 cases. Amer. J. Med. 22:883, 1957.

Dubos, R. J.: Bacterial and Mycotic Infections of Man. Philadelphia, J. B. Lippincott Co., 1958.

Felson, B.: Fundamentals of Chest Roentgenology. Philadelphia, W. B. Saunders Co., 1960.

Ferris, B. G., Jr.: Studies of pulmonary function. New England J. Med. 262:557, 609, 1960.

Fraser, R. G., and Bates, D. V.: Body section roentgenography in the evaluation and differentiation of chronic hypertrophic emphysema and asthma. Amer. J. Roentgen. 82:39, 1959.

Fraser, R. G., and Paré, J. A. P.: Diagnosis of Diseases of the Chest (Vols. I and II). Philadelphia, W. B. Saunders Co., 1970.

Fred, H. L., Burdine, J. A., Jr., Gonzalez, D. A., Lockhart, R. W., Peabody, C. A., and Alexander, J. K.: Arteriographic assessment of lung scanning in the diagnosis of pulmonary thromboembolism. New Eng. J. Med. 275:1025–1032, 1966.

Gaensler, E. A.: Clinical pulmonary physiology. New England J. Med. 252:177, 221, 264, 1955.

Gaensler, E. A.: Evaluation of pulmonary function: methods. Ann. Rev. Med. 12:385, 1961.

Gell, P. G. H., and Coombs, R. R. A.: Clinical Aspects of Immunology. Oxford, Blackwell Scientific Publication, 1968.

Hackney, J. D., Sears, C. H., and Collier, C. R.: Estimation of arterial CO_2 tension by rebreathing technique. J. Appl. Physiol. 12:425, 1958.

Hapke, E. J., Seal, R. M. E., and Thomas, G. O.: Farmer's lung. A clinical, radiographic, functional and serological correlation of acute and chronic stages. Thorax 23:451–468, 1968.

Hargreave, F. E., Pepys, J., Longbottom, J. L., and Wraith, D. G.: Bird breeder's (fancier's) lung. Lancet 1:445–449, 1966.

Hessen, I.: Roentgenogen examination of pleural fluid: a study of the localization of free effusions, the potentialities of diagnosing minimal quantities of fluid and its existence under physiological conditions. Acta Radiol. Suppl. 86, 1951.

Jefferson, K. E.: The normal pulmonary angiogram and some changes seen in chronic non-specific lung disease. I. The pulmonary vessels in the normal pulmonary angiogram. Proc. Roy. Soc. Med. 58:677–681, 1965.

Johnson, J. E.: Farmer's lung in Maryland, Clinical microbiological, and immunological studies. Ann. Intern. Med. 64:860–872, 1966.

Kane, I. J.: Sectional Radiography of the Chest. New York, Springer, 1953.

Laurenzi, G. A., Potter, R. T., and Kass, E. H.: Bacteriologic flora of the lower respiratory tract. New Eng. J. Med. 265:1273–1278, 1961.

Leopold, S. S.: The Principles and Methods of Physical Diagnosis. Philadelphia, W. B. Saunders Co., 1957.

MacBryde, C. M.: Signs and Symptoms. Philadelphia, J. B. Lippincott Co., 1957.

Milne, E. N. C., and Bass, H.: Roentgenologic and functional analysis of combined chronic obstructive pulmonary disease and congestive cardiac failure. Invest. Radiol. 4:129, 1969.

Naimark, A., and Cherniack, R. M.: The compliance of the respiratory system and its components in health and obesity. J. Appl. Physiol. 15:377, 1960.

Page, L. R., and Culver, P. J.: A Syllabus of Laboratory Examinations in Clinical Diagnosis. Cambridge, Harvard University Press, 1960.

Pepys, J., and Jenkins, P. A.: Precipitin (FLH) test in farmer's lung. Thorax 20:21, 1965.

Pepys, J., Riddell, R. W., Citron, K. M., and Clayton, Y. M.: Precipitins against extracts of hay and moulds in the serum of patients with farmer's lung, aspergillosis, asthma, and sarcoidosis. Thorax 17:366, 1962.

Prior, J. A., and Silberstein, J. S.: Physical Diagnosis. St. Louis, C. V. Mosby Co., 1959.

Robertson, A. J., and Coope, R.: Rales, rhonchi and Laennec. Lancet 2:417, 1957.

Rosenblatt, G., and Stein, M.: Clinical value of the forced expiratory time measured during auscultation. New Eng. J. Med. 267:432–435, 1962.

Salvin, S. B.: Current concepts of diagnostic serology and skin hypersensitivity in the mycoses. Amer. J. Med. 27:97–114, 1959.

Sasahara, A. A., and Stein, M.: Pulmonary Embolic Disease. New York, Grune and Stratton, 1965.

Schwartz, I., and Small, M. J.: Preliminary studies in the use of superheated saline nebulization in the bacteriologic diagnosis of pulmonary tuberculosis. Amer. Rev. Resp. Dis. 84:279–280, 1961.

Smart, J.: Transbronchial pulmonary biopsy. Thorax 21:444, 1966.

Smyllie, H. C., Blendis, L. M., and Armitage, P.: Observer disagreement in physical signs of the respiratory system. Lancet 2:412–413, 1965.

Somner, A. R., Hillis, B. R., Douglas, A. C., Marks, B. L., and Grant, I. W. B.: Value of bronchoscopy in clinical practice. A review of 1,109 examinations. Brit. Med. J. 1:1079–1084, 1958.

Wacker, W. E. C., Rosenthal, M., Snodgrass, P. J., and Amador, E.: A triad for the diagnosis of pulmonary embolism and infarction. J.A.M.A. 178:8–13, 1961.

Wagner, H. N., Jr., Sabiston, D. C., Jr., McAfee, J. G., Tow, D., and Stern, H. S.: Diagnosis of massive pulmonary embolism in man by radioisotope scanning. New Eng. J. Med. 271:377–384, 1964.

Wells, B. B.: Clinical Pathology. Application and Interpretation. Philadelphia, W. B. Saunders, Co., 1956.

Woolmer, R.: Symposium on Acid Base Balance. London, J & A Churchill, Ltd. 1960.

SECTION 4.   The Patterns of Respiratory Disease

Adams, W., and Veith, I.: Pulmonary Circulation. New York, Grune & Stratton, 1959.

Baldwin, E. deF., Cournand, A., and Richards, D. W., Jr.: Pulmonary insufficiency. II. A study of 39 cases of pulmonary fibrosis. Medicine 28:1, 1949.

Baldwin, E. deF., Cournand, A., and Richards, D. W., Jr.: Pulmonary insufficiency. III. A study of 122 cases of chronic pulmonary emphysema. Medicine 28:201, 1949.

Barach, A. L., and Bickerman, H. A.: Pulmonary Emphysema. Baltimore, Williams & Wilkins, 1956.

Bass, H., Henderson, J. A. M., Heckscher, T., Oriol, A., and Anthonisen, N. R.: Regional structure and function in bronchiectasis. A correlative study using bronchography and Xe.[133] Amer. Rev. Resp. Dis. 97:598–609, 1968.

Bates, D. V.: Chronic bronchitis and emphysema. New Eng. J. Med. 278:546–551, 600–604, 1968.

Bates, D. V., Knott, J. M. S., and Christie, R. V.: Respiratory function in emphysema in relation to prognosis. Quart. J. Med. 25:137, 1956.

Bates, D. V., Macklem, P. T., and Christie, R. V.: Respiratory Function in Disease. 2nd ed. Philadelphia, W. B. Saunders Co., 1971.

Beresford, O. D.: Hereditary haemorrhagic telangiectasia with pulmonary arterio-venous fistula. Brit. J. Dis. Chest. 61:219–220, 1967.

Bowden, D. H., Fisher, V. W., and Wyatt, J. P.: Cor pulmonale in cystic fibrosis; morphometric analysis. Amer. J. Med. 38:226–232, 1965.

Briscoe, W. A., Kueppers, F., Davis, A. L., and Bearn, A. G.: Case of inherited deficiency of serum alpha-1-antitrypsin associated with pulmonary emphysema. Amer. Rev. Resp. Dis. 94:529–539, 1966.

Brunner, S.: Lung cysts. A clinical radiological study. Thesis. Munksgaard, Copenhagen, 1964.

Buchsbaum, H. W., Martin, W. A., Turino, G. M., and Rowland, L. P.: Chronic alveolar hypoventilation due to muscular dystrophy. Neurology 18:319–327, 1968.

Burrows, B.: Chronic obstructive lung disease (bronchitis-emphysema syndrome). Diagnosis and physiologic effects. Postgrad. Med. 39:105–112, 1966.

Burrows, B., Fletcher, C. M., Heard, B. E., Jones, N. L., and Wootliff, J. S.: Emphysematous and bronchial types of chronic airways obstruction: clinicopathological study of patients in London and Chicago. Lancet 1:830–835, 1966.

Burwell, C. S., Robin, E. D., Whaley, R. D., and Bickelmann, A. G.: Extreme obesity associated with alveolar hypoventilation—a Pickwickian syndrome. Amer. J. Med. 21:811, 1956.

Cherniack, N. S., and Carton, R. W.: Factors associated with respiratory insufficiency in bronchiectasis. Amer. J. Med. 41:562–571, 1966.

Cherniack, R. M.: Respiratory effects of obesity. C.M.A.J. 80:613, 1959.

Cherniack, R. M.: The oxygen consumption and efficiency of the respiratory muscles in health and emphysema. J. Clin. Invest. 38:494, 1959.

Cherniack, R. M.: The physical properties of the lung in chronic obstructive pulmonary emphysema. J. Clin. Invest. 35:394, 1956.

Cherniack, R. M., Cuddy, T. E., and Armstrong, J. B.: The significance of pulmonary elastic and viscous resistance in orthopnea. Circulation 15:859, 1957.

Cooke, F. N., and Blades, B.: Cystic disease of the lungs. J. Thorac. Surg. 23:546, 1952.

Crofton, J., and Douglas, A.: Respiratory Diseases. Oxford, Blackwell Scientific Publications, 1969.

Dale, W. A., and Rahn, H.: Rate of gas absorption during atelectasis. Amer. J. Physiol. 170:606, 1952.

di Sant'Agnese, P. A., and Talamo, R. C.: Pathogenesis and physiopathology of cystic fibrosis of the pancreas. New Eng. J. Med. 277:1287–1294, 1344–1352, 1399–1408, 1967.

Dollery, C. T., Gillam, P. M. S., Hugh-Jones, P., and Zorab, P. A.: Regional lung function in kyphoscoliosis. Thorax 20:175–181, 1965.

Ebert, R. V.: Pulmonary emphysema. Ann. Rev. Med. 7:123, 1956.

Eriksson, S.: Studies in alpha antitrypsin deficiency. Acta Med. Scand. *177*:(Suppl. 432):1–85, 1965.

Fishman, A. P., Turino, G. M., and Bergofsky, E. H.: The syndrome of alveolar hypoventilation. Amer. J. Med. *23*:33, 1957.

Fleischner, F. G.: The pathogenesis of bronchiectasis. Radiology *53*:818, 1949.

Fletcher, C. M.: Chronic bronchitis. Its prevalence, nature, and pathogenesis. Amer. Rev. Resp. Dis. *80*:483, 1959.

Forster, R. E.: Rate of gas uptake by red blood cells. *In* Fenn, W. O., and Rahn, H. (Eds.): Handbook of Physiology. Vol. 1, Sec. 3. Washington, D. C., American Physiological Society, 1964, pp. 827–837.

Fowler, N. O., Black-Schaffer, B., Scott, R. C., and Gueron, M.: Idiopathic and thromboembolic pulmonary hypertension. Amer. J. Med. *40*:331–345, 1966.

Fraser, R. G., and Bates, D. V.: Body section roentgenography in the evaluation and differentiation of chronic hypertrophic emphysema and asthma. Amer. J. Roentgen. *82*:39, 1959.

Fraser, R. G., and Paré, J. A. P.: Diagnosis of Diseases of the Chest. (2 vols.) Philadelphia, W. B. Saunders Co., 1970, p. 1388.

Gell, P. G. H., and Coombs, R. R. A.: Clinical Aspects of Immunology. Oxford, Blackwell Scientific Publications, 1968.

Gould, D. M., and Torrance, D. J.: Pulmonary edema. Amer. J. Roentgen. *73*:366, 1955.

Hammon, L., and Rich, A. R.: Fulminating diffuse interstitial fibrosis of the lungs. Trans. Amer. Clin. Climat. Ass. *51*:154–163, 1935.

Hamman, L., and Rich, A. R.: Acute diffuse interstitial fibrosis of the lungs. Bull. Johns Hopkins Hosp., *74*:177–212, 1944.

Harley, H. R. S.: Subphrenic abscess. Thorax *4*:1, 1949.

Heard, B. E.: Pathology of Chronic Bronchitis and Emphysema. London, J. and A. Churchill Ltd., 1969.

Heppleston, A. G.: Chronic diffuse interstitial fibrosis of the lungs. Thorax 6:426, 1951.

Heppleston, A. G.: Pathology of honeycomb lung. Thorax *11*:77, 1956.

Hickam, J. B., and Ross, J. C.: Respiratory acidosis in chronic pulmonary heart disease: pathogenesis, clinical features and management. Progr. Cardiovasc. Dis. *1*:309, 1959.

Hogg, J. C., Macklem, P. T., and Thurlbeck, W. M.: Site and nature of airway obstruction in chronic obstructive lung disease. New Eng. J. Med. *278*:1355–1360, 1968.

Holley, H. S., Milic-Emili, J., Becklake, M. R., and Bates, D. V.: Regional distribution of pulmonary ventilation and perfusion in obesity. J. Clin. Invest. *46*:475–481, 1967.

Hughes, J. M. B., Glazier, J. B., Maloney, J. E., and West, J. B.: Effect of interstitial pressure on pulmonary blood-flow. Lancet *1*:192–193, 1967.

Hugh-Jones, P.: The functional pathology of emphysema. Brit. J. Anaesth. *30*:107, 1958.

Ishikawa, S., Bowden, D. H., Fisher, V., and Wyatt, J. P.: The emphysema profile in two midwestern cities in North America. Arch. Environ. Health *18*:660–666, 1969.

Jeresaty, R. M., Knight, H. F., and Hart, W. E.: Pulmonary arteriovenous fistulas in childhood. Amer. J. Dis. Child. *111*:256–261, 1966.

Jones, N. L., Burrows, B., and Fletcher, C. M.: Serial studies of 100 patients with chronic airway obstruction in London and Chicago. Thorax *22*:327–335, 1967.

Jones, N. L., and Goodwin, J. F.: Respiratory function in pulmonary thromboembolic disorders. Brit. Med. J. *1*:1089–1093, 1965.

Kaufman, B. J., Ferguson, M. H., and Cherniack, R. M.: Hypoventilation in obesity. J. Clin. Invest. *38*:500, 1959.

Keltz, H.: The effect of respiratory muscle dystunction on pulmonary function. Amer. Rev. Resp. Dis. *91*:934–938, 1965.

Kueppers, F., Briscoe, W. A., and Bearn, A. G.: Hereditary deficiency of serum alpha-1-antitrypsin. Science *146*:1678, 1964.

Lawther, P. J.: Air pollution and chronic bronchitis. Med. Thorac. *24*:44–52, 1967.

Lieberman, J.: Clinical syndromes associated with deficient lung fibrinolytic activity. New Eng. J. Med. *260*:619–626, 1959.

Liebow, A. A., Hales, M. R., Harrison, W., Bloomer, W., and Lindskog, G. E.: The genesis and functional implications of collateral circulation of lungs. Yale J. Biol. & Med. *22*:637, 1950.

Leigh, T. F., and Weens, H. S.: The Mediastinum. Springfield, Ill., Charles C Thomas, 1959.

Lilienthal, J. L., Jr., and Riley, R. L.: Circulation through the lung and diffusion of gases. Ann. Rev. Med. *5*:237, 1954.

MacKay, I. R., and Ritchie, B.: Diffuse fibrosing alveolitis (diffuse interstitial fibrosis of the lungs): two cases with autoimmune features. Thorax *20*:200–205, 1965.

Macklem, P. T.: Airway obstruction and collateral ventilation. Physiol. Rev. *51*:(No. 2)368–436, 1971.

Marshall, R.: The physiology and pharmacology of the pulmonary circulation. Progr. Cardiovasc. Dis. *1*:341, 1959.

McLean, K. H.: The pathogenesis of pulmonary emphysema. Amer. J. Med. *25*:62, 1958.

Mitchell, R. S.: A summary of the Third Conference on Research in Emphysema. Air pollution and chronic pulmonary insufficiency. Amer. Rev. Resp. Dis. *83*:402, 1961.

Mitchell, R. S., and Filley, G.: Symposium on Emphysema and the "Chronic Bronchitis" Syndrome. Amer. Rev. Resp. Dis. *80*:(Suppl.), 1959.

Naimark, A., and Cherniack, R. M.: The compliance of the respiratory system and its components in health and obesity. J. Appl. Physiol. *15*:377, 1960.

Niden, A. H.: The acute effects of atelectasis on the pulmonary circulation. J. Clin. Invest. *43*:810–824, 1964.

Norris, R. M., Jones, J. G., and Bishop, J. M.: Respiratory gas exchange in patients with spontaneous pneumothorax. Thorax *23*:427–433, 1968.

Oswald, N. C.: Recent Trends in Chronic Bronchitis. London, Lloyd-Luke, 1959.

Parker, B. M., and Smith, J. R.: Pulmonary embolism and infarction. A review of the physiologic consequences of pulmonary arterial obstruction. Amer. J. Med. *24*:402, 1958.

Pepys, J.: Pulmonary hypersensitivity disease due to inhaled organic antigens (editorial). Ann. Intern. Med. *64*:943–947, 1966.

Pepys, J.: Hypersensitivity diseases of the lungs due to fungi and organic dusts. Basel, Switzerland, S. Karger, 1969, p. 147.

Polgar, G., and Denton, R.: Cystic fibrosis in adults. Studies of pulmonary function and some physical properties of bronchial mucus. Amer. Rev. Resp. Dis. *85*:319, 1962.

Race, G. A., Scheifly, C. H., and Edwards, J. E.: Hydrothorax in congestive heart failure. Amer. J. Med. *22*:83, 1957.

Rankin, J., Jaeschke, W. H., Callies, Q. C., and Dickie, A.: Farmer's lung. Physiopathologic features of the acute interstitial granulomatous pneumonitis of agricultural workers. Ann. Int. Med. *57*:606, 1962.

Reid, J. M., Cuthbert, J., and Craik, J. E.: Chronic diffuse idiopathic fibrosing alveolitis. Brit. J. Dis. Chest. *59*:194–201, 1965.

Reid, L.: Measurement of the bronchial mucous gland layer: A diagnostic yardstick in chronic bronchitis. Thorax *15*:132, 1960.

Reid, L.: The Pathology of Emphysema. Chicago, Year Book Medical Publishers, 1967.

Reid, L., and Simon, G.: Pathological findings and radiological changes in chronic bronchitis and emphysema. Brit. J. Radiol. 32:291, 1959.

Riley, R. L.: The work of breathing and its relation to respiratory acidosis. Ann. Int. Med. 41:172, 1954.

Rottenberg, L. A., and Golden, R.: Spontaneous pneumothorax. A study of 105 cases. Radiology 53:157, 1949.

Roughton, F. J. W.: Transport of oxygen and carbon dioxide. In Fenn, W. O., and Rahn, H. (Eds.): Handbook of Physiology. Vol. 1, Sec. 3. Washington, D. C., American Physiological Society, 1964, 767–825.

Rushmer, R. F.: Cardiovascular Dynamics. Philadelphia, W. B. Saunders Co., 1961.

Sasahara, A. A., and Stein, M.: Pulmonary Embolic Disease. New York, Grune and Stratton, 1965.

Scadding, J. G., and Hinson, K. F. W.: Diffuse fibrosing alveolitis (diffuse interstitial fibrosis of the lungs). Correlation of histology at biopsy with prognosis. Thorax 22:291–304, 1967.

Sharma, O. P., Colp, C., and Williams, M. H., Jr.: Course of pulmonary sarcoidosis with and without corticosteroid therapy as determined by pulmonary function studies. Amer. J. Med. 41:541–551, 1966.

Sharp, J. T., Henry, J. P., Sweany, S. K., Meadows, W. R., and Pietras, R. J.: Inertance and its gas and tissue components in normal and obese men. J. Clin. Invest. 43:503–510, 1964.

Sharp, J. T., Sweany, S. K., Henry, J. P., Pietras, R. J., Meadows, W. R., Amaral, E., and Rubinstein, H. M.: Lung and thoracic compliances in ankylosing spondylitis. J. Lab. Clin. Med. 63:254–263, 1964.

Simon, G.: Radiology and emphysema. Clin. Radiol. 15:293–306, 1964.

Spain, D. M.: Patterns of pulmonary fibrosis as related to pulmonary function. Ann. Int. Med. 33:1150, 1950.

Staub, N. C., Nagano, H., and Pearce, M. E.: Pulmonary edema in dogs, especially sequence of fluid accumulation in lungs. J. Appl. Physiol. 22:227–240, 1967.

Stringer, C. J., Stanley, A. L., Bates, R. C., and Summers, J. E.: Pulmonary arteriovenous fistula. Amer. J. Surg. 89:1054, 1955.

Talamo, R. C., Blennerhassett, J. B., and Austen, K. F.: Current concepts: familial emphysema and alpha-1-antitrypsin deficiency. New Eng. J. Med. 275:1301–1304, 1966.

Thurlbeck, W. M.: Chronic obstructive lung disease. In Somers, S. (Ed.): Pathology Annual, 1968, pp. 367–398.

Thurlbeck, W. M.: The pathology of pulmonary emphysema. In Gordon, B. L., Carleton, R. A., Faber, L. P. (Eds.): Clinical Cardiopulmonary Physiology. 3rd ed. New York, Grune and Stratton Inc., 1969, p. 555.

Thurlbeck, W. M., Henderson, J. A. M., Fraser, R. G., and Bates, D. V.: Chronic obstructive lung disease: a comparison between clinical, roentgenologic, functional, and morphologic criteria in chronic bronchitis, emphysema, asthma, and bronchiectasis. Medicine 49:81–145, 1970.

Tysinger, D. S., Jr., and Meneely, G. R.: Spontaneous pneumothorax; clinical diagnosis and management. Amer. J. Surg. 89:360, 1955.

West, J. R., and di Sant'Agnese, P. A.: Studies of pulmonary function in cystic fibrosis of the pancreas. Amer. J. Dis. Child. 86:496, 1953.

William, J. V., Tierney D. F., and Parker, H. R.: Surface forces in the lung, atelectasis, and transpulmonary pressure. J. Appl. Physiol. 21:819–827, 1966.

Wood, P.: Pulmonary hypertension. Brit. M. Bull. 8:348, 1952.

Xalabarder, C.: What is atelectasis? Tubercle 30:266, 1949.

SECTION 5. Respiratory Failure and Its Management

Aber, G. M., Bayley, T. J., Bishop, J. M.: Interrelationships between renal and cardiac function and respiratory gas exchange in obstructive airways disease. Clin. Sci. 25:159–170, 1963.

Addington, W. W., Kettel, L. J., and Cugell, D. W.: Alkalosis due to mechanical hyperventilation in patients with chronic hypercapnia. Amer. Rev. Resp. Dis. 93:736–741, 1966.

Ambiavagar, M., Robinson, J. S., Morrison, I. M., and Jones, E. S.: Intermittent positive pressure ventilation in the treatment of severe crushing injuries of the chest. Thorax 21:359–366, 1966.

Anthonisen, N. R., and Smith, H. J.: Respiratory acidosis as a consequence of pulmonary edema. Ann. Intern. Med. 62:991–999, 1965.

Avery, M. E.: The Lung and Its Disorders in the Newborn Infant. 2nd ed. Philadelphia, W. B. Saunders Co., 1968.

Bendixen, H. H., Egbert, L. D., Hedley-White, J., Laver, M. B., and Pontoppidan, H.: Respiratory Care. St. Louis, C. V. Mosby Co., 1965, p. 252.

Bigelow, D. B., Petty, T. L., Ashbaugh, D. G., Levine, B. E., Nett, L. M., and Tyler, S. W.: Acute respiratory failure: experiences of a respiratory care unit. Med. Clin. N. Amer. 51:323, 1967.

Bowden, D. H., Adamson, I. Y. R., and Wyatt, J. P.: Reaction of lung cells to high concentrations of oxygen. Arch. Path. 86:671–675, 1968.

Brewis, R. A. L.: Oxygen toxicity during artificial ventilation. Thorax 24:656–666, 1969.

Caldwell, P. R. B., Lee, W. L., Jr., Schildkraut, H. S., and Archibald, E. R.: Changes in lung volume, diffusing capacity, and blood gases in men breathing oxygen. J. Appl. Physiol. 21:1477–1483, 1966.

Campbell, E. J. M.: A method of controlled oxygen administration which reduces the risk of carbon dioxide retention. Lancet 2:12, 1960.

Campbell, E. J. M.: Respiratory failure. The relation between oxygen concentrations of inspired air and arterial blood. Lancet 2:10, 1960.

Campbell, E. J. M.: The J. Burns Amberson Lecture. The management of acute respiratory failure in chronic bronchitis and emphysema. Amer. Rev. Resp. Dis. 96: 626–639, 1967.

Campbell, E. J. M., and Gebbie, T.: Masks and tent for providing controlled oxygen concentrations. Lancet 1:468–469, 1966.

Campbell, E. J. M., and Short, D. S.: The cause of edema in cor pulmonale. Lancet 1:1184, 1960.

Cherniack, R. M.: The management of acute respiratory failure. Chest 58:(Suppl. 2) 427–436, 1970.

Cherniack, R. M.: The management of respiratory failure in chronic obstructive lung disease. Ann. N.Y. Acad. Sci. 121:942, 1965.

Cherniack, R. M.: The management of respiratory insufficiency in myocardial infarction. Illinois Med. J. 135:559, May, 1969.

Cherniack, R. M., and Cuddy, T. E.: Respiratory insufficiency in acute myocardial infarction. C.M.A.J. 101:478–482, 1969.

Cherniack, R. M., and Goldberg, I.: The effect of nebulized bronchodilator delivered with and without IPPB on ventilatory function in chronic obstructive emphysema. Amer. Rev. Resp. Dis. 91:13, 1965.

Cherniack, R. M., and Hakimpour, K.: The rationale use of oxygen in respiratory insufficiency. J.A.M.A. 199:178–182, 1967.

Cherniack, R. M., Handford, R. G., and Svanhill, E.: Home Care of Chronic Respiratory Disease. J.A.M.A. 208:821–824, 1969.

Cherniack, R. M., and Kirk, B. W.: Acute Respiratory Failure. *In* Conn. H. F. (Ed.): Current Therapy—1972. Philadelphia, W. B. Saunders Co., 1972.

Cherniack, R. M., and Young, G.: An evaluation of ethamivan as a respiratory stimulant in barbiturate intoxication, and alveolar hypoventilation in emphysema and obesity. Ann. Intern. Med. *60*:631–640, 1964.

Cullen, J. H., and Kaemmerlen, J. T.: Acute ventilatory failure in chronic obstructive lung disease. Amer. Rev. Resp. Dis. *98*:998–1002, 1968.

Filley, G. F.: Pulmonary Insufficiency and Respiratory Failure. Philadelphia, Lea and Febiger, 1967.

Flenley, D. C.: Respiratory Failure. Scot. Med. J. *15*:61–72, 1970.

Flenley, D. C., Hutchison, D. C. S., and Donald, K. W.: Behaviour of apparatus for oxygen administration. Brit. Med. J. *2*:1081, 1963.

Fowler, W. S., Helmholz, H. F., Jr., and Millder, R. D.: Treatment of pulmonary emphysema with aerosolized bronchodilator drugs and intermittent positive pressure breathing. Proc. Mayo Clin *28*:743, 1953.

Fyles, T. W., Hildes, J. P., Gemmell, J. P., and Handford, R. G.: The home care medical program of the Winnipeg General Hospital. C.M.A.J. *85*:1097, 1961.

Gilbert, R., Keighley, J., and Auchincloss, J. H., Jr.: Mechanisms of chronic carbon dioxide retention in patients with obstructive pulmonary disease. Amer. J. Med. *38*:217–225, 1965.

Gregory, G. A., Kitterman, J. A., Phibbs, R. H., Tooley, W. H., and Hamilton, W. K.: Treatment of idiopathic respiratory distress syndrome with continuous positive airway pressure. New Eng. J. Med. *284*:1333, 1971.

Hackney, J. D., Sears, C. H., and Collier, C. R.: Estimation of arterial CO_2 tension by rebreathing technique. J. Appl. Physiol. *12*:425, 1958.

Harris, P.: Principles of management of cor pulmonale. Chest 58(Suppl. 2)437–440, 1970.

Harris, P., Segel, N., Bishop, J. M.: The relation between pressure and flow in the pulmonary circulation in normal subjects and in patients with chronic bronchitis and mitral stenosis. Cardiovasc. Res. *2*:73–83, 1968.

Harris, P., Segel, N., Green, I., and Hausley, E.: The influence of the airways resistance and alveolar pressure on the pulmonary vascular resistance in chronic bronchitis. Cardiovasc. Res. *2*:84–92, 1968.

Hatcher, J. D., and Jennings, D. B. (Eds.): International Symposium on the Cardiovascular and Respiratory Effects of Hypoxia. New York, S. Karger, 1966.

Heath, D., Edwards, J. E.: The pathology of hypertensive pulmonary vascular disease. Circulation *18*:533–547, 1958.

Hickam, J. B., and Ross, J. C.: Respiratory acidosis in chronic pulmonary heart disease: Pathogenesis, clinical features and management. Progr. Cardiovasc. Dis. *1*:309, 1959.

Hutchison, D. C. S., Flenley, D. C., and Donald, K. W.: Controlled oxygen therapy in respiratory failure. Brit. Med. J. *2*:1159–1166, 1964.

Ishikawa, S., and Cherniack, R. M.: The effect of nebulized bronchodilators on air flow resistance in chronic airways obstruction. Amer. Rev. Resp. Dis. *99*:703–710, 1969.

Jessen, O., Kristensen, H. S., and Rasmussen, K.: Tracheostomy and artificial ventilation in chronic lung disease. Lancet *2*:9–12, 1967.

Kory, R. C., Bergmann, J. C., Sweet, R. D., and Smith, J. R.: Comparative evaluation of oxygen therapy techniques. J.A.M.A. *179*:767–772 (March 10), 1962.

Lane, D. J., Howell, J. B. L., and Giblin, B.: Relation between airways obstruction and CO_2 tension in chronic obstructive airways disease. Brit. Med. J. *2*:707–709, 1968.

Laurenzi, G.: Adverse effect of oxygen on mucociliary clearance. New Eng. J. Med. *279*:333, 1968.

Levine, B. E., Bigelow, D. B., Petty, T. L., Hamstra, R. H., Beckuitt, H. J., and Mitchell, R. S.: The role of long-term continuous oxygen administration in patients with chronic airway obstruction with hypoxemia. Ann. Intern. Med. 66:639, 1967.

McLelland, R. M. A.: Complications of tracheostomy. Brit. Med. J. 2:567–569, 1965.

Milic-Emili, J., and Tyler, J. M.: Relation between work output of the respiratory muscles and end-tidal CO_2 tension. J. Appl. Physiol. 18:497–504, 1963.

Miller, W. F.: Physical therapeutic measures in the treatment of chronic bronchopulmonary disorders. Amer. J. Med. 24:929, 1958.

Miller, W. F.: Rehabilitation of patients with chronic obstructive lung disease. Med. Clin. N. Amer. 51:349, 1967.

Moore, F. E., Lyons, J. H., Pierce, E. C., Morgan, A. P., Drinker, P. A., MacArthur, J. D., and Dammin, G. J.: Post-Traumatic Pulmonary Insufficiency. Philadelphia, W. B. Saunders Co., 1969, p. 234.

Motley, H. L., Cournand, A., Werko, L., Himmelstein, A., and Dresdale, D.: The influence of short periods of induced hypoxia upon pulmonary artery pressures in man. Amer. J. Physiol. 150:315–320, 1947.

National Academy of Sciences – National Research Council, Committee on Anesthesia: Workshop on intensive care units, Washington, 1963. Anesthesiology, 25/2:192, 1964.

Noble, M. I. M., Trenchard, D., and Guz, A.: The value of diuretics in respiratory failure. Lancet 2:257–260, 1966.

Pain, M. C. F., Charlton, G. C., and Read, J.: Effect of intravenous aminophylline on distribution of pulmonary blood flow in obstructive lung disease. Amer. Rev. Resp. Dis. 95:1005–1014, 1967.

Petty, T. L.: Ambulatory Care for Emphysema and Chronic Bronchitis. Chest 58: (Suppl. 2)441–448, 1970.

Petty, T. L., Bigelow, D. B., Nett, L. M.: The intensive respiratory care unit: an approach to the care of acute respiratory failure. Calif. Med. 107:381, 1967.

Petty, T. L., and Finigan, M. M.: The clinical evaluation of prolonged ambulatory oxygen therapy in patients with chronic airway obstruction. Amer. J. Med. 45:242, 1968.

Petty, T. L., Nett, L. M., Finigan, M. M., Brink, G. A., and Carsello, P. R.: A comprehensive care program for chronic airway obstruction: methods and preliminary evaluation of symptomatic and functional improvement. Ann. Intern. Med. 70:1109, 1969.

Pierce, A. K., Taylor, H. F., Archer, R. K., and Miller, W. F.: Responses to exercise training in patients with emphysema. Arch. Intern. Med. 113:78, 1964.

Rees, H. A., Millar, J. S., and Donald, K. W.: A study of the clinical course and arterial blood gas tensions of patients in status asthmaticus. Quart. J. Med. 38:541–561, 1968.

Refsum, H. E.: Relationship between state of consciousness and arterial hypoxemia and hypercapnia in patients with pulmonary insufficiency, breathing air. Clin. Sci. 25:361, 1963.

Reynolds, E. O. R., Roberton, N. R. C., and Wigglesworth, J. S.: Hyaline membrane disease, respiratory distress and surfactant deficiency. Pediatrics 42:758–768, 1968.

Robin, E. D., and O'Neill, R. P.: The fighter versus the nonfighter. Control of ventilation in chronic obstructive pulmonary disease. Arch. Environ. Health 7:125, 1963.

Rotheram, E. B., Safar, P., and Robin, E. D.: CNS Disorder during mechanical ventilation in chronic pulmonary disease. J.A.M.A. 189:993–996, 1964.

Safar, P. (Ed.): Respiratory Therapy. Philadelphia, F. A. Davis Co., 1965.

Sieker, H. O., and Hickam, J. B.: Carbon dioxide intoxication, the clinical syndrome, etiology and management with particular reference to the use of mechanical respirators. Medicine 35:389, 1956.

Stahlman, M. T., Young, W. C., Gray, J., and Shephard, F. M.: The management of respiratory failure in idiopathic respiratory distress syndrome of prematurity. Ann. N.Y. Acad. Sci. *121*:930–941, 1965.

Sykes, M. K., McNicol, M. W., and Campbell, E. J. M.: Respiratory Failure. Oxford, Blackwell Scientific Publications, 1969.

Tai, E., and Read, J.: Response of blood gas tensions to aminophylline and isoprenalin in patients with asthma. Thorax 22:543–550, 1967.

Therapy of acute respiratory failure: A statement by the committee on therapy of the American Thoracic Society. Amer. Rev. Resp. Dis. 93:475–480, 1966.

Valentine, P. A., Fluck, D. C., Mousney, J. P. D., Reid, D., Shillingford, J. P., and Steiner, R. E.: Blood-gas changes after acute myocardial infarction. Lancet 2:837–841, 1966.

Vidyasagar, D., and Chernick, V.: Continuous positive transpulmonary pressure in hyaline membrane disease. A simple method. Pediatrics *48*:296, 1971.

Waddell, J. A., Emerson, P. A., and Gunstone, R. F.: Hypoxia in bronchial asthma. Brit. Med. J. 2:402–404, 1967.

Wolfsdorf, J., Swift, D. L., and Avery, M. E.: Mist therapy reconsidered; an evaluation of the respiratory deposition of labelled water aerosols produced by jet and ultrasonic nebulizers. Pediatrics *43*:799–808, 1969.

INDEX